WITHDRAWAL

Allergy Information for Teens

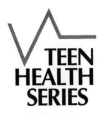

**TEEN
HEALTH
SERIES**

First Edition

Allergy Information for Teens

Health Tips about Allergic Reactions Such as Anaphylaxis, Respiratory Problems, and Rashes

Including Facts about Identifying and Managing Allergies to Food, Pollen, Mold, Animals, Chemicals, Drugs, and Other Substances

◆

Edited by Karen Bellenir

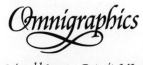

Omnigraphics

615 Griswold Street • Detroit, MI 48226

Bibliographic Note

Because this page cannot legibly accommodate all the copyright notices, the Bibliographic Note portion of the Preface constitutes an extension of the copyright notice.

Edited by Karen Bellenir

Teen Health Series

Karen Bellenir, *Managing Editor*
David A. Cooke, M.D., *Medical Consultant*
Elizabeth Barbour, *Permissions Associate*
Dawn Matthews, *Verification Assistant*
Laura Pleva Nielsen, *Index Editor*
EdIndex, Services for Publishers, *Indexers*

* * *

Omnigraphics, Inc.

Matthew P. Barbour, *Senior Vice President*
Kay Gill, *Vice President—Directories*
Kevin Hayes, *Operations Manager*
Leif Gruenberg, *Development Manager*
David P. Bianco, *Marketing Director*

* * *

Peter E. Ruffner, *Publisher*

Frederick G. Ruffner, Jr., *Chairman*

Copyright © 2006 Omnigraphics, Inc.

ISBN 0-7808-0799-5

Library of Congress Cataloging-in-Publication Data

Allergy information for teens : health tips about allergic reactions such as anaphylaxis, respiratory problems, and rashes, including facts about identifying and managing allergies to food, pollen, mold, animals, chemicals, drugs, and other substances / edited by Karen Bellenir.
    p. cm. -- (Teen health series)
    Summary: "Provides basic consumer health information for teens on allergies, types of allergic reactions, testing and treatments. Includes index, resource information and recommendations for further reading" -- Provided by publisher.
    Includes bibliographical references and index.
    ISBN 0-7808-0799-5 (hardcover : alk. paper)
    1. Allergy. 2. Allergy in children. 3. Food allergy. 4. Insect allergy. I. Bellenir, Karen. II. Title. III. Series.
    RC584.A45 2006
    616.97--dc22
                                                                    2005031765

The information in this publication was compiled from the sources cited and from other sources considered reliable. While every possible effort has been made to ensure reliability, the publisher will not assume liability for damages caused by inaccuracies in the data, and makes no warranty, express or implied, on the accuracy of the information contained herein.

∞

This book is printed on acid-free paper meeting the ANSI Z39.48 Standard. The infinity symbol that appears above indicates that the paper in this book meets that standard.

Printed in the United States

Table of Contents

Preface ix

Part I: Understanding Allergies

Chapter 1—Allergies: The Basic Facts 3
Chapter 2—The Immune System And Its Role In Allergies 13
Chapter 3—Allergy Testing 33
Chapter 4—Allergy Shots (Immunotherapy) 37
Chapter 5—Allergy Medications 41
Chapter 6—Epinephrine 53
Chapter 7—Alternative Therapies For Allergy Patients 59
Chapter 8—Allergy-Related Research 65

Part II: Allergic Reactions

Chapter 9—Anaphylaxis: The Most Dangerous Allergic Reaction 75
Chapter 10—You And Your Stuffy Nose 85
Chapter 11—Rhinitis 93
Chapter 12—Sinusitis 99
Chapter 13—Conjunctivitis (Pink Eye) 109
Chapter 14—Rashes: The Itchy Truth 115
Chapter 15—Eczema 119
Chapter 16—Contact Dermatitis 127
Chapter 17—Urticaria (Hives) And Angioedema 131
Chapter 18—Headaches May Be Caused By Allergies 139
Chapter 19—Allergic Diseases And Cognitive Impairment 143

Part III: Food Allergies And Intolerances

Chapter 20—Food Allergy: An Overview 149

Chapter 21—Problem Foods: Is It An Allergy Or An Intolerance?...... 165

Chapter 22—Food Challenges Identify True Food Allergies 171

Chapter 23—Egg Allergy 177

Chapter 24—Milk Allergy 183

Chapter 25—Lactose Intolerance 189

Chapter 26—Nut And Peanut Allergies 195

Chapter 27—Seafood Allergies 203

Chapter 28—Wheat Allergy Or Gluten Intolerance? 207

Chapter 29—Learning To Take Control Of Your Food Allergies 215

Chapter 30—Decoding Food Labels 219

Chapter 31—Food Allergies And Your Social Life.............................. 233

Chapter 32—Will Food Proteins In Cosmetics And
               Bath Products Cause Allergic Reactions? 241

Part IV: Allergens In The Air

Chapter 33—Are You Allergic To Something In The Air? 245

Chapter 34—Pollen Allergies 265

Chapter 35—Allergies To Mold 275

Chapter 36—Cockroach Allergy 283

Chapter 37—Dust Mite Allergy 287

Chapter 38—Allergies To Pets 295

Chapter 39—Pets Can Have Allergies, Too 305

Part V: Environmental, Chemical, And Drug Allergies

Chapter 40—Insect Venom Allergies 313

Chapter 41—Poison Ivy And Other Problematic Plants 321

Chapter 42—Allergies And Cosmetics 327

Chapter 43—Fragrance Allergies 335

Chapter 44—Allergy To Wool Alcohols (Lanolin) 341

Chapter 45—Allergy To Paraphenylenediamine (Hair Dyes) 345

Chapter 46—Nickel Allergy 351

Chapter 47—Latex Allergies 355
Chapter 48—Drug Allergies.. 361
Chapter 49—Chemical Sensitivities....................................... 367

Part VI: If You Need More Information

Chapter 50—Resources For More Information About Allergies 375
Chapter 51—Additional Reading About Allergies 383

Index 393

Preface

About This Book

According to the National Institute of Allergy and Infectious Diseases, more than 50 million Americans suffer from allergic diseases. Allergies occur when the immune system responds to a false alarm. In an allergic person, a material that is normally harmless—such as grass pollen, household dust, or a type of food—is mistaken for a threat and attacked. Symptoms may include sniffles, sneezes, itchy rashes, or watery eyes. Sufferers endure chronic misery that can affect all aspects of family, school, and social life. Allergies can also be deadly. Every year approximately 150 Americans, usually adolescents and young adults, die from food-induced anaphylaxis—a sudden, severe allergic reaction that can overwhelm the body's respiratory and cardiovascular systems.

Allergy Information For Teens describes the various different types of allergic reactions—including anaphylaxis, rhinitis and sinusitis, conjunctivitis (pink eye), rashes, hives, and more—and discusses the substances that commonly trigger them, such as various foods, pollen, mold, dust, pets, insect venom, latex, medications, and other chemicals. It describes the immune system's role in allergic disease and provides facts about allergy testing and treatment. A directory of resources for more information about allergies is included along with suggestions for additional reading.

Readers seeking further information about asthma and the role allergies play in its development and course may wish to consult *Asthma Information For Teens*, a separate volume in the *Teen Health Series*.

How To Use This Book

This book is divided into parts and chapters. Parts focus on broad areas of interest; chapters are devoted to single topics within a part.

Part I: Understanding Allergies provides fundamental facts about allergies and the immune system abnormalities that cause them. It describes the tests most frequently used to diagnose allergies or to identify specific allergens. The use of allergy shots (immunotherapy), medications, and alternative therapies to help relieve symptoms is also explained.

Part II: Allergic Reactions begins with a discussion of anaphylaxis, a type of allergic response that is rare, but potentially fatal. Other types of reactions that can affect the respiratory tract, eyes, and skin are explained, and the part concludes with facts about allergy-related headaches and cognitive impairment.

Part III: Food Allergies And Intolerances describes the types of allergic reactions that are related to food items and explains the differences between true food allergies and food intolerances. It offers specific facts about such common allergies as eggs, milk, nuts, and seafood, and provides tips for managing them. A chapter focused on coping with food allergies in social situations is also included.

Part IV: Allergens In The Air describes the types of allergens commonly found circulating in the air, both indoors and out-of-doors, including pollens, molds, dust, and pet dander. It explains the types of symptoms commonly associated with airborne allergens and offers tips for managing them. Because pets can have allergies (as well as be a source of allergens), the part concludes with a chapter about allergies in pets.

Part V: Environmental, Chemical, And Drug Allergies provides information about other common types of allergens encountered in the outdoor environment or related to medications or chemicals. These include allergies to insect venom, cosmetics, fragrances, hair dyes, nickel, latex, penicillin, and anesthetics. The various types of reactions associated with chemical sensitivities are also discussed.

Part VI: If You Need More Information offers a directory of sources for additional information about allergies and a list of related reading material, including books, cookbooks for people with food allergies, magazine and journal articles, and web-based resources.

Bibliographic Note

This volume contains documents and excerpts from publications issued by the following government agencies: National Cancer Institute; National Institute of Allergy and Infectious Diseases; National Institute of Environmental Health Sciences; U.S. Department of Labor, Occupational Safety and Health Administration; and the U.S. Food and Drug Administration.

In addition, this volume contains copyrighted documents and articles produced by the following organizations: A.D.A.M., Inc.; Access Media Group, LLC; Allergy and Asthma Network Mothers of Asthmatics; American Academy of Allergy, Asthma, and Immunology; American Academy of Dermatology; American Academy of Otolaryngology–Head and Neck Surgery; American Animal Hospital Association; American College of Allergy, Asthma and Immunology; American Lung Association; American Osteopathic College of Dermatology; Asthma and Allergy Foundation of America; Better Health Channel (Victoria, Australia); Cleveland Clinic Foundation; DEY, L.P.; Food Allergy and Anaphylaxis Network; International Food Information Council Foundation; National Jewish Medical and Research Center; Nemours Foundation; New Zealand Dermatological Society; Science in Africa; University of Cincinnati, NetWellness; University of Florida, Institute of Food and Agricultural Sciences; University of Maine, Cooperative Extension; WebMD; and the World Allergy Organization.

Full citation information is provided on the first page of each chapter. Every effort has been made to secure all necessary rights to reprint the copyrighted material. If any omissions have been made, please contact Omnigraphics to make corrections for future editions.

Acknowledgements

In addition to the organizations listed above, special thanks are due to verification assistant Dawn Matthews, permission specialist Liz Barbour, and illustrator Alison DeKleine.

About The *Teen Health Series*

At the request of librarians serving today's young adults, the *Teen Health Series* was developed as a specially focused set of volumes within Omnigraphics' *Health Reference Series*. Each volume deals comprehensively with a topic selected according to the needs and interests of people in middle school and high school.

Teens seeking preventive guidance, information about disease warning signs, medical statistics, and risk factors for health problems will find answers to their questions in the *Teen Health Series*. The *Series*, however, is not intended to serve as a tool for diagnosing illness, in prescribing treatments, or as a substitute for the physician/patient relationship. All people concerned about medical symptoms or the possibility of disease are encouraged to seek professional care from an appropriate health care provider.

If there is a topic you would like to see addressed in a future volume of the *Teen Health Series*, please write to:

Editor
Teen Health Series
Omnigraphics, Inc.
615 Griswold Street
Detroit, MI 48226

Locating Information Within The *Teen Health Series*

The *Teen Health Series* contains a wealth of information about a wide variety of medical topics. As the *Series* continues to grow in size and scope, locating the precise information needed by a specific student may become more challenging. To address this concern, information about books within the *Teen Health Series* is included in *A Contents Guide to the Health Reference Series*. The *Contents Guide* presents an extensive list of more than 10,000 diseases, treatments, and other topics of general interest compiled from the Tables of Contents and major index headings from the books of the *Teen Health Series* and *Health Reference Series*. To access *A Contents Guide to the Health Reference Series*, visit www.healthreferenceseries.com.

Our Advisory Board

We would like to thank the following advisory board members for providing guidance to the development of this *Series*:

Dr. Lynda Baker
Associate Professor of Library and Information Science,
Wayne State University, Detroit, MI

Nancy Bulgarelli
William Beaumont Hospital Library, Royal Oak, MI

Karen Imarisio
Bloomfield Township Public Library, Bloomfield Township, MI

Karen Morgan
Mardigian Library, University of Michigan-Dearborn, Dearborn, MI

Rosemary Orlando
St. Clair Shores Public Library, St. Clair Shores, MI

Medical Consultant

Medical consultation services are provided to the *Teen Health Series* editors by David A. Cooke, M.D. Dr. Cooke is a graduate of Brandeis University, and he received his M.D. degree from the University of Michigan. He completed residency training at the University of Wisconsin Hospital and Clinics. He is board-certified in internal medicine. Dr. Cooke currently works as part of the University of Michigan Health System and practices in Ann Arbor, MI. In his free time, he enjoys writing, science fiction, and spending time with his family.

Part 1

Understanding Allergies

Chapter 1

Allergies: The Basic Facts

Questions About Allergies

Your eyes itch, your nose is running, you're sneezing, and you're covered in hives. The enemy known as allergies has struck again—and all you want to do is curl up into a ball of misery.

There has to be something you can do to feel better. After all, doctors seem to have a cure for everything, right? Not for allergies. There are, however, things that you can do to relieve allergy symptoms or avoid getting the symptoms, even though you can't actually get rid of the allergies themselves.

What are allergies?

Allergies are abnormal immune system reactions to things that are typically harmless to most people. When you're allergic to something, your immune system mistakenly believes that this substance is harmful to your body. (Substances that cause allergic reactions, such as certain foods, dust, plant pollen, or medicines, are known as allergens.) In an attempt to protect the

About This Chapter: This chapter begins with text under the headings "Questions About Allergies" and "Dealing With Allergies." This information was provided by TeensHealth, one of the largest resources online for medically reviewed health information written for parents, kids, and teens. For more articles like this one, visit www.TeensHealth.org, or www.KidsHealth.org. © 2004 The Nemours Center for Children's Health Media, a division of The Nemours Foundation. "Allergy Statistics" is a fact sheet from the National Institute of Allergy and Infectious Diseases, December 2004.

body, the immune system produces IgE antibodies to that allergen. Those antibodies then cause certain cells in the body to release chemicals into the bloodstream, one of which is histamine. The histamine then acts on a person's eyes, nose, throat, lungs, skin, or gastrointestinal tract and causes the symptoms of the allergic reaction. Future exposure to that same allergen will trigger this antibody response again. This means that every time you come into contact with that allergen, you'll have an allergic reaction.

Allergic reactions can be mild, like a runny nose, or they can be severe, like difficulty breathing. An asthma attack, for example, is often an allergic reaction to something that is breathed into the lungs in a person who is susceptible.

Some types of allergies produce multiple symptoms, and in rare cases, an allergic reaction can become very severe— this severe reaction is called anaphylaxis. Some of the signs of anaphylaxis are difficulty breathing, difficulty swallowing,

---

♣ It's A Fact!!
Allergy Quiz

Answer these questions to test your knowledge about allergies.

1. What are allergies?
   A. Infectious diseases
   B. Abnormal immune system reactions

2. What should you do if you're allergic to milk?
   A. Read food labels carefully
   B. Don't get close to cows
   C. Neither of these

3. Some allergic teens have asthma. Which of these things is known to trigger attacks in some people with asthma?
   A. Homework
   B. Cockroaches

4. What are some things that teens might be allergic to?
   A. Dogs and cats
   B. Nuts
   C. Cleaning their rooms
   D. All of the above

5. What should you do if you think you have a food allergy?
   A. Make your little brother taste everything before you eat it
   B. Stop eating the foods you believe give you problems
   C. See your doctor

Answers can be found at the end of this chapter (Source: © 2003 The Nemours Center for Children's Health Media, a division of The Nemours Foundation.)

swelling of the lips, tongue, and throat or other parts of the body, and dizziness or loss of consciousness. Anaphylaxis usually occurs minutes after exposure to a triggering substance, such as a peanut, but some reactions may be delayed by as long as four hours. Luckily, anaphylactic reactions don't occur often, and they can be treated successfully if proper medical procedures are followed.

Why do people get allergies?

The tendency to develop allergies is often hereditary, which means it can be passed down through your genes. (Thanks a lot, Mom and Dad!) However, just because a parent or sibling might have allergies, that doesn't mean you will definitely get them, too. A person usually doesn't inherit a particular allergy, just the likelihood of having allergies.

What are some things that people are allergic to?

Some of the most common allergens are:

Foods: Food allergies are most common in infants and often go away as a child gets older. Although some food allergies can be serious, many simply cause annoying symptoms like an itchy rash, a stuffy nose, and diarrhea. Most allergy specialists agree that the foods that people are most commonly allergic to are milk and other dairy products, eggs, wheat, soy, peanuts and tree nuts, and seafood.

Insect bites and stings: The venom (poison) in insect bites and stings causes allergic reactions in many people. These allergies can be severe and may cause an anaphylactic reaction in some people.

Airborne particles: These are often called environmental allergens, and they're the most common allergens. Some examples of airborne particles that can cause allergies in people are dust mites (tiny bugs that live in house dust); mold spores; animal dander (flakes of scaly, dried skin, and dried saliva from your pets); and pollen from grass, ragweed, and trees.

Medicines: Antibiotics—medications used to treat infections—are the most common types of medicines that cause allergic reactions. Many other medicines, including over-the-counter medications (those you can buy without a prescription), can also cause allergic reactions.

Chemicals: Some cosmetics or laundry detergents can cause people to break out in an itchy rash (hives). Usually, this is because the person has a reaction to the chemicals in these products. Dyes, household cleaners, and pesticides used on lawns or plants can also cause allergic reactions in some people.

How do doctors diagnose and treat allergies?

If your family doctor suspects you might have an allergy, he or she might refer you to an allergist, a person who specializes in allergy treatment, for further testing. The allergy specialist will ask you questions both about your own allergy symptoms (such as how often they occur and when) and about whether any family members have allergies. The allergist will also perform tests to confirm an allergy—these will depend on the type of allergy a person has and may include a skin test or blood test.

The most complete way to avoid allergic reactions is to stay away from the substances that cause them (called avoidance). Doctors can also treat some allergies using medications and shots.

Avoidance: In some cases, like food allergies, avoiding the allergen is a life-saving necessity. That's because, unlike allergies to airborne particles that can be treated with shots or medications, the only way to treat food allergies is to avoid the allergen entirely. For example, people who are allergic to peanuts

♣ It's A Fact!!

In 1902, two French scientists injected dogs with a small amount of extract from the sea anemone. Nothing happened. A week later, they repeated the procedure in exactly the same way—and watched, amazed, as the animals developed severe reactions.

The dogs had somehow become sensitive to the formerly harmless substance. The researchers had discovered allergy.

Source: Excerpted from "How Was Allergy Discovered?" © Copyright 2005 National Jewish Medical and Research Center. All rights reserved. For additional information, visit http://asthma.national jewish.org or call 1-800-222 LUNG.

should avoid not only peanuts, but also any food that might contain even tiny traces of them.

Avoidance can help protect people against non-food or chemical allergens, too. In fact, for some people, eliminating exposure to an allergen is enough to prevent allergy symptoms and they don't need to take medicines or go through other allergy treatments.

Here are some things that can help you avoid airborne allergens:

- Keep family pets out of certain rooms, like your bedroom, and bathe them if necessary.

- Remove carpets or rugs from your room (hard floor surfaces don't collect dust as much as carpets do).

- Don't hang heavy drapes, and get rid of other items that allow dust to accumulate.

- Clean frequently (if your allergy is severe, you may be able to get someone else to do your dirty work!)

- Use special covers to seal pillows and mattresses if you're allergic to dust mites.

- If you're allergic to pollen, keep windows closed when pollen season's at its peak, change your clothing after being outdoors—and don't mow lawns.

- Avoid damp areas, such as basements, if you're allergic to mold, and keep bathrooms and other mold-prone areas clean and dry.

Medications: Medications such as pills or nasal sprays are often used to treat allergies. Although medications can control the allergy symptoms (such as sneezing, headaches, or a stuffy nose), they are not a cure and can't make the tendency to have allergic reactions go away. Many effective medications are available to treat common allergies, and your doctor can help you to identify those that work for you.

Another type of medication that some severely allergic people will need to have on hand is a shot of epinephrine, a fast-acting medicine that can help offset an anaphylactic reaction. This medicine comes in an easy-to-carry container that looks like a pen. Epinephrine is available by prescription only.

☞ Remember!!

Allergic individuals can exhibit a variety of reactions depending on the allergen and the way it was absorbed into the body.

1. Seasonal allergic rhinitis sometimes called "hay fever" is caused by an allergy to the pollen of trees, grasses, weeds or mold spores. Depending on what you are allergic to, the section of the country and the pollination periods, seasonal allergic rhinitis may occur in the spring, summer or fall and may last until the first frost. The sufferer has spells of sneezing, itching and watery eyes, runny nose, burning palate and throat. Seasonal allergies also can trigger asthma.

2. Allergic rhinitis is a general term used to apply to anyone who has symptoms of nasal congestion, sneezing and a runny nose due to allergies. This may be a seasonal problem as with hay fever, or it may be a year-round problem caused by indoor allergens such as dust mite droppings, animal dander, cockroach droppings or indoor molds/mildew. Frequently, this problem is complicated by sinusitis. Patients with constant nasal symptoms should consult their allergist.

3. Eczema or atopic dermatitis is a non-contagious, itchy rash that often occurs on the hands, arms, legs and neck, although it can cover the entire body. This condition is frequently associated with allergies, and substances to which a person is sensitive may aggravate it.

4. Contact dermatitis is a reaction affecting areas of the skin which become red, itchy and inflamed after contact with allergens or irritants such as plants, cosmetics, medications, metals and chemicals.

5. Urticaria or hives are red, itchy, swollen areas of the skin that can vary in size and appear anywhere on the body. Approximately 25% of the U.S. population will experience an episode of hives at least once in their lives. Most common are acute cases of hives, where the cause is readily identifiable as a reaction to a viral infection, medication, food, or latex. Some people have chronic hives that occur almost daily for months to years, with no identifiable trigger. Angioedema is a swelling of the deeper layers of the skin. It is not red or itchy, and most often occurs in soft tissue, such as the eyelids or mouth. Hives and angioedema may appear together or separately on the body.

Source: Excerpted from "Frequently Asked Questions," © 2004 American Academy of Allergy, Asthma and Immunology. All rights reserved.

If you have a severe allergy and your doctor thinks you should carry it, he or she will give you instructions on how to use it.

Shots: Allergy shots are also referred to as allergen immunotherapy. By receiving injections of small amounts of an allergen, your body can gradually develop antibodies and undergo other immune system changes. These changes help block the reaction caused by the substance to which you're allergic. Immunotherapy is only recommended for specific allergies, such as allergic rhinitis, and doesn't help with some allergies, like food allergies.

Although a lot of people find the thought of allergy shots unsettling, shots can be highly effective—and it doesn't take long to get used to them. In many cases, the longer a person receives allergy shots, the more they help the body build up antibodies that fight the allergies. Although the shots don't cure allergies, they do tend to raise a person's tolerance when exposed to the allergen, which means fewer or less severe symptoms.

If you're severely allergic to bites and stings, talk to a doctor about getting venom immunotherapy (shots) from an allergist.

Is it a cold or allergies?

If the spring and summer seasons leave you sneezing and wheezing, you may suffer from allergies. Colds, on the other hand, are more likely to occur at any time (though they're more common in the colder months). Although colds and allergies produce similar symptoms, colds usually last only a week or so. And although both may cause your nose and eyes to itch, colds and other viral infections may also give you a fever and aches and pains. Cold symptoms often worsen as the days go on and then gradually improve, but allergies begin immediately after exposure to the offending allergen and last as long as that exposure continues. If you're not sure whether your symptoms are being caused by allergies or a cold, talk with your doctor.

Dealing With Allergies

So once you know you have allergies, how do you deal with them? First and foremost, try to avoid things you're allergic to! If you have a food allergy, that means avoiding foods that trigger symptoms and learning how to read food labels to make sure you're not consuming even tiny amounts of allergens.

For people with environmental allergies, keeping your house clean of dust and pet dander and watching the weather for those days when pollen is high can help. Switch to perfume-free and dye-free detergents, cosmetics, and beauty products (you may see non-allergenic ingredients listed as hypoallergenic on product labels). Avoid contact with household cleaners and yard chemicals whenever possible.

If you're taking medication, be sure to follow the directions carefully and make sure your regular doctor is aware of anything an allergist gives you (like shots or prescriptions). If you have a severe allergy, you may want to consider wearing a medical emergency ID (such as a MedicAlert bracelet), which will explain your allergy and who to contact in case of an emergency.

If you've been diagnosed with allergies, you have a lot of company. The National Institutes of Health (NIH) report that more than 50 million Americans are affected by allergic diseases. The good news is that doctors and scientists are working to better understand allergies, to improve treatment methods, and to possibly prevent allergies altogether.

♣ It's A Fact!!
Things You May Be Allergic To

Allergens that you breathe in from:
- House dust mites
- Cockroaches
- Pets
- Pollens from trees, grasses and weeds
- Mold spores
- Dusts and fumes at work

Allergens that you ingest:
- Foods
- Medications

Allergens from insect stings and bites:
- Bees, wasps, yellow jackets, hornets and ants
- Mosquitoes
- Biting flies

Allergens that you put on the skin: These allergens can cause a poison-ivy type rash or contact dermatitis. The allergic reaction is a cell-mediated reaction and not caused by IgE.

- Cosmetics
- Shampoos and conditioners
- Rubber products
- Metals such as jewelry

Source: Reprinted with permission from "What Are You Allergic To?" © 2005 World Allergy Organization (www.worldallergy.org). All rights reserved.

Allergy Statistics

- More than 50 million Americans suffer from allergic diseases.

- Allergies are the 6th leading cause of chronic disease in the United States, costing the health care system $18 billion annually.

- Two estimates of prevalence of allergic rhinoconjunctivitis (hay fever) in the United States are nine percent and 16 percent. The prevalence of allergic rhinitis has increased substantially over the past 15 years.

- In 2002, approximately 14 million office visits to health care providers were attributed to allergic rhinitis.

- Estimates of the prevalence of allergy to latex allergens in the general population vary widely, from less than one percent to six percent.

- Certain individuals, including health care workers who wear latex gloves and children with spina bifida who have had multiple surgical procedures, are at particularly high risk for allergic reactions to latex. Atopic individuals (those with allergies) are at an increased risk of developing latex allergy.

- Atopic dermatitis is one of the most common skin diseases, particularly in infants and children. The estimated prevalence in the United States varies from 9 to 30 percent. The prevalence of atopic dermatitis appears to be increasing.

- Health care provider visits for contact dermatitis and other eczemas, which include atopic dermatitis, are 7 million per year.

- Chronic sinusitis is the most commonly reported chronic disease, affecting 16.3 percent of people (nearly 32 million) in the United States in 1997.

- In 1996, estimated U.S. health care expenditures attributable to sinusitis were approximately $5.8 billion.

- Experts estimate food allergy occurs in six to eight percent of children four years of age or under, and in four percent of adults. Approximately

150 Americans, usually adolescents and young adults, die annually from food-induced anaphylaxis.

• Peanut or tree nut allergies affect approximately 0.6 percent and 0.4 percent of Americans, respectively, and cause the most severe food-induced allergic reactions.

• Allergic drug reactions account for five to ten percent of all adverse drug reactions, with skin reaction being the most common form.

• Penicillin is a common cause of drug allergy. Approximately seven percent of normal volunteers react to penicillin allergy skin tests (IgE antibodies). While the true number of deaths from drug reactions is unknown, anaphylactic reactions to penicillin occur in 32 of every 100,000 exposed patients.

• Acute urticaria (hives) is common, affecting 10 to 20 percent of the population at some time in their lives. Half of those affected continue to have symptoms for more than six months.

• Allergy to venom of stinging insects (honeybees, wasps, hornets, yellow jackets, and fire ants) is relatively common, with prevalence of systemic reactions in three percent of American and one percent of children. Between 40 and 100 Americans have been reported to die annually from anaphylaxis to insects, although this number may be markedly underestimated.

Allergy Quiz: Answers

1. B;   2. A;   3. B;   4. D;   5. C

Source: This information was provided by TeensHealth, one of the largest resources online for medically reviewed health information written for parents, kids, and teens. For more articles like this one, visit www.TeensHealth.org, or www.KidsHealth.org. © 2003 The Nemours Center for Children's Health Media, a division of The Nemours Foundation.

Chapter 2

The Immune System And Its Role In Allergies

Introduction

The immune system is a network of cells, tissues, and organs that work together to defend the body against attacks by "foreign" invaders. These are primarily microbes (germs)—tiny, infection-causing organisms such as bacteria, viruses, parasites, and fungi. Because the human body provides an ideal environment for many microbes, they try to break in. It is the immune system's job to keep them out or, failing that, to seek out and destroy them.

When the immune system hits the wrong target or is crippled, however, it can unleash a torrent of diseases, including allergy, arthritis, or AIDS.

The immune system is amazingly complex. It can recognize and remember millions of different enemies, and it can produce secretions and cells to match up with and wipe out each one of them.

The secret to its success is an elaborate and dynamic communications network. Millions and millions of cells, organized into sets and subsets, gather like clouds of bees swarming around a hive and pass information back and forth. Once immune cells receive the alarm, they undergo tactical changes

About This Chapter: Excerpted from "Understanding the Immune System: How It Works," National Institute of Allergy and Infectious Diseases and the National Cancer Institute, NIH Pub. No. 03-5423, September 2003.

and begin to produce powerful chemicals. These substances allow the cells to regulate their own growth and behavior, enlist their fellows, and direct new recruits to trouble spots.

✎ What's It Mean?

Allergen: Any substance that causes an allergy.

Allergy: A harmful response of the immune system to normally harmless substances.

Antibodies: Molecules (also called immunoglobulins) produced by a B cell in response to an antigen. When an antibody attaches to an antigen, it helps the body destroy or inactivate the antigen.

Antigen: A substance or molecule that is recognized by the immune system. The molecule can be from foreign material such as bacteria or viruses.

Basophils: White blood cells that contribute to inflammatory reactions. Along with mast cells, basophils are responsible for the symptoms of allergy.

Complement: A complex series of blood proteins whose action "complements" the work of antibodies. Complement destroys bacteria, produces inflammation, and regulates immune reactions.

Complement Cascade: A precise sequence of events, usually triggered by antigen-antibody complexes, in which each component of the complement system is activated in turn.

Inflammatory Response: Redness, warmth, and swelling produced in response to infection, as the result of increased blood flow and an influx of immune cells and secretions.

Mast Cell: A granulocyte found in tissue. The contents of mast cells, along with those of basophils, are responsible for the symptoms of allergy.

Memory Cells: A subset of T cells and B cells that have been exposed to antigens and can then respond more readily when the immune system encounters those same antigens again.

Self And Nonself

The key to a healthy immune system is its remarkable ability to distinguish between the body's own cells—self—and foreign cells—nonself. The body's immune defenses normally coexist peacefully with cells that carry distinctive "self" marker molecules. But when immune defenders encounter cells or organisms carrying markers that say "foreign," they quickly launch an attack.

Anything that can trigger this immune response is called an antigen. An antigen can be a microbe such as a virus, or even a part of a microbe. Tissues or cells from another person (except an identical twin) also carry nonself markers and act as antigens. This explains why tissue transplants may be rejected.

In abnormal situations, the immune system can mistake self for nonself and launch an attack against the body's own cells or tissues. The result is called an auto-immune disease. Some forms of arthritis and diabetes are auto-immune diseases. In other cases, the immune system responds to a seemingly harmless foreign substance such as ragweed pollen. The result is allergy, and this kind of antigen is called an allergen.

♣ **It's A Fact!!**

An allergy is the result of an immune system response to an otherwise harmless substance.

The Structure Of The Immune System

The organs of the immune system are positioned throughout the body. They are called lymphoid organs because they are home to lymphocytes, small white blood cells that are the key players in the immune system.

Bone marrow, the soft tissue in the hollow center of bones, is the ultimate source of all blood cells, including white blood cells destined to become immune cells. The thymus is an organ that lies behind the breastbone; lymphocytes known as T lymphocytes, or just "T cells," mature in the thymus.

Lymphocytes can travel throughout the body using the blood vessels. The cells can also travel through a system of lymphatic vessels that closely parallels the body's veins and arteries. Cells and fluids are exchanged between blood and lymphatic vessels, enabling the lymphatic system to monitor the body for invading microbes. The lymphatic vessels carry lymph, a clear fluid that bathes the body's tissues.

Small, bean-shaped lymph nodes are laced along the lymphatic vessels, with clusters in the neck, armpits, abdomen, and groin. Each lymph node contains specialized compartments where immune cells congregate, and where they can encounter antigens.

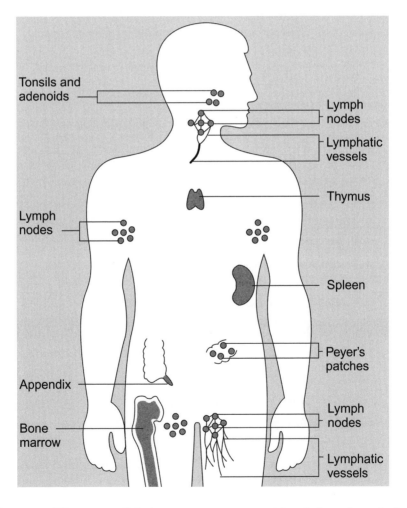

Figure 2.1. The organs of the immune system are positioned throughout the body

Immune cells and foreign particles enter the lymph nodes via incoming lymphatic vessels or the lymph nodes' tiny blood vessels. All lymphocytes exit lymph nodes through outgoing lymphatic vessels. Once in the bloodstream, they are transported to tissues throughout the body. They patrol everywhere for foreign antigens, then gradually drift back into the lymphatic system, to begin the cycle all over again.

The spleen is a flattened organ at the upper left of the abdomen. Like the lymph nodes, the spleen contains specialized compartments where immune cells gather and work, and serves as a meeting ground where immune defenses confront antigens.

Clumps of lymphoid tissue are found in many parts of the body, especially in the linings of the digestive tract and the airways and lungs—territories that serve as gateways to the body. These tissues include the tonsils, adenoids, and appendix.

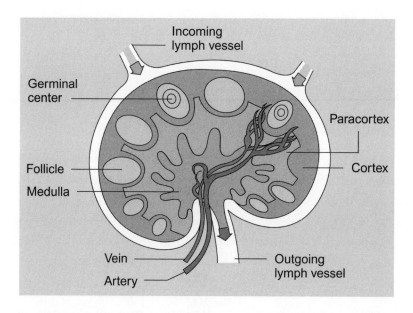

Figure 2.2. *The lymph node contains numerous specialized structures. T cells concentrate in the paracortex, B cells in and around the germinal centers, and plasma cells in the medulla.*

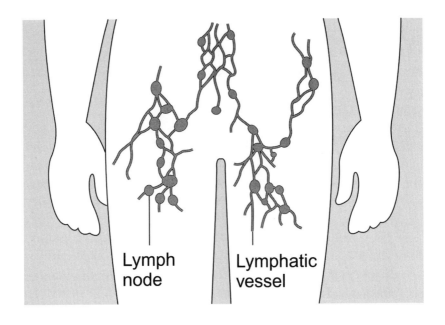

Figure 2.3. Immune cells and foreign particles enter the lymph nodes via incoming lymphatic vessels or the lymph nodes' tiny blood vessels.

Immune Cells And Their Products

The immune system stockpiles a huge arsenal of cells, not only lymphocytes but also cell-devouring phagocytes and their relatives. Some immune cells take on all comers, while others are trained on highly specific targets. To work effectively, most immune cells need the cooperation of their comrades. Sometimes immune cells communicate by direct physical contact, sometimes by releasing chemical messengers.

The immune system stores just a few of each kind of the different cells needed to recognize millions of possible enemies. When an antigen appears, those few matching cells multiply into a full-scale army. After their job is done, they fade away, leaving sentries behind to watch for future attacks.

B Lymphocytes

B cells and T cells are the main types of lymphocytes.

B cells work chiefly by secreting substances called antibodies into the body's fluids. Antibodies ambush antigens circulating the bloodstream. They are powerless, however, to penetrate cells. The job of attacking target cells—either cells that have been infected by viruses or cells that have been distorted by cancer—is left to T cells or other immune cells.

Each B cell is programmed to make one specific antibody. For example, one B cell will make an antibody that blocks a virus that causes the common cold, while another produces an antibody that attacks a bacterium that causes pneumonia.

When a B cell encounters its triggering antigen, it gives rise to many large cells known as plasma cells. Every plasma cell is essentially a factory for producing an antibody. Each of the plasma cells descended from a given B cell manufactures millions of identical antibody molecules and pours them into the bloodstream.

An antigen matches an antibody much as a key matches a lock. Some match exactly; others fit more like a skeleton key. But whenever antigen and antibody interlock, the antibody marks the antigen for destruction.

T Cells

Unlike B cells, T cells do not recognize free-floating antigens. Rather, their surfaces contain specialized antibody-like receptors that see fragments of antigens on the surfaces of

♣ **It's A Fact!!**

All immune cells begin as immature stem cells in the bone marrow. They respond to different cytokines and other signals to grow into specific immune cell types, such as T cells, B cells, or phagocytes. Because stem cells have not yet committed to a particular future, they are an interesting possibility for treating some immune system disorders. Researchers currently are investigating if a person's own stem cells can be used to regenerate damaged immune responses in autoimmune diseases and immune deficiency diseases.

♣ **It's A Fact!!**

Antibodies belong to a family of large molecules known as immunoglobulins. Different types play different roles in the immune defense strategy.

- Immunoglobulin G, or IgG, works efficiently to coat microbes, speeding their uptake by other cells in the immune system.

- IgM is very effective at killing bacteria.

- IgA concentrates in body fluids—tears, saliva, the secretions of the respiratory tract and the digestive tract—guarding the entrances to the body.

- IgE, whose natural job probably is to protect against parasitic infections, is the villain responsible for the symptoms of allergy.

- IgD remains attached to B cells and plays a key role in initiating early B-cell response.

infected or cancerous cells. T cells contribute to immune defenses in two major ways: some direct and regulate immune responses; others directly attack infected or cancerous cells.

Helper T cells, or Th cells, coordinate immune responses by communicating with other cells. Some stimulate nearby B cells to produce antibody, others call in microbe-gobbling cells called phagocytes, still others activate other T cells.

Killer T cells—also called cytotoxic T lymphocytes or CTLs—perform a different function. These cells directly attack other cells carrying certain foreign or abnormal molecules on their surfaces. CTLs are especially useful for attacking viruses because viruses often hide from other parts of the immune system while they grow inside infected cells. CTLs recognize small fragments of these viruses peeking out from the cell membrane and launch an attack to kill the cell.

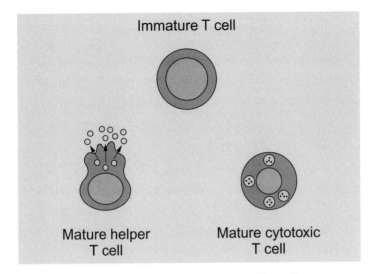

Figure 2.4. Some T cells are helper cells, others are killer cells.

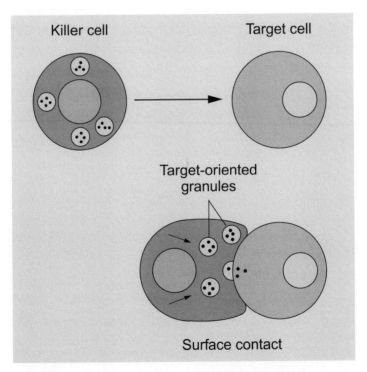

Figure 2.5. Killer cell makes contact with target cell, trains its weapons on the target, then strikes.

In most cases, T cells only recognize an antigen if it is carried on the surface of a cell by one of the body's own MHC, or major histocompatibility complex, molecules. MHC molecules are proteins recognized by T cells when distinguishing between self and nonself. A self MHC molecule provides a recognizable scaffolding to present a foreign antigen to the T cell.

Although MHC molecules are required for T-cell responses against foreign invaders, they also pose a difficulty during organ transplantations. Virtually every cell in the body is covered with MHC proteins, but each person has a different set of these proteins on his or her cells. If a T cell recognizes a nonself MHC molecule on another cell, it will destroy the cell. Therefore, doctors must match organ recipients with donors who have the closest MHC makeup. Otherwise the recipient's T cells will likely attack the transplanted organ, leading to graft rejection.

Natural killer (NK) cells are another kind of lethal white cell, or lymphocyte. Like killer T cells, NK cells are armed with granules filled with potent chemicals. But while killer T cells look for antigen fragments bound to self-MHC molecules, NK cells recognize cells lacking self-MHC molecules. Thus NK cells have the potential to attack many types of foreign cells.

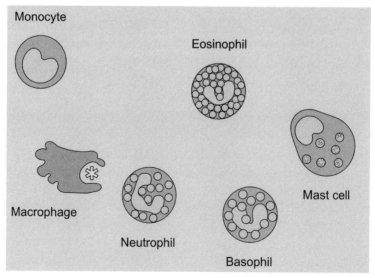

Figure 2.6. Phagocytes, granulocytes, and mast cells, all with different methods of attack, demonstrate the immune system's versatility.

Both kinds of killer cells slay on contact. The deadly assassins bind to their targets, aim their weapons, and then deliver a lethal burst of chemicals.

Phagocytes And Their Relatives

Phagocytes are large white cells that can swallow and digest microbes and other foreign particles. Monocytes are phagocytes that circulate in the blood. When monocytes migrate into tissues, they develop into macrophages. Specialized types of macrophages can be found in many organs, including lungs, kidneys, brain, and liver.

Macrophages play many roles. As scavengers, they rid the body of worn-out cells and other debris. They display bits of foreign antigen in a way that draws the attention of matching lymphocytes. And they churn out an amazing variety of powerful chemical signals, known as monokines, which are vital to the immune responses.

Granulocytes are another kind of immune cell. They contain granules filled with potent chemicals, which allow the granulocytes to destroy microorganisms. Some of these chemicals, such as histamine, also contribute to inflammation and allergy.

One type of granulocyte, the neutrophil, is also a phagocyte; it uses its prepackaged chemicals to break down the microbes it ingests. Eosinophils and basophils are granulocytes that "degranulate," spraying their chemicals onto harmful cells or microbes nearby.

The mast cell is a twin of the basophil, except that it is not a blood cell. Rather, it is found in the lungs, skin, tongue, and linings of the nose and intestinal tract, where it is responsible for the symptoms of allergy.

A related structure, the blood platelet, is a cell fragment. Platelets, too, contain granules. In addition to promoting blood clotting and wound repair, platelets activate some of the immune defenses.

Cytokines

Components of the immune system communicate with one another by exchanging chemical messengers called cytokines. These proteins are secreted by cells and act on other cells to coordinate an appropriate immune response. Cytokines include a diverse assortment of interleukins, interferons, and growth factors.

Some cytokines are chemical switches that turn certain immune cell types on and off.

One cytokine, interleukin 2 (IL-2), triggers the immune system to produce T cells. IL-2's immunity-boosting properties have traditionally made it a promising treatment for several illnesses. Clinical studies are ongoing to test its benefits in other diseases such as cancer, hepatitis C, and HIV infection and AIDS. Other cytokines also are being studied for their potential clinical benefit.

Other cytokines chemically attract specific cell types. These so-called chemokines are released by cells at a site of injury or infection and call other immune cells to the region to help repair the damage or fight off the invader. Chemokines often play a key role in inflammation and are a promising target for new drugs to help regulate immune responses.

Complement

The complement system is made up of about 25 proteins that work together to "complement" the action of antibodies in destroying bacteria. Complement also helps to rid the body of antibody-coated antigens (antigen-antibody complexes). Complement proteins, which cause blood vessels to become dilated and then leaky, contribute to the redness, warmth, swelling, pain, and loss of function that characterize an inflammatory response.

Complement proteins circulate in the blood in an inactive form. When the first protein in the complement series is activated—typically by antibody that has locked onto an antigen—it sets in motion a domino effect. Each component takes its turn in a precise chain of steps known as the complement cascade. The end product is a cylinder inserted into—and puncturing a hole in—the cell's wall. With fluids and molecules flowing in and out, the cell swells and bursts. Other components of the complement system make bacteria more susceptible to phagocytosis or beckon other cells to the area.

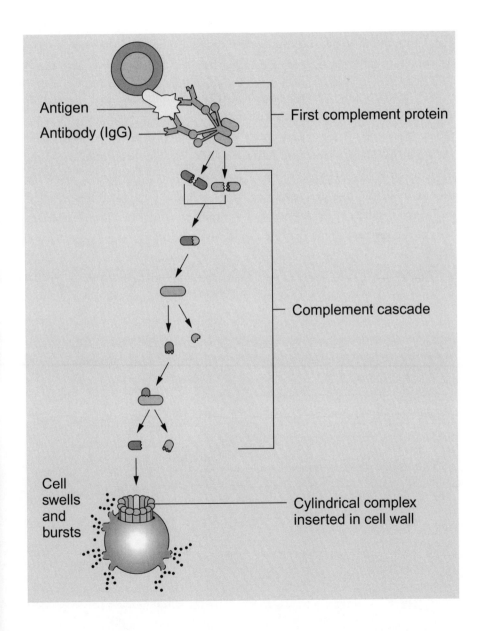

Antigen

Antibody (IgG)

First complement protein

Complement cascade

Cell swells and bursts

Cylindrical complex inserted in cell wall

Figure 2.7. The interlocking steps of the complement cascade end in cell death.

Mounting An Immune Response

Infections are the most common cause of human disease. They range from the common cold to debilitating conditions like chronic hepatitis to life-threatening diseases such as AIDS. Disease-causing microbes (pathogens) attempting to get into the body must first move past the body's external armor, usually the skin or cells lining the body's internal passageways.

The skin provides an imposing barrier to invading microbes. It is generally penetrable only through cuts or tiny abrasions. The digestive and respiratory tracts—both portals of entry for a number of microbes—also have their own levels of protection. Microbes entering the nose often cause the nasal surfaces to secrete more protective mucus, and attempts to enter the nose or lungs can trigger a sneeze or cough reflex to force microbial invaders out of the respiratory passageways. The stomach contains a strong acid that destroys many pathogens that are swallowed with food.

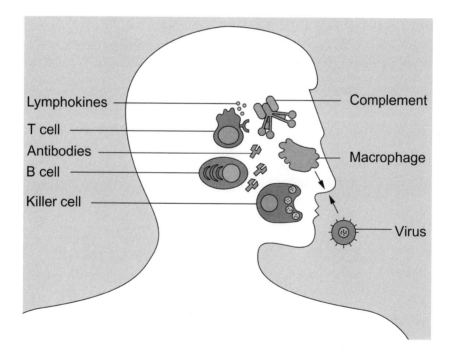

Figure 2.8. When challenged, the immune system has many weapons to choose.

If microbes survive the body's front-line defenses, they still have to find a way through the walls of the digestive, respiratory, or urogenital passageways to the underlying cells. These passageways are lined with tightly packed epithelial cells covered in a layer of mucus, effectively blocking the transport of many organisms. Mucosal surfaces also secrete a special class of antibody called IgA, which in many cases is the first type of antibody to encounter an invading microbe. Underneath the epithelial layer a number of cells, including macrophages, B cells, and T cells, lie in wait for any germ that might bypass the barriers at the surface.

Next, invaders must escape a series of general defenses, which are ready to attack, without regard for specific antigen markers. These include patrolling phagocytes, NK cells, and complement.

Microbes that cross the general barriers then confront specific weapons tailored just for them. Specific weapons, which include both antibodies and T cells, are equipped with singular receptor structures that allow them to recognize and interact with their designated targets.

Bacteria, Viruses, And Parasites

The most common disease-causing microbes are bacteria, viruses, and parasites. Each uses a different tactic to infect a person, and, therefore, each is thwarted by a different part of the immune system.

Most bacteria live in the spaces between cells and are readily attacked by antibodies. When antibodies attach to a bacterium, they send signals to complement proteins and phagocytic cells to destroy the bound microbes. Some bacteria are eaten directly by phagocytes, which signal to certain T cells to join the attack.

All viruses, plus a few types of bacteria and parasites, must enter cells to survive, requiring a different approach. Infected cells use their MHC molecules to put pieces of the invading microbes on the cell's surface, flagging down cytotoxic T lymphocytes to destroy the infected cell. Antibodies also can assist in the immune response, attaching to and clearing viruses before they have a chance to enter the cell.

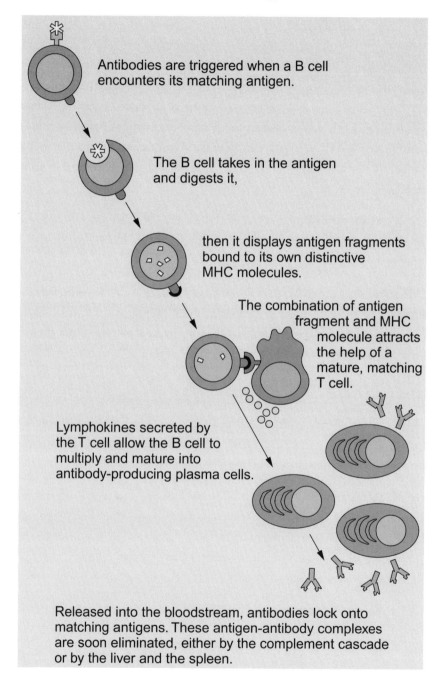

Antibodies are triggered when a B cell encounters its matching antigen.

The B cell takes in the antigen and digests it,

then it displays antigen fragments bound to its own distinctive MHC molecules.

The combination of antigen fragment and MHC molecule attracts the help of a mature, matching T cell.

Lymphokines secreted by the T cell allow the B cell to multiply and mature into antibody-producing plasma cells.

Released into the bloodstream, antibodies lock onto matching antigens. These antigen-antibody complexes are soon eliminated, either by the complement cascade or by the liver and the spleen.

Figure 2.9. B-cells play an important role in the immune system.

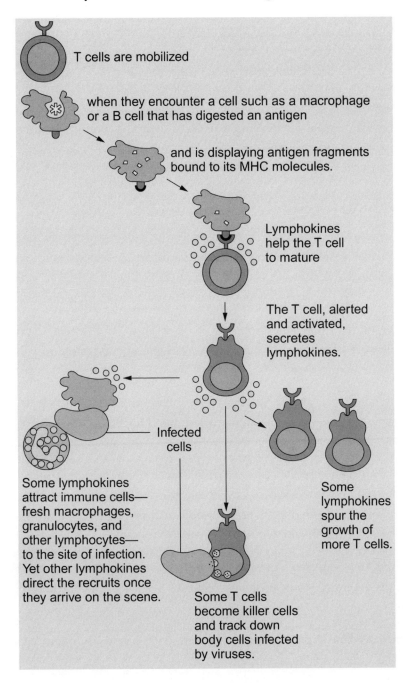

T cells are mobilized

when they encounter a cell such as a macrophage or a B cell that has digested an antigen

and is displaying antigen fragments bound to its MHC molecules.

Lymphokines help the T cell to mature

The T cell, alerted and activated, secretes lymphokines.

Infected cells

Some lymphokines attract immune cells—fresh macrophages, granulocytes, and other lymphocytes—to the site of infection. Yet other lymphokines direct the recruits once they arrive on the scene.

Some lymphokines spur the growth of more T cells.

Some T cells become killer cells and track down body cells infected by viruses.

Figure 2.10. T-cells play an important role in the immune system.

Parasites live either inside or outside cells. Intracellular parasites such as the organism that causes malaria can trigger T-cell responses. Extracellular parasites are often much larger than bacteria or viruses and require a much broader immune attack. Parasitic infections often trigger an inflammatory response when eosinophils, basophils, and other specialized granular cells rush to the scene and release their stores of toxic chemicals in an attempt to destroy the invader. Antibodies also play a role in this attack, attracting the granular cells to the site of infection.

Immunity: Natural And Acquired

Long ago, physicians realized that people who had recovered from the plague would never get it again—they had acquired immunity. This is because some of the activated T and B cells become memory cells. The next time an individual meets up with the same antigen, the immune system is set to demolish it.

Immunity can be strong or weak, short-lived or long-lasting, depending on the type of antigen, the amount of antigen, and the route by which it enters the body.

Immunity can also be influenced by inherited genes. When faced with the same antigen, some individuals will respond forcefully, others feebly, and some not at all.

An immune response can be sparked not only by infection but also by immunization with vaccines. Vaccines contain microorganisms—or parts of microorganisms—that have been treated so they can provoke an immune response but not full-blown disease.

Immunity can also be transferred from one individual to another by injections of serum rich in antibodies against a particular microbe (antiserum).

For example, immune serum is sometimes given to protect travelers to countries where hepatitis A is widespread. Such passive immunity typically lasts only a few weeks or months.

Infants are born with weak immune responses but are protected for the first few months of life by antibodies received from their mothers before birth. Babies who are nursed can also receive some antibodies from breast milk that help to protect their digestive tracts.

Immune Tolerance

Immune tolerance is the tendency of T or B lymphocytes to ignore the body's own tissues. Maintaining tolerance is important because it prevents the immune system from attacking its fellow cells. Scientists are hard at work trying to understand how the immune system knows when to respond and when to ignore.

Tolerance occurs in at least two ways. Central tolerance occurs during lymphocyte development. Very early in each immune cell's life, it is exposed to many of the self molecules in the body. If it encounters these molecules before it has fully matured, the encounter activates an internal self-destruct pathway and the immune cell dies. This process, called clonal deletion, helps ensure that self-reactive T cells and B cells do not mature and attack healthy tissues.

Because maturing lymphocytes do not encounter every molecule in the body, they must also learn to ignore mature cells and tissues. In peripheral tolerance, circulating lymphocytes might recognize a self molecule but cannot respond because some of the chemical signals required to activate the T or B cell are absent. So-called clonal anergy, therefore, keeps potentially harmful lymphocytes switched off. Peripheral tolerance may also be imposed by a special class of regulatory T cells that inhibits helper or cytotoxic T-cell activation by self antigens.

Vaccines

Medical workers have long helped the body's immune system prepare for future attacks through vaccination. Vaccines consist of killed or modified microbes, components of microbes, or microbial DNA that trick the body into thinking an infection has occurred. An immunized person's immune system attacks the harmless vaccine and prepares for subsequent invasions. Vaccines remain one of the best ways to prevent infectious diseases and have an excellent safety record. Previously devastating diseases such as smallpox, polio, and whooping cough have been greatly controlled or eliminated through worldwide vaccination programs.

Allergic Diseases

The most common types of allergic diseases occur when the immune system responds to a false alarm. In an allergic person, a normally harmless material such as grass pollen or house dust is mistaken for a threat and attacked. Allergies such as pollen allergy are related to the antibody known as IgE. Like other antibodies, each IgE antibody is specific; one acts against oak pollen, another against ragweed.

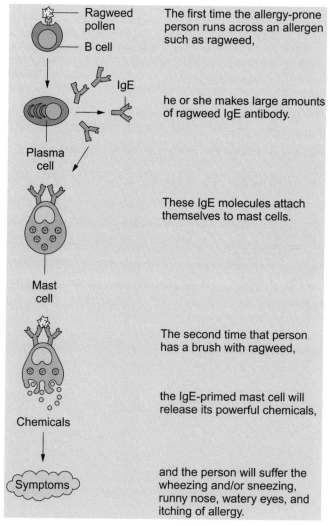

Figure 2.11. The development of an allergy.

Chapter 3

Allergy Testing

Allergy testing is the only way to find out if you're allergic. It is also the only way to find out which allergens are causing your allergic condition. Once you know what you are allergic to, it is much easier to avoid your allergens and treat your symptoms.

What types of allergy testing can be done?

Prick Skin Testing: A reliable test for allergies is the prick skin test. A small amount of each thing you may be allergic to (allergen) is placed on the skin—often the back. The skin is then pricked. If you are allergic to an allergen, you will get a bump and redness where the skin is pricked. After a short time, each skin test reaction is measured for swelling and redness. If there is a large enough skin reaction, it means that you may be allergic to the allergen placed at that site. The information from your prick skin test results and your history of symptoms will help your doctor to determine if you have an allergy.

Antihistamines can affect the skin test results. Your doctor may tell you to stop these medications for days to weeks before the testing is done. Other medicines can also affect the results and may need to be avoided. Ask your healthcare provider what medicines to avoid before your prick skin tests are done.

✤ It's A Fact!!
How are allergies diagnosed?

First, your doctor will ask you questions about your health and symptoms. Make sure to tell your doctor if anyone in your family has allergies. If family members have allergies, your chances of having allergies increase. Your doctor uses the following information to make a diagnosis of allergy:

• Physical exam

• History of your symptoms and family history

• Allergy tests (not always needed)

Allergy tests can be done to help identify if you are allergic and what you are allergic to. Once allergies are identified, specific avoidance and treatment measures can be recommended. There are several types of allergy testing.

Source: © Copyright 2005 National Jewish Medical and Research Center. All rights reserved.

Intradermal Skin Testing: Another form of skin testing for allergy is by intradermal skin testing. This method is not as reliable as prick skin testing. It is most often used when prick skin testing is negative and there is a strong suspicion of allergy from the history. A small amount of each thing you may be allergic to (allergen) is placed under the skin with a needle, usually on the arm. If you are allergic to an allergen, you will get a bump and redness where the needle has gone under the skin. After a short time, each skin test reaction is measured for swelling and redness. If there is a large enough skin reaction, it means that you may be allergic to the allergen placed at that site. The information from these test results and your history of symptoms will help your doctor to determine if you have an allergy.

Antihistamines and other medicines can also affect these skin test results. Ask your healthcare provider what medicines to avoid before your skin tests are done.

Blood Testing: A blood test is another kind of test that can be done to help find out if you have allergies. There is some evidence that blood tests are not as sensitive as prick skin tests in determining allergies. However, a blood test may be done if you have skin problems or, if there is concern that someone will have a severe reaction to a skin test (this is very rare). There are many types of blood tests that can be used to detect allergies. The most common one is called RAST testing.

Patch Skin Testing: Patch skin testing may be used to find out if a rash is from direct contact with an allergen. Small amounts of allergens are placed on the skin, often the back. The skin is covered with a watertight bandage for several days. After several days the patch is removed and the skin reactions are measured to find out if you may have a contact allergy.

Food Challenge: If you have a positive skin test to foods, your doctor may consider a food challenge. In some cases, this test is the only way to make a diagnosis of food allergy. Increasing doses of the suspected food are given and you are checked for symptoms. The food challenge may be double blind. This means neither the patient, nor the person giving the test knows the type of food being challenged. Only the doctor prescribing the challenge knows the food. Food challenges are done in a medical setting where emergency care is available. This test is rarely done if there is a history of a life-threatening reaction to a food.

Alternative (Unproven) Methods: There are many other tests to diagnose allergies. Many have not been scientifically proven to be effective and accurate. Talk with your doctor or a board-certified allergist about the best way to determine your allergies.

✎ What's It Mean?

RAST: RAST is an abbreviation for RadioAllergoSorbent Test, a trademark of Pharmacia Diagnostics, which originated the test. RAST is a laboratory test used to detect IgE antibodies to specific allergens.

Source: Excerpted from "Allergy-Immunology Glossary," © 2005 American College of Allergy, Asthma, and Immunology. All rights reserved. Reprinted with permission.

Should you see an allergy expert?

Many people with allergies see a family doctor for allergy care. You may choose to visit a doctor who is an expert in allergies. These doctors are called board-certified allergists. Here are a few reasons to see an allergy expert:

- Your symptoms make daily activities hard.

- Your symptoms are getting worse.

- You are concerned about side effects of medicine.

- Your regular doctor refers you to an expert for tests.

Allergy tests can be done to help identify if you are allergic, and what you are allergic to. Once allergies are identified, specific avoidance and treatment measures can be recommended. Talk with you doctor if you think you may have allergies.

✔ **Quick Tip**

Are there other allergy tests?

You may hear of allergy tests that are unproven or not universally accepted. If your health care provider suggests one of these tests, consider getting a second opinion about allergy testing:

- cytotoxicity blood test

- electroacupuncture biofeedback

- urine autoinjection

- skin titration

- sublingual provocative testing

- candidiasis allergy theory

- basophil histamine release

Source: Excerpted from "Allergy Testing For Children," and reprinted with permission from the Asthma and Allergy Foundation of America, © 2005. All rights reserved.

Chapter 4

Allergy Shots (Immunotherapy)

Though not a cure, allergy shots can significantly reduce allergy symptoms in some people who are unable to avoid allergens, and who do not respond well to other medications.

What is immunotherapy?

Immunotherapy (commonly called allergy shots) is a form of treatment to reduce your allergic reaction to allergens. Allergens are substances to which you are allergic. Research has shown that allergy shots can reduce symptoms of allergic rhinitis (hay fever) and allergic asthma. Remember, not all asthma is due to allergies. Allergy shots can be effective against grass, weed and tree pollens, house dust mites, cat and dog dander and insect stings. Allergy shots are less effective against molds and are not a useful method for the treatment of food allergy.

Immunotherapy consists of a series of injections (shots) with a solution containing the allergens that cause your symptoms. Treatment usually begins with a weak solution given once or twice a week. The strength of the solution is gradually increased with each dose. Once the strongest dosage is reached, the injections are often given once a month to control your symptoms. At this point, you have decreased your sensitivity to the allergens. You have reached your maintenance level. Allergy shots should always be given at your healthcare provider's office.

✎ What's It Mean?

Immunotherapy: Immunotherapy ("allergy shots") is a form of preventive and anti-inflammatory treatment of allergy to substances such as pollens, house dust mites, fungi, and stinging insect venom. Immunotherapy involves giving gradually increasing doses of the substance, or allergen, to which the person is allergic. The incremental increases of the allergen cause the immune system to become less sensitive to the substance, perhaps by causing production of a particular "blocking" antibody, which reduces the symptoms of allergy when the substances is encountered in the future.

Source: Excerpted from "Allergy-Immunology Glossary," © 2005 American College of Allergy, Asthma, and Immunology. All rights reserved. Reprinted with permission.

When is immunotherapy recommended?

If you are thinking of allergy shots, ask your healthcare provider about a referral to a board certified allergist. A board certified allergist will follow a number of steps to evaluate if allergy shots are right for you.

First, the allergist will ask you questions about your environment and symptoms. This will help determine if skin testing is needed. Prick skin testing may be done. This will help identify the specific allergens that are causing your symptoms. Skin testing should only be done under the supervision of a board certified allergist.

Once an allergy has been identified, the next step is to decrease or eliminate exposure to the allergen. This is called environmental control. Evidence shows that allergy and asthma symptoms may improve over time, if the recommended environmental control changes are made. For example, removing furry or feathered pets or following control measures for house dust mites and cockroaches may decrease symptoms. Preventing your contact with grasses, weeds and tree pollen may be more difficult. Closing outside doors and windows and using air conditioning decreases exposure in the home.

Next, your healthcare provider may recommend medication. Antihistamines and nasal medications may be recommended. Allergy shots may be recommended for people with severe allergic rhinitis. They may also be recommended for people with allergic asthma when the allergen cannot be avoided. Allergy shots should be prescribed only by a board certified allergist.

How long are allergy shots given?

Six months to a year of allergy shots may be required before you notice any improvement in symptoms. If your symptoms do not improve after this time, ask you allergist to review your overall treatment program. If the treatment is effective, the shots often continue three to five years, until the person is symptom-free or until symptoms can be controlled with mild medications for one year. In general, allergy shots should be stopped if they are not effective within two to three years.

What is rush immunotherapy?

Rush immunotherapy is a series of allergy shots. They are given over two to three days in a row. This "rushes" the initial phase of the treatment. Increasing doses of allergen extract are given every 30 minutes to hourly instead of every few days or weeks. There is an increased risk of a reaction with this procedure. Therefore, rush immunotherapy should only be done in a hospital or high risk procedure area under very close supervision.

Are there other therapies?

There are a number of alternative treatments that claim to "cure" allergies. These methods are not supported by scientific studies. They are not approved by the American Academy of Allergy and Immunology. Unapproved alternative treatments include:

- High-dose vitamin and mineral therapy;

- Urine injections;

- Bacterial vaccines;

- Exotic diets.

It is easy to feel overwhelmed or confused by the many different methods of allergy testing and treatment. We encourage you to work with a board certified allergist to evaluate and determine what is appropriate for you.

♣ It's A Fact!!

- Allergy shots are an effective and safe treatment for people who suffer from a variety of allergic diseases, including allergic rhinitis (hay fever), asthma, and insect stings.

- The treatment—also known as immunotherapy or allergy immunization—works by introducing small amounts of purified substances to which the person is allergic, in gradually increasing amounts. The allergy shots improve the patient's natural resistance to the allergens and minimize or eliminate the need for medications.

- Allergy shots usually must be continued for several years, but sometimes can be discontinued with immunity maintained for a lifetime.

- Allergy shots have been available since the early part of the century. The treatment has been continuously improved and refined.

- Performed by a trained and experienced physician, allergy shots are very safe. However, because the treatment involves introducing a substance to which the person is allergic, in rare cases severe reactions can occur. It is recommended that only allergists, or other physicians with special training, administer or supervise allergy shots.

- Allergy shots are one component of the treatment of allergies and asthma. Others are avoidance of the allergens that cause symptoms, and appropriate medications to control symptoms.

- Research continues to show that besides decreasing symptoms, allergy shots may also prevent the development of asthma in some patients with allergic rhinitis and, if begun early, may prevent future allergies.

Source: From "Immunotherapy (Allergy Shots)," © 2005 American College of Allergy, Asthma, and Immunology (ACAAI). All rights reserved. Reprinted with permission. More information on allergy shots is available in a free brochure created by the American College of Allergy, Asthma and Immunology entitled "You Can Have a Life Without Allergies." It is available on the ACAAI website http://www.acaai.org or by calling 800-842-7777.

Chapter 5

Allergy Medications

What You Need to Know about Allergy Medications

There is no cure for allergies, but there are several types of medicines available—both over-the-counter and prescription—to help ease annoying symptoms like congestion and runny nose. These include antihistamines, decongestants, combination medicines, corticosteroids, and others.

Allergy shots, which gradually increase your ability to tolerate allergens, are also available.

Antihistamines

Antihistamines have been used for years to treat allergy symptoms. They can be taken as pills, liquid, nasal spray, or eye drops. Over-the-counter antihistamine eye drops can relieve red itchy eyes, while nasal sprays can be used to treat the symptoms of seasonal or year-round allergies.

Examples of antihistamines include:

About This Chapter: This chapter begins with "What You Need to Know about Allergy Medications" from "Allergy Medications," © 2005 Cleveland Clinic Foundation, 9500 Euclid Avenue, Cleveland, OH 44195, www.clevelandclinic.org. Additional information is available from the Cleveland Clinic Health Information Center, 216-444-3771, tollfree 800-223-2273 extension 43771, or at http://www.clevelandclinic.org/health. Text under the heading "Over-the-Counter Medications" is reprinted with permission from the Asthma and Allergy Foundation of America, © 2005. All rights reserved.

- **Over-the-counter:** Benadryl, Claritin, Chlor-Trimeton, Dimetane, and Tavist. Ocu-Hist is an OTC eye drop.

- **Prescription:** Clarinex, Allegra, and Zyrtec. Atarax is a prescription nasal spray. Eye drops include Emadine and Livostin.

How do antihistamines work?

When you are exposed to an allergen—like ragweed pollen—it triggers your immune system to go into action. Immune system cells known as "mast cells" release a substance called histamine, which attaches to receptors in blood vessels causing them to enlarge. Histamine also binds to other receptors causing redness, swelling, itching, and changes in secretions. By blocking histamine receptors, antihistamines prevent these symptoms.

What are the side effects?

Many over-the-counter antihistamines cause drowsiness. Non-sedating antihistamines are available by prescription.

Decongestants

Decongestants relieve congestion and are often prescribed along with antihistamines. They come in nasal spray, eye drop, or pill form.

Nasal spray and eye drop decongestants can be used for only a few days, since long-term use can make symptoms worse. Pills may be taken longer safely.

Some examples of decongestants include:

- **Over-the-counter:** Sudafed tablets, Neo-Synephrine, and Afrin nasal sprays, and Visine eye drops.

- **Prescription:** Prescription decongestants include drugs like Claritin-D that combine a decongestant with another allergy medicine.

How do decongestants work?

During an allergic reaction, tissues in your nose swell in response to contact with the allergen. That swelling produces fluid and mucous. Blood vessels in the eyes also swell, causing redness. Decongestants shrink swollen nasal tissues and blood vessels to relieve the symptoms of nasal swelling, congestion, mucous secretion, and redness.

What are the side effects?

Decongestants may raise blood pressure, so they are not recommended for people who have blood pressure problems or glaucoma. They may also cause insomnia or irritability and restrict urinary flow.

✎ What's It Mean?

Antihistamines: Antihistamines are a group of drugs that block the effects of histamine, a chemical released in body fluids during an allergic reaction. In rhinitis, antihistamines reduce itching, sneezing, and runny nose.

Anti-inflammatories: Anti-inflammatory drugs reduce the symptoms and signs of inflammation. Although not a drug, immunotherapy ("allergy shots") reduces inflammation in both allergic rhinitis and allergic asthma.

Bronchodilators: Bronchodilators are a group of drugs that widen the airways in the lungs.

Corticosteroids: Corticosteroids are a group of anti-inflammatory drugs similar to the natural corticosteroid hormones produced by the cortex of the adrenal glands. Among the disorders that often improve with corticosteroid treatment include asthma, allergic rhinitis, eczema, and rheumatoid arthritis.

Theophylline: Theophylline is a bronchodilator drug, given by mouth, that widens the airways to the lung. It also is used to prevent attacks of apnea (cessation of breathing) in premature infants and to treat heart failure because it stimulates heart rate and increases urine excretion.

Source: Excerpted from "Allergy-Immunology Glossary," © 2005 American College of Allergy, Asthma, and Immunology. All rights reserved. Reprinted with permission.

Combination Medicines

Some allergy medicines contain both an antihistamine and a decongestant to relieve multiple symptoms. There are also other combinations, such as those between an allergy medicine and asthma medicine and an antihistamine eye drop with a mast cell stabilizer drug.

The following are some examples of combination medicines:

- **Over-the-counter:** Benadryl Allergy and Sinus, Tylenol Allergy and Sinus, and Dimetapp.

- **Prescription:** Allegra-D, Claritin-D, Semprex-D, and Zyrtec-D for nasal allergies. Naphcon, Vasocon, Zaditor, Patanol, and Optivar for allergic conjunctivitis.

Corticosteroids

Corticosteroids reduce inflammation associated with allergies. They prevent and treat nasal stuffiness, sneezing, and itchy, runny nose due to seasonal or year-round allergies. They can also decrease inflammation and swelling from other types of allergic reactions.

Corticosteroids are available as pills for serious allergies or asthma, inhalers for asthma, nasal sprays for seasonal or year-round allergies, creams for skin allergies, or as an eye drop for allergic conjunctivitis. Often, a doctor will prescribe a corticosteroid in addition to other allergy medications, for treatment of severe allergy symptoms.

The drugs are highly effective, but they must be taken daily to be of benefit—even when you aren't feeling symptoms. In addition, it may take one to two weeks before the full effect of the medicine can be felt.

Some corticosteroids include the following:

- **Nasal corticosteroids:** Beconase, Rhinocort, Flonase, Nasonex, and Nasacort, used to treat nasal allergy symptoms.

- **Inhaled corticosteroids:** Beclovent, Pulmicort, Flovent, and Azmacort, used to treat asthma. Advair is an inhaled drug that combines a corticosteroid with another drug to treat asthma. Inhaled corticosteroids are available only with a prescription.

- **Eye drops:** Dexamethasone, Alrex.

- **Oral steroid:** Deltasone, also called prednisone.

What are the side effects?

Corticosteroids have many potential side effects, especially when given orally and for a long period of time.

Side effects with short-term use include the following:

- Weight gain

- Fluid retention

- High blood pressure

Side effects with long-term use include the following:

- Growth suppression

- Diabetes

- Cataracts of the eyes

- Bone thinning osteoporosis

- Muscle weakness

Side effects of inhaled corticosteroids may also cause cough and yeast infections of the mouth.

Bronchodilators

Bronchodilators are inhaled medicines used to control asthma symptoms and are available only with a prescription. A short-acting bronchodilator is used to provide quick relief for asthma symptoms during an attack. Long-acting bronchodilators can provide up to 12-hours of relief from asthma symptoms, which is helpful to people who suffer from nighttime asthma problems.

How do bronchodilators work?

Bronchodilators relax the muscle bands that tighten around the airways. This rapidly opens the airways, letting more air in and out of the lungs, improving breathing.

Bronchodilators also help clear mucus from the lungs. As the airways open, the mucus moves more freely and can be coughed out more easily.

Generally one or two puffs of the inhaler relieve the wheezing and chest tightness associated with a mild attack. It may be necessary to take more puffs for severe attacks.

Some types of bronchodilators include the following:

- Ventolin, Proventil, Volmax
- Brethaire
- Tornalate
- Xopenex
- Alupent, Metaprel
- Maxair

What are the side effects?

Bronchodilators are potent drugs. If overused, they can cause dangerous side effects such as high blood pressure and a fast heartbeat.

✔ **Quick Tip**
Prescription Pointers

Before giving or taking any medications, take a minute to examine your prescription. First make sure the name on the prescription is correct. Then read the label carefully and look closely at the medication. Notify your pharmacist if you notice any of these warning signs:

- The tablets or capsules are a different size or color from what you usually take; or liquids look or smell different.

- The medication name on the label is different from what your physician prescribed.

- Instructions on the label are different from previous instructions or the instructions given by your physician.

- The pills in the bottle are not all the same.

- Some pills in the same package show a variation in color or appear darker or lighter than others.

- Capsules are deformed.

- Imprints on capsules or tablets appear smeared.

- The medication has expired or will expire prior to completion of the prescription (usually only the manufacturer's bottle will contain the expiration date).

Source: Reprinted courtesy of Allergy & Asthma Network Mothers of Asthmatics (AANMA), 800-878-4403, www.breatherville.org, © 2002.

Mast Cell Stabilizers

Mast cell stabilizers can be used to treat mild to moderate inflammation in the bronchial tubes and other symptoms of allergic reactions. These medications can also be used to prevent asthma symptoms during exercise and can be given before exposure to an allergen when it cannot be avoided.

Mast cell stabilizers are available as inhalers for asthma, eyedrops for allergic conjunctivitis, and nasal sprays for nasal allergy symptoms. Like many drugs it may take several weeks before the full effects are felt.

Some examples of mast cell stabilizers include the following:

- Intal
- Crolom
- Alocril
- Alamast
- Tilade
- Alomide
- Opticrom
- Nasalcrom

How do mast cell stabilizers work?

Mast cell stabilizers work by stopping the release of histamine from mast cells (cells that make and store histamine). Some of these drugs also have important anti-inflammatory effects.

What are the side effects?

Throat irritation, coughing, or skin rashes sometimes can occur with inhaled treatment. Some people say that Tilade has a bad taste. Using a spacer to take the medicine and drinking juice following treatment may decrease the taste. Eye drops may cause burning, stinging, or blurred vision.

Leukotriene Modifiers

Leukotriene modifiers are used to treat asthma and nasal allergy symptoms. They are often prescribed along with an inhaled corticosteroid for treatment of mild and moderate persistent asthma.

These medications are available only with a doctor's prescription and come as pills or chewable tablets.

Some brand names include the following:

- Accolate
- Zyflo
- Singulair

How do they work?

Leukotriene modifiers block the effects of leukotrienes, chemicals produced in the body in response to an allergy.

What are the side effects?

- Stomach pain or stomach upset
- Heartburn

- Fever
- Stuffy nose
- Cough

- Rash
- Headache

Immunotherapy

Immunotherapy, or allergy shots, may be the most effective form of treatment if you suffer from allergies more than three months of the year. These shots expose you to gradually increasing levels of the offending allergen to help your immune system build tolerance.

Over-The-Counter Medications

It's the beginning of your "allergy season"—that time of year when there is something in the air that causes you to have hay fever. You sneeze, have a runny nose and watery eyes, and just feel miserable. You are probably not looking forward to the many days and nights of discomfort to come.

You can do something to make your allergies easier to bear, though. There are a number of medications you can purchase "over-the-counter"—without a prescription—that will reduce your symptoms.

What over-the-counter medications can I use for treating allergies?

The two major classes of over-the-counter (OTC) medications for treating allergies are antihistamines and decongestants.

Antihistamines help relieve sneezing, itching, and runny nose. They work best if you take them routinely during the allergy season rather than waiting until you feel miserable.

Most antihistamines cause few side effects. About one in five people do become drowsy, though, which affects mental alertness. This often becomes less of a problem with continued use. Other side effects include dry mouth, constipation, blurred vision, and difficulty urinating. These effects usually occur with higher doses. Children may have nightmares and be nervous, restless, and irritable.

There are three classes of antihistamines:

• Alkylamines, including pheniramine maleate (Triaminic); brompheniramine maleate (Bromfed, Dimetane, Dimetapp); chlorpheniramine maleate (Atrohist, Chlor-Trimeton, etc.); and triprolidine hydrochloride (Actifed).

• Ethanolamines, including clemastine fumarate (Tavist) and diphenhydramine hydrochloride (Benadryl).

• Ethylenediamines, including pyrilamine maleate (Triaminic).

Each class works to block the affect of histamine, a substance that the body makes during an allergic reaction. The ethanolamines cause the most

✔ Quick Tip
Tips For OTC Medication Use

• Do not drive or use machinery that requires mental alertness when you first take antihistamines. They often cause drowsiness.

• Check with your doctor before taking OTC medications with other prescription drugs. They may interact.

• Do not use out-of-date medication. Check the expiration date on the label. If out of date, flush the medication down the toilet.

• Do not keep medication in the bathroom. The supply will keep its full strength longer when stored in a cool, dry spot with no direct light.

• Avoid storing the product in temperatures that are very hot or very cold.

• Keep all medication out of reach of children—preferably in bottles with a safety-lock top.

Source: Reprinted with permission from the Asthma and Allergy Foundation of America, © 2005. All rights reserved.

♣ It's A Fact!!
FDA Approves OTC Claritin

FDA has approved Claritin (loratadine) as an over-the-counter (OTC) allergy drug product. Previously available only as a prescription drug, Claritin is approved for seasonal allergic rhinitis—a condition that causes runny nose, nasal congestion, sneezing, and itchy nose, throat, eyes, and ears.

"By making it easier to get this widely-used drug, today's action will enable many people to get less-sedating, effective relief for their allergy symptoms more quickly and at a lower cost," said Mark B. McClellan, M.D., Ph.D., Commissioner of Food and Drugs. "This approval reflects FDA's commitment to bringing prescription drugs to the over-the-counter market when they can be safely used without a prescription."

Claritin's approval for OTC marketing was based on FDA's criteria for determining appropriate drugs for OTC use—namely that the drug in question treats a condition that consumers can diagnose and manage themselves; that the drug is sufficiently safe for use by consumers without direct prescriber supervision; and that the drug's label explains potential adverse effects and conditions of use with clear and understandable directions. When drugs move from prescription to OTC status the price typically declines.

The action also marks a milestone in FDA's work with the National Transportation Safety Board to improve public awareness of the concerns about possible impairment caused by certain prescription and OTC drug products that cause drowsiness. Because OTC antihistamines already on the market may cause drowsiness, the FDA requires them to carry warnings about using them while driving or operating machinery. This new approval offers many consumers a potentially safer alternative to currently available OTC drugs that may contribute to driving impairment.

Approximately 10 to 30 percent of adults in the United States suffer from seasonal allergy symptoms. In April 1993, Claritin was approved as one of the first new generation antihistamines developed to be less sedating than traditional antihistamines.

Source: From *FDA News*, U. S. Food and Drug Administration (FDA), November 27, 2002.

drowsiness, and the alkylamines are least sedating. Try one of each class to find out which works best for you.

If you become drowsy when you take OTC antihistamines, you may find that taking a single large dose at bedtime will provide enough relief of symptoms. The drowsy side effect will occur while you sleep.

Another antihistamine, which doesn't fit into these classes, is phenindamine tartrate (Nolahist). It offers another choice for people with allergies.

Long-acting, 8- to 12-hour antihistamines give longer relief and can help you get through the night with fewer allergy symptoms. If you need prompt relief, the 4-hour type begins working faster, often within 20 minutes.

When antihistamines work well, they typically reduce symptoms by 50 percent to 80 percent, but they rarely relieve all symptoms.

Do not take antihistamines if you have angle-closure glaucoma. They can raise your eye pressure. Do not use them if you have trouble urinating because of prostate problems. Avoid them if you have emphysema or chronic bronchitis. The medications may dry the mucus in your chest and cause breathing problems. It is safer not to take them along with antidepressants, tranquilizers, sleeping pills, or alcohol.

Some antihistamines may make you drowsy, or there may be other reasons not to take them. Your work may require clear thinking and alertness, such as when using dangerous machinery or driving vehicles. In that case, talk to your doctor about the newer, nonsedating antihistamines.

Decongestants come as topical eye and nose drops and sprays and as oral tablets and liquid. They narrow blood vessels and reduce blood flow in the affected area, which helps clear congestion and improve breathing.

The topical products are applied to the surfaces of the nose or eyes. Oral products work systemically. They have a slower onset of action, but they usually last longer than many topical products.

The nose drops and sprays should be used for no more than three days to avoid rebound swelling in the nose. Congestion increases and can become difficult to treat.

Eye drops are safer, but those that can be bought over the counter do not contain antihistamines. They are much less effective than prescription combination antihistamine/decongestant eye drops.

The oral decongestants relieve stuffy nose and drainage, but do nothing for itching and sneezing. They sometimes cause headache, nervousness, tremors, sleeplessness, fast heartbeat, and rapid pulse. They should not be used by people who have high blood pressure, heart problems, thyroid disease, diabetes, or prostate problems unless they are under a doctor's care. Because the drugs can interact with some other medications, consult your doctor before taking them with other medications.

Antihistamine/decongestant combinations are best for nasal and eye allergies. The combination products may also reduce the sedating effects of antihistamine taken alone. Beware of combinations that also contain a pain reliever, such as acetaminophen or aspirin. Chronic use can lead to an inflamed liver and bleeding from the stomach or intestine.

An antiinflammatory medication, cromolyn sodium (Nasalcrom), is now available over the counter. It is a nasal spray that works by preventing mast cells from releasing histamine and other triggers of inflammation. It is effective in treating watery eyes, runny nose, and sneezing.

Cromolyn sodium does not stop inflammation once it has begun. For it to help, it should be started before the allergy season begins and used daily during the season. There are few side effects, although some people get nasal stinging or burning.

When should I see a doctor?

It is usually okay to treat nasal and eye allergies with OTC medications. Sometimes, though, problems develop such as repeated sinus infections, ear infections, headaches, cough, and wheezing or difficulty with exercise. Call your doctor immediately to discuss these problems and how to manage them.

The doctor may prescribe medications that may make you feel better or suggest you see an allergy specialist. Specialists often can stop the allergic condition from getting worse and can reverse the problems.

Chapter 6

Epinephrine

Epinephrine by injection is the treatment of choice for anaphylactic reactions because it quickly begins working to reverse symptoms of an anaphylactic reaction. Epinephrine constricts blood vessels, relaxes smooth muscles in the lungs to improve breathing, stimulates the heartbeat, and works to reverse hives and swelling around the face and lips. The effects of epinephrine usually last 10 to 20 minutes.

The EpiPen® auto-injector is a disposable drug delivery system featuring spring activation and a concealed needle. It is designed for self-administration of epinephrine in acute allergic emergencies (anaphylaxis). It provides a rapid, convenient dose of epinephrine for individuals needing protection from potentially fatal allergic reactions.

EpiPen® Dosing

Epinephrine dosing is based on body weight. Your doctor will prescribe what is right for you. The EpiPen® auto-injector (0.3 mg) is for individuals weighing 66 lbs. or more. The EpiPen® JR auto-injector (0.15 mg) is for individuals weighing between 33 and 66 lbs. Both strengths deliver a single dose.

Sometimes a single dose of epinephrine may not be enough to completely reverse the effects of an anaphylactic reaction. For that reason, your physician may prescribe more than one auto-injector.

About The Self-Injection Procedure

The injection itself is relatively painless, and the beneficial effects of the drug will be felt soon after injection. The most common changes you may feel are a rapid heartbeat and slight nervousness, "like a shot of adrenaline." As with any epinephrine product, you may also experience palpitations (irregular pulsing of the heart), sweating, dizziness, and headache. The EpiPen® auto-injector should only be used on the fleshy outer portion of the thigh and can be used through clothing.

Directions For Use

- Follow these directions only when ready to use.
- Never put thumb, fingers, or hand over black tip.
- Do not remove gray activation cap until ready to use.

1. Familiarize yourself with the unit.

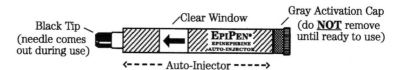

Figure 6.1. The EpiPen auto-injector.

2. Grasp unit, with the black tip pointing downward.

3. Form a fist around the auto-injector (black tip down).

4. With your other hand, pull off the gray activation cap.

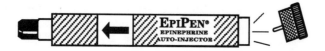

Figure 6.2. When ready to use, pull off the gray activation cap.

5. Hold black tip near outer thigh.

6. Swing and jab firmly into outer thigh so that auto-injector is perpendicular (at a 90° angle) to the thigh.

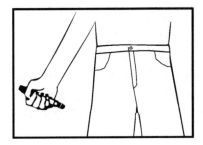 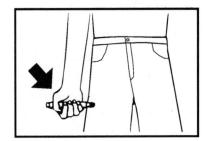

Figure 6.3. Jab firmly into the outer thigh.

7. Hold firmly in thigh for several seconds.

8. Remove unit, massage injection area for several seconds.

9. Check black tip:

   • if needle is exposed, you received the dose

   • if not, repeat steps #5–8

10. Note: most of the liquid (about 90%) stays in the auto-injector and cannot be reused.

11. Bend the needle back against a hard surface.

12. Carefully put the unit (needle first) back into the carrying tube (without the gray activation cap).

13. Recap the carrying tube.

14. Immediately after use:

   • go immediately to the nearest hospital emergency room. You may need further medical attention.

   • tell the physician that you have received an injection of epinephrine (show your thigh).

• give your used EpiPen/EpiPen® Jr to the physician for inspection and proper disposal.

♣ It's A Fact!!

Know The Facts

Some teens tell us they've heard the needle in an epinephrine auto-injector (EpiPen®) is thick and several inches long. Actually, the needle is small, about ½ inch or so. People who have used the epinephrine auto-injector report that the injection isn't very painful, and that the shot helped give immediate relief of the symptoms of an allergic reaction.

Practice, Practice, Practice

The EpiPen® trainer, which contains neither the medicine nor a needle, is a great tool for practicing how to use the auto-injector. The more you practice giving an injection, the easier it will be to do so in an emergency. You may also want to encourage others (for example, family members, friends, and school staff) to practice.

Satisfy Your Curiosity

Instead of throwing away an expired EpiPen®, inject it into an orange or a grapefruit. Individuals who have administered the EpiPen®, and have also practiced on fruit, say that it gave them a good idea of the amount of pressure they need to use to activate an auto-injector.

Once you've fired the auto-injector, be sure to properly dispose of the unit afterward. DEY, the manufacturer of EpiPen®, suggests throwing away the activation cap (gray cap) and then placing the used unit, needle first, into the amber carrying tube. Take the unit to the hospital or to your doctor's office for disposal.

Studies have shown that a delay in receiving epinephrine is most often the cause of fatal anaphylaxis. If you are worried that you won't know when to administer medication, talk to your doctor. He or she can help you work through your fear and give you some examples of when it would be necessary for you to use epinephrine.

EpiPen® Is Not Reusable

Each EpiPen® auto-injector delivers a single dose of epinephrine. Even though liquid remains inside an auto-injector after use, the unit cannot be used again.

Disposing Of EpiPen® After Use

Do not throw the EpiPen® auto-injector away after use. Instead, bend the needle back against a hard surface and carefully re-insert the fired unit, without replacing the safety cap—needle first—into the amber carrying tube. Re-cap the amber tube. Go immediately to the nearest hospital emergency room, since you may need further medical attention. Tell the doctor that you have received an injection of epinephrine and give the doctor your used EpiPen® auto-injector for inspection and proper disposal.

✔ Quick Tip

Are there any special tips I should know?

- Keep your EpiPen® at room temperature. Do not refrigerate.
- Do not expose your EpiPen® to direct sunlight.
- Do not keep your EpiPen® in a vehicle during hot weather.
- Store your EpiPen® in the plastic tube it comes in.
- Occasionally inspect your EpiPen® through the viewing window of the unit. Make sure the solution is clear and colorless. If it is brown, replace with a fresh unit.
- Be sure to have multiple units available in case you cannot reach a hospital within minutes.

Source: Excerpted from "About EpiPen: Common Questions and Answers," reprinted with permission from http://www.epipen.com, an informational website from DEY, L.P. © 2005 DEY. All rights reserved.

Safety Information

EpiPen® (epinephrine) Auto-Injector 0.3/0.15 mg is indicated for emergency treatment of allergic reactions (anaphylaxis) for people with a history of an anaphylactic reaction.

EpiPen® should be used with extreme caution in people who have heart disease. Side effects of EpiPen® may include fast or irregular heartbeat, nausea, and breathing difficulty. Certain side effects may be increased if EpiPen® is used while taking tricyclic antidepressants or MAOIs (monoamine oxidase inhibitors).

Chapter 7

Alternative Therapies For Allergy Patients

What is alternative medicine?

Any unproven treatment for an illness or disease is considered an alternative medical approach by most American medical doctors. "Unproven" means there is not enough acceptable scientific evidence to show that the treatment works. The term alternative medicine refers to a wide variety of treatments considered outside "mainstream" or "usual" medical approaches in the United States today.

Many people turn to alternative medicine to help alleviate their asthma or allergy symptoms. These treatment approaches may include, but are not limited to, one or more of the following:

- Acupuncture
- Ayurvedic medicine
- Biofeedback; mental imaging; stress reduction; relaxation techniques
- Chiropractic spinal manipulation
- Diet, exercise, yoga, lifestyle changes
- Herbal medicine, vitamin supplements

About This Chapter: "Alternative Therapies," reprinted with permission from the Asthma and Allergy Foundation of America, © 2005. All rights reserved.

- Folk medicine from various cultures

- Laser therapy

- Massage

- Hypnosis

- Art or music therapy

Why people use alternative medicine?

Recent statistics show that nearly 40 percent of Americans try some form of alternative medicine. Medical and scientific experts do believe that some remedies may be worth a try, providing they are not harmful. In some cases, specific alternative medical treatment may improve or relieve symptoms of a specific illness or disease. Risks should not outweigh the potential benefits.

If you believe a particular alternative medical approach might help reduce your asthma or allergy symptoms, talk with your doctor about it, and how you could integrate that treatment into your overall asthma/allergy management plan.

No one should use alternative medicine without first consulting a board-certified physician. Any alternative medical approach should be used in addition to your normal asthma or allergy management plan.

You should not substitute an alternative medical treatment for your regular medications or treatments. Be especially careful about use of alternative medicine on children. Approaches that are harmless for adults may not be harmless for children.

Does health insurance cover alternative medical treatment?

Health plans vary in what alternative medicine expenses they will pay. Many plans provide coverage for some but not all alternative therapies. If your doctor writes you a prescription for a specific treatment such as acupuncture or massage, you may be more likely to get partial or full reimbursement of the expense. Always check with your insurance provider before assuming the coverage is available.

What are cautions or considerations for people who use alternative medicine?

Beware the placebo effect: If you really want an alternative medical treatment to work, you may think it is working, even if it really isn't. This "placebo effect" often occurs for people using alternative medicine. Symptoms of asthma or allergy also may improve on their own as an illness (like a cold or flu) runs its course. If you use prescribed medications for your allergy or asthma symptoms, it may take time for them to "kick in." So you may simply be feeling better because your medications started working—not because the alternative medicine is working.

Read between the label lines: The federal government requires labels to state how an herb or vitamin may affect the body but labels are not required to carry health warnings. Labels also cannot claim any medical or health benefit. Products often are not properly labeled, especially those imported from other countries. Many people experience toxic—and sometimes deadly—effects from improperly using labeled herbs. Some products contain unnamed medicines such as steroids, anti-inflammatories or sedatives that act to reduce your symptoms. Other "hidden ingredients" in various products can be dangerous or even lethal. Use products tested for safety and effectiveness.

Follow directions: Never increase the amount or frequency of a dose or use a treatment or device in a different way than recommended. Do not use herbs in combinations. Do not take herbs if you are pregnant or breast feeding.

Beware of developing allergy symptoms: Allergies to specific plants and other substances (such as latex or nickel) can build up over time. Products you've used for years may suddenly cause mild to serious allergy symptoms, especially if you already are allergic to something. Check to see if new herbs, foods or other products you plan to use are in the same "family" as your known allergens.

Use quality products and services: Lack of quality standards is a serious problem for people who use various alternative medical treatments. Look for products that list the amount of the active ingredient(s). Make sure people giving you any kind of treatment are properly certified. Ask your pharmacist or health product store manager for recommendations. Research the product or service before you use it.

Consult with your physician before starting any new treatment: This point cannot be stressed enough. If you have symptoms of asthma or allergy, but you have not been diagnosed, consult a board-certified doctor for a proper diagnosis. Do not rely on health product store personnel to help treat undiagnosed symptoms. If you know you have asthma or allergies, again, talk with your doctor about the alternative medicine you want to use—before you try it.

Are there useful alternative therapies for people who have asthma or allergies?

Keep in mind: alternative therapy is medical treatment for which there is no conclusive, supporting scientific evidence. This does not necessarily mean the treatment is useless or ineffective. You simply must be careful in what you choose and how you use it.

Acupuncture: A technique that involves inserting needles into key points of the body. Evidence suggests that acupuncture may signal the brain to release endorphins. These are hormones made by the body. When released, endorphins can help reduce pain and create a sense of well being. People with asthma or allergy may experience more relaxed or calmer breathing. Users should be aware of the risk of contaminated needles or punctured organs.

Biofeedback: A technique that helps people control involuntary physical responses. Results are mixed, with children and teenagers showing the greatest benefit.

Chiropractic spinal manipulation: A technique that emphasizes manipulation of the spine in order to help the body heal itself. People who get chiropractic treatment for allergies or asthma may find it easier to breathe after treatment. There is no evidence that this treatment impairs the underlying disease or pulmonary function.

Hypnosis: An artificially induced dream state that leaves the person open to suggestion, hypnosis is a legitimate technique to help people manage various conditions. Hypnosis might give people with asthma or allergies more self-discipline to follow good health practices.

♣ It's A Fact!!

Individuals who may have allergies to various pollens, including weeds and grasses, should be quite cautious in using certain herbal supplements. Use caution in taking herbs when you have seasonal, year-round or food allergies. For example, individuals who are sensitive to ragweed/weed pollens may "cross-react" to compounds such as Echinacea due to their similar plant families. If you are sensitive to sunflower seeds and/or various types of melons, you may also react to Echinacea. Researchers have reportedly identified several dozen cases in which Echinacea has been associated with asthma attacks and/or allergic reactions. Thus, one may use this supplement to fight a cold and wind up with worsening allergy-type symptoms.

Source: Excerpted and reprinted with permission from "Risks of Herbal Medicine," by Clifford W. Bassett, M.D., © 2003 American Academy of Allergy, Asthma and Immunology. All rights reserved.

Laser treatment: A technique that uses high intensity light to shrink swollen tissue or unblock sinuses. Laser therapy may provide temporary relief, but it may also cause scarring or other long-term physical problems.

Massage, relaxation techniques, art/music therapy, yoga: Stress and anxiety may cause your airways to constrict more if you have asthma or allergies. Various techniques can help you relax, reduce anxiety or control your breathing. The results may provide some benefit in helping you cope with asthma or allergy symptoms. However, evidence is not conclusive that these techniques improve lung function.

Chapter 8

Allergy-Related Research

Scientists Identify Genes That Regulate Allergic Response To Diesel Fumes

The risk of developing respiratory allergies from exposure to diesel emissions depends largely on genetics, according to a study funded by the National Institute of Allergy and Infectious Diseases (NIAID), part of the National Institutes of Health (NIH). Given their findings, researchers estimate that up to 50 percent of the United States population could be in jeopardy of experiencing health problems related to air pollution. The study is published in the January 10, 2004 issue of the British journal *The Lancet*.

"This important study adds to previous data that suggest how modern environmental factors interact with the body's defenses to produce 'airway' diseases considered rare before the advent of industrialized society," says Anthony S. Fauci, M.D., director of NIAID.

"The knowledge provided by this work will help us identify people who are susceptible to the deleterious effects of diesel emissions on the clinical

About This Chapter: This chapter includes text from the following National Institute of Allergy and Infectious Diseases (NIAID) News Releases: "Scientists Identify Genes that Regulate Allergic Response to Diesel Fumes," January 8, 2004; "Early Fevers Associated with Lower Allergy Risk Later in Childhood," February 9, 2004; "Chronic Sinusitis Sufferers Have Enhanced Immune Responses to Fungi," October 8, 2004; and "Novel Therapy Tested in Mice Could Chase away Cat Allergies," March 27, 2005.

course of asthma and hay fever," says Kenneth Adams, Ph.D., who oversees asthma research funded by NIAID. "It will also help accelerate development of drugs to treat and prevent these diseases."

This study also received support from the National Institute of Environmental Health Sciences, another NIH component.

The authors of the study examined how a family of antioxidant-related genes—GSTM1, GSTT1 and GSTP1—reacts to diesel exhaust particles, a common air pollutant. The body generates antioxidants to detoxify harmful particles and limit the corresponding allergic reaction.

Researchers sampled the DNA of volunteers who are allergic to ragweed to find which forms of the genes they had. The participants were then given doses of ragweed through the nose, followed by either a placebo or quantities of diesel exhaust particles equivalent to breathing the air in Los Angeles, California, for 40 hours.

The mix of ragweed and diesel exhaust triggered greater allergic responses than ragweed alone. Additionally, the diesel particles caused volunteers who lacked the antioxidant-producing form of the GSTM1 gene to have significantly greater allergic responses, compared to the other participants. Up to 50 percent of the U.S. population does not have this form of the GSTM1 gene. Within the group that lacked GSTM1, those who had a particular variant of the GSTP1 gene experienced even greater allergic reactions. Researchers estimate that 15 to 20 percent of the U.S. population falls into this category.

"Diesel emissions can trigger allergic symptoms, but the genetic factors involved in the process are quite complex," says David Diaz-Sanchez, Ph.D., assistant professor in the Division of Immunology and Allergy at the University of California Los Angeles, who co-authored the study with scientists from the University of Southern California. "Our findings suggest that people who lack the genes to make key antioxidants may have difficulty fighting the harmful effects of air pollution."

Dr. Diaz-Sanchez says that he and the other researchers will work to find other genes involved in pollution-related health problems such as asthma, lung cancer and heart disease, with the goal of discovering possible treatments and preventions. "We are focused on investigating ways we can overcome this genetic deficiency," he says. "This may be accomplished by either giving people drugs that replace the role of the genes or by boosting the body's natural defenses."

Reference: F Gilliland et al. Effect of glutathione-S-transferase M1 and P1 genotypes on xenobiotic enhancement of allergic responses: randomised, placebo-controlled crossover study. *The Lancet* 363 (9403): 119–25 (2004).

Early Fevers Associated With Lower Allergy Risk Later In Childhood

Infants who experience fevers before their first birthday are less likely to develop allergies by ages six or seven, according to a new study funded by the National Institute of Allergy and Infectious Diseases (NIAID), part of the National Institutes of Health (NIH). The study, published February 9, 2004, in the *Journal of Allergy and Clinical Immunology*, lends support to the well-known "hygiene hypothesis," which contends that early exposure to infections might protect children against allergic diseases in later years.

"The prevalence of asthma and allergies has increased dramatically world-wide in recent years," says Anthony S. Fauci, M.D., director of NIAID. "This study provides evidence that diminished exposure to early immunological challenges could be one of the reasons for this trend."

"The hygiene hypothesis is widely recognized but largely unproven," says Kenneth Adams, Ph.D., who oversees asthma research funded by NIAID. "The findings of this study strengthen the hypothesis and, after more research, could lead to preventative therapies for asthma and allergies."

The authors of the study followed the medical records of 835 children from birth to age one, documenting any fever-related episodes. Fever was defined as a rectal temperature of 101 degrees Fahrenheit or above. At age six to seven years, more than half of the children were evaluated for their sensitivity to common allergens, such as dust mites, ragweed and cats.

Researchers found that, of the children who did not experience a fever during their first year, 50.0 percent showed allergic sensitivity. Of those who had one fever, 46.7 percent became allergy-prone. The children who suffered two or more fevers in their infancy had greater protection, with only 31.3 percent showing allergic sensitivity by ages six to seven.

In particular, fever-inducing infections involving the eyes, ears, nose, or throat appeared to be associated with a lower risk of developing allergies, compared with similar infections that did not result in fevers.

"We didn't expect fever to relate with such a consistent effect," says Christine C. Johnson, Ph.D, M.P.H., senior research epidemiologist of the Henry Ford Health System in Detroit, Michigan, and one of the co-authors of the study. "It also was interesting that the more fevers an infant had, the less likely it was that he or she would be sensitive to allergies."

Dr. Johnson says that more research is needed to establish if early fevers have a direct effect on allergic development in children. Additionally, she and the other authors are working to determine if early exposure to pets as well as high levels of bacteria could also lower allergy risk. "If we can uncover which environmental factors affect allergic development and why, it may be possible to immunize children against these conditions," she says.

Reference: L Keoki Williams et al. The relationship between early fever and allergic sensitization at age 6 to 7 years. *Journal of Allergy and Clinical Immunology* 113(2): 291–296 (2004).

Chronic Sinusitis Sufferers Have Enhanced Immune Responses To Fungi

Scientists supported by the National Institute of Allergy and Infectious Diseases (NIAID), part of the National Institutes of Health, have discovered that people with chronic sinus inflammation have an exaggerated immune response to common airborne fungi. The results of their study appeared online October 8, 2004 in *The Journal of Allergy and Clinical Immunology*.

"This study is the first to show a possible immunologic basis for chronic sinusitis, an important starting point to better understand the etiology of the illness," says Marshall Plaut, M.D., chief of NIAID's allergic mechanisms section. Despite the enormous health impact of chronic sinusitis—nearly 30 million people were diagnosed with sinusitis in 2002, according to U.S. Centers for Disease Control and Prevention, and direct costs of the illness exceed $5.6 billion per year—the condition is very poorly understood, he says.

The researchers, led by Hirohito Kita, M.D., of the Mayo Clinic in Rochester, Minnesota, compared blood samples taken from 18 people diagnosed with chronic sinusitis with blood samples from 15 healthy volunteers. Nasal secretions from the two groups were also examined for the presence of fungal proteins and inflammation-causing immune system molecules.

Airborne microscopic fungi spores abound indoors and out. People may inhale a million or more fungal spores each day, notes Dr. Kita. The mere presence of such fungi in the airways, however, is not enough to cause sinusitis because these spores can be found in the upper respiratory tracts of both sinusitis sufferers and non-sufferers. Indeed, in this study, levels of fungal proteins in nasal secretions were similar in both groups.

The Mayo Clinic scientists looked for evidence that people with sinusitis respond abnormally to these harmless fungi. The investigators exposed immune cells derived from the blood samples to extracts of four common airborne fungi: Alternaria, Aspergillus, Penicillium and Cladosporium. The cells of chronic sinusitis sufferers released significant amounts of three immune-modulating chemicals, called cytokines, specifically interferon-gamma, interleukin-5 (IL-5) and IL-13. In contrast, cells from healthy volunteers released very little interferon-gamma and no IL-5 or IL-13. The most dramatic responses occurred after exposure to Alternaria.

Importantly, says Dr. Kita, the released cytokines represent both major classes of cytokines-interferon-gamma is in the Th1 group and IL-5 and IL-13 are in the Th2 class. This is notable because scientists have thought that allergic reactions involve only Th2 cytokines, Dr. Kita explains. (While chronic sinusitis is not considered to be an allergic disease, people with the condition also often have asthma and allergic rhinitis, giving scientists reason to suspect a link.) The current findings add to an evolving understanding of allergic diseases that suggests symptoms may stem from a combination of Th1 and Th2 cytokines.

The combined effect of excess Th2 and Th1 cytokines released in the presence of fungi may explain a number of chronic sinusitis symptoms, including persistent inflammation of sinus and nasal mucous passages, say the scientists.

Previously, Mayo clinic scientists used intranasal antifungal agents to successfully treat patients with chronic sinusitis. While those studies generated controversy, in part because other researchers were unable to replicate the findings, Dr. Kita says today's report supports the rationale of treating chronic sinusitis with antifungals. Clinical trials to further test antifungal therapy for chronic sinusitis are being planned, adds Dr. Kita.

Reference: S-H Shin et al. Chronic rhinosinusitis: An enhanced immune response to ubiquitous airborne fungi. *The Journal of Allergy and Clinical Immunology*. Published online Oct. 8, 2004. doi: 10.1016/j.jaci.2004.06.012.

Novel Therapy Tested In Mice Could Chase Away Cat Allergies

A molecule designed to block cat allergies successfully prevented allergic reactions in laboratory mice, as well as in human cells in a test tube, University of California, Los Angeles (UCLA) researchers report in the April 2005 issue of *Nature Medicine*, available online now. In the future, the investigators say, these promising results could lead to a new therapy not only for human cat allergies, but also possibly for severe food allergies such as those to peanuts.

The National Institute of Allergy and Infectious Diseases (NIAID), part of the National Institutes of Health, funded the research. "This novel approach to treating cat allergies is encouraging news for millions of cat-allergic Americans. Moreover, these results provide proof-of-concept for using this approach to develop therapies to prevent deadly food allergy reactions as well," says NIAID Director Anthony S. Fauci, M.D.

The injectable treatment puts a brake on the release of a key chemical from cells involved in cat allergy reactions. That chemical, histamine, brings on allergy symptoms such as sneezing, wheezing, itching, watery eyes and sometimes asthma. When a cat-allergic person touches or inhales a protein found in cat saliva or dander (small scales from skin or hair), key immune system cells respond by spewing out histamine. Allergy experts estimate that 14 percent of children 6 to 19 years old are allergic to cats.

The treatment comprises a molecule that loosely tethers a feline and a human protein together. The feline end is the notorious protein (called Fel d1) found in cat dander and saliva that causes so much misery in allergy sufferers. On the other end sits a piece of human antibody (called IgG Fcg1) that docks to a cell receptor that can be recruited to stop allergic reactions.

The investigators named the chimeric molecule GFD, or gamma Feline domesticus, for its human and feline parts, explains principal investigator Andrew Saxon, M.D., of UCLA. The cat allergen end of GFD binds to antibodies on the surface of the cell. The human end of GFD links to a different cell surface protein (called FcgRIIB) that interrupts the allergic response.

Dr. Saxon and his colleagues first tested GFD in blood donated by people allergic to cats. They cultured blood cells with either GFD or with a purified human antibody as a control. Then they added the cat protein that triggers allergic reactions to all the blood cell cultures.

"We measured more than 90 percent less histamine in the cultures with GFD," says Dr. Saxon. "Those results suggested that GFD successfully prevented the immune cells from reacting to cat allergen. The next step was to test GFD in mice that we had made allergic to the allergenic protein found in cat saliva and dander."

The researchers tested GFD in two different types of allergic mice. One set was genetically engineered to have human cat-allergy cell receptors. These mice were "passively allergic" to cats: they would react to cat protein only after the scientists first injected them with human allergic antibodies to cats. When these mice were then injected with cat allergen, GFD blocked the allergic reaction involving the human cell receptors, an indication that it might also work in people.

Scientists made another set of mice allergic to cats by injecting them with cat protein and an immune system booster. These mice became "actively allergic" to cats: their reactions to cat allergen would be comparable to reactions in a cat-allergic person. Scientists injected some of these mice with GFD, and then injected cat allergen into the windpipes of all the mice, including a control group that was not allergic to cats. GFD damped asthma-like and other allergic reactions in the cat-allergic mice: reactions in the mice that received GFD were similar to the control group mice that were not allergic to cats.

The molecule has the potential to prevent allergic reactions long after injections cease, Dr. Saxon says. However, further research and clinical testing would be required before it might be used in humans. He also is interested in applying this approach to develop a preventive treatment for serious food allergies.

Reference: D. Zhu et al. A chimeric human-cat fusion protein blocks cat-induced allergy. *Nature Medicine* DOI: 10.1038/nm1219 (2005).

Part 2

Allergic Reactions

Chapter 9

Anaphylaxis: The Most Dangerous Allergic Reaction

Commonly Asked Questions About Anaphylaxis

What is anaphylaxis?

Anaphylaxis is a sudden, severe, potentially fatal, systemic allergic reaction that can involve various areas of the body (such as the skin, respiratory tract, gastrointestinal tract, and cardiovascular system). Symptoms occur within minutes to two hours after contact with the allergy-causing substance, but in rare instances may occur up to four hours later. Anaphylactic reactions can be mild to life-threatening. The annual incidence of anaphylactic reactions is about 30 per 100,000 persons, and individuals with asthma, eczema, or hay fever are at greater relative risk of experiencing anaphylaxis.

Common causes of anaphylaxis include the following:

• Food

• Medication

- Insect stings

- Latex

Less common causes include the following:

- Food-dependent exercise-induced anaphylaxis

- Idiopathic anaphylaxis

Anaphylaxis To Food: Peanuts, tree nuts (walnuts, cashews, etc.), shell-fish, fish, milk, and eggs commonly cause anaphylactic reactions. Only a trace amount of a problem food can cause a reaction in some individuals.

In the U.S., food-induced anaphylaxis is believed to cause about 30,000 trips to the emergency room and between 150 to 200 deaths each year. Individuals who are allergic to foods and have asthma are believed to be at a higher risk for developing an anaphylactic reaction.

A recent study of 32 cases of fatal food-allergy induced anaphylaxis showed that adolescents who have peanut and tree nut allergy and asthma and don't have quick access to epinephrine, EpiPen®, during a reaction, are at highest risk for a fatal reaction.

Strict avoidance of the allergen is necessary for avoiding a severe reaction. Read food labels for every food each and every time you eat it. Ask questions about ingredients and preparation methods when eating away from home.

Anaphylaxis To Medication: Anaphylactic reactions to medication will typically occur within an hour after taking the drug, however reactions may occur several hours later. It is estimated that up to 10 percent of the population may be at risk for allergic reactions to medications.

According to literature from the American Academy of Allergy, Asthma and Immunology, "The chances of developing an allergic reaction may be increased if the drug is given frequently, in large doses, or by injection rather than by pill. The most important factor may be an inherited genetic tendency of the immune system to develop allergies. Contrary to popular myth, however, a family history of allergy to a specific drug does not mean that a patient has an increased chance of reacting to the same drug."

If you experience symptoms of an allergic reaction after taking medication, speak to your doctor. If symptoms are severe, or resemble anaphylaxis, get emergency medical help immediately.

Anaphylaxis To Insect Sting: Honeybees, bumblebees, yellow jackets, hornets, wasps, fire ants, and harvester ants are the most common causes of insect stings in the United States. The symptoms of anaphylactic reactions to insect stings usually occur within minutes of the sting.

Insect sting reactions can range from local to mild to life threatening. Local reactions can involve swelling of an area larger than the sting site; for example, the entire arm can be swollen after a sting on the hand. This type of reaction may also include nausea and low-grade fever. Insect stings account for about 50 deaths each year.

To minimize the risk of an insect sting, avoid brightly colored clothing and/or scented cosmetics, perfumes, etc., avoid walking barefoot, use caution when cooking outdoors, and keep insecticide handy when working outdoors.

Anaphylaxis To Latex: Latex allergy is most commonly diagnosed in individuals who are exposed to latex frequently, such as those employed in the health care or rubber industry fields, and in children with spina bifida and other congenital diseases requiring multiple surgeries. An estimated one percent of the U.S. population has latex allergy. Approximately 10 to 17 percent of those employed in the health care occupations have this allergy.

Some individuals with latex allergy will also develop reactions when eating foods that cross react with latex. These foods commonly include bananas, kiwi, avocados, and European chestnuts; and less commonly include potatoes; tomatoes; and peaches, plums, cherries, and other pitted fruits.

Food-Dependent Exercise-Induced Anaphylaxis: Food-dependent exercise-induced anaphylaxis is very rare and occurs only when an individual eats a specific food and exercises within three to four hours after eating. Individuals experiencing this type of reaction typically have asthma and other allergic conditions. Although any food may contribute to this form of anaphylaxis, foods that have been reported include wheat, shellfish, fruit, milk, celery, and fish.

✔ **Quick Tip**

3 R's For Treating Anaphylaxis

- Recognize symptoms
- React quickly
- Review what happened and be sure to prevent it from reoccurring

Steps For Treating An Anaphylactic Reaction

If you suspect an anaphylactic reaction is occurring, don't lose precious time. Do the following:

- Act quickly!
- Follow your physician's instructions for treatment.
- Call Emergency Medical Services (or 911) and request epinephrine. Do not attempt to drive yourself to a medical facility. Get to a hospital as soon as possible and plan to stay at least four to six hours in case symptoms return.

How You Can Protect Yourself

- Speak to your doctor or allergist if you've had a severe reaction to a food, insect sting, medication, latex, or after exercising.

- If prescribed, carry a supply of epinephrine (EpiPen®) at all times. Teach yourself and others how to use it. Practice with an expired EpiPen® by injecting it into an orange. Additionally, EpiPen®s are available in Twin Paks™ that include an EpiPen® trainer, the same device as the EpiPen® without the needle or medication. Practice using the EpiPen® until it becomes second nature.

- Educate others about your allergy; for example, what you need to avoid, the symptoms of an allergic reaction, and how others can help during an allergic emergency.

- Wear a MedicAlert® bracelet or necklace noting your allergy.

Source: © 2005 The Food Allergy & Anaphylaxis Network.

Food-dependent exercise-induced anaphylaxis appears to be twice as common in females than in males and is common in individuals who are in their late teens to thirties.

Idiopathic Anaphylaxis: Idiopathic anaphylaxis is a severe reaction in which no cause can be determined. It can affect individuals of all ages although females are affected much more frequently than males. As with other forms of anaphylaxis, idiopathic anaphylaxis can be life threatening. Prophylactic daily treatment with a combination of medications can control the symptoms, and most episodes of idiopathic anaphylaxis subside spontaneously after several months or years.

Who is at risk for having an anaphylactic reaction?

Anyone with a previous history of anaphylactic reactions is at risk for another severe reaction. Individuals with food allergies (particularly shellfish, peanuts, and tree nuts) and asthma may be at increased risk for having a life-threatening anaphylactic reaction. A recent study showed that teens with food allergy and asthma appear to be at highest risk for a reaction because they are more likely to dine away from home; they are less likely to carry medications, and may ignore or not recognize symptoms.

What are the symptoms of an anaphylactic reaction?

An anaphylactic reaction may begin with a tingling sensation, itching, or metallic taste in the mouth. Other symptoms can include hives, a sensation of warmth, asthma symptoms, swelling of the mouth and throat area, difficulty breathing, vomiting, diarrhea, cramping, a drop in blood pressure, and loss of consciousness. These symptoms may begin in as little as five to 15 minutes to up to two hours after exposure to the allergen, but life-threatening reactions may progress over hours.

Some individuals have a reaction, and the symptoms go away only to return two to three hours later. This is called a bi-phasic reaction. Often the symptoms occur in the respiratory tract and take the individual by surprise.

If you have an anaphylactic reaction, seek professional medical help quickly. Stay in the hospital for four to six hours to be sure you can get help if you have a bi-phasic reaction. More than one individual's life has been saved because he or she was in the hospital when this second reaction occurred. If the hospital staff discharges you, sit in the lobby and read a magazine. Do not leave and assume you can get back to the hospital on time.

What medication is used to treat an anaphylactic reaction?

Epinephrine is the drug of choice for treating an anaphylactic reaction. It works to reverse the symptoms of an anaphylactic reaction and helps prevent the progression of it. It is available via prescription as an EpiPen® or EpiPen® Jr. Epinephrine Auto-Injector. It is important to administer epinephrine as soon as one detects the symptoms of anaphylaxis. Individuals who have been prescribed epinephrine must carry it with them at all times because accidents are never planned.

Antihistamines, such as Benadryl®, and steroids are often used to further improve the

✔ Quick Tip
How To Use An Epinephrine Auto-Injector

1. Pull off gray safety cap.

2. Place black tip on outer thigh (always apply to thigh).

3. Using a swing and jab motion, press hard into thigh until Auto-Injector mechanism functions. Hold in place and count to ten. The EpiPen® unit should then be removed and discarded. Massage the injection area for ten seconds.

4. Once EpiPen® is used, call the Rescue Squad. State additional epinephrine may be needed. Take the used unit with you to the Emergency Room. Plan to stay for observation at the Emergency Room for at least four hours.

How To Dispose An EpiPen®

After using an EpiPen®, throw away the gray cap. Place a penny in the bottom of the plastic tube, slip the EpiPen® into the tube, and close it. Return the used EpiPen® to your doctor for disposal.

Source: © 2005 The Food Allergy & Anaphylaxis Network.

recovery of a person with an anaphylactic reaction. Antihistamines and asthma medications may be administered with epinephrine, but never instead of epinephrine because they cannot reverse many of the symptoms of anaphylaxis.

Common Myths About Anaphylaxis

There is no doubt that anaphylaxis is a very real and serious threat for many people with food allergies. Patients and families who are at risk for anaphylaxis must be on guard at all times to deal with a reaction. However, as with most things in medicine, there are a number of common myths about anaphylaxis that lead to confusion and—in some cases—unnecessary fear and anxiety. Here we will try to dispel some of the more common myths about anaphylaxis.

Myth: Each episode of anaphylaxis will become increasingly severe.

Fact: There is no predictable pattern of anaphylaxis. Future episodes may be the same, more severe, or less severe. With food allergy, this depends on the dose of allergen you eat and whether you have become more or less allergic.

Myth: All cases of anaphylaxis are life-threatening.

Fact: Some cases of anaphylaxis are mild and will go away even without treatment. However, since it is not possible to predict how a reaction will progress, each episode must be taken very seriously.

Myth: Anaphylaxis can occur hours or days after eating a food.

Fact: Although anaphylactic reactions may persist for several hours, almost all episodes will begin within hours of eating the problem food.

Myth: Anaphylaxis takes at least 20 minutes to begin, so there is always time to get to treatment.

Fact: Reactions can begin very suddenly, sometimes even within seconds of eating a food. In addition, it is important to remember that treatment may be less effective if it is delayed.

✔ Quick Tip
Anaphylaxis Case Scenario

Imagine you are spending a winter day snow boarding with your friends. After a while, you have worked up an appetite. Someone runs back to their car and returns with some snacks for the group.

Your friend offers you a package of crackers. You think about it for a minute, and then decide that you really don't want to call it quits for the day to go home and eat, and the crackers are the exact same kind of crackers that you've eaten without a problem in the past. So, you eat them.

Soon your skin begins to itch and your throat feels scratchy and tight. You realize that an allergic reaction is occurring. You know that you should give yourself the EpiPen® you keep stored in your car.

You quietly slip away from the group and make your way down to your car, which is parked at the bottom of the hill and across a field. When you get there, the EpiPen® is so cold it doesn't work. While trying to warm it up, you collapse. The next thing you remember is being helped by an ambulance crew.

How could this situation have been better handled?

1. Keep your medicine, especially your EpiPen®, with you at all times. You might not think you'll need it, but accidents are never planned.

2. Never leave or store your EpiPen® in a car. The EpiPen® needs to be stored at room temperature, between 59 and 85 degrees Fahrenheit. Extreme cold can cause the auto-injector mechanism not to work properly. It can also affect the effectiveness of the medicine.

3. Never leave your friends and go off alone if you think you are having an allergic reaction. Tell them what is going on and how they can help (for example, call 911).

4. Read labels for all foods, even if you've eaten the same food safely in the past. Manufacturers sometimes change the ingredients in a food, so it is never safe to assume a food is okay to eat because you've had it before.

Source: Excerpted from "Featured Topics and Articles," © 2005 The Food Allergy & Anaphylaxis Network. All Rights Reserved. Reprinted with permission. For additional information, visit http://www.foodallergy.org or http://www.fankids.org.

Myth: Anaphylaxis will go away within one to two hours.

Fact: About one-fourth of the anaphylaxis cases will have ongoing symptoms or a second wave of symptoms three to four hours after the initial exposure.

Myth: All cases of anaphylaxis have hives or swelling.

Fact: About 20 percent of cases of anaphylaxis will not have any hives or other skin symptoms. In fact, many of the worst episodes do not have any hives or swelling.

Myth: Taking Benadryl® or other medications before eating a problem food can prevent anaphylaxis.

Fact: Although it may be possible to block a mild allergic reaction with medicine, preventing anaphylaxis usually is not possible. In fact, the medicine might prevent the early phase of the reaction, such as hives, that could serve as a warning sign to get help, thereby leaving you even more at risk for a dangerous reaction.

Myth: Epinephrine is dangerous.

Fact: Epinephrine is safe for most people. The risks of anaphylaxis far outweigh the risks of epinephrine for the majority of patients.

Myth: Anaphylaxis is easy to avoid as long as you know what you are allergic to and take care to avoid it.

Fact: Most cases of anaphylaxis occur because of accidental exposure. It is therefore never safe to be without medication if you are at risk for anaphylaxis.

Myth: Contact reactions are a common cause of anaphylaxis.

Fact: Although contact reactions, such as getting peanut or milk on your hands from a dirty table, can cause anaphylaxis, they are much more likely to cause only a local reaction where the contact occurred.

Myth: All peanut reactions cause severe anaphylaxis.

Fact: Although peanut allergy may have the greatest potential to cause severe anaphylaxis, many patients with this allergy only experience mild reactions. They should still be prepared to deal with a more severe reaction.

Myth: You can predict the severity of a patient's' reaction based on their allergy tests.

Fact: Although allergy tests are helpful in determining what someone is allergic to, they cannot be used to predict how severe a reaction that person might have. Someone with a smaller skin test or a lower blood test (RAST; radioallergosorbent test) result may have just as severe a reaction as someone with an extremely high level of allergy.

Myth: There are new treatments available to desensitize people with food allergy.

Fact: There are currently no such treatments available. Be very careful of anyone who claims that food allergy can be cured.

✎ What's It Mean?

Anaphylaxis: Anaphylaxis, or anaphylactic shock, is a severe, frightening, and life-threatening allergic reaction. The reaction, although rare, can occur after an insect sting or as a reaction to an injected drug—for example, penicillin or antitetanus (horse) serum. Less commonly, the reaction occurs after a particular food or drug has been taken by mouth.

Epinephrine: Epinephrine is a naturally occurring hormone, also called adrenaline. It is one of two chemicals (the other is norepinephrine) released by the adrenal gland. Epinephrine increases the speed and force of heart beats and thereby the work that can be done by the heart. It dilates the airways to improve breathing and narrows blood vessels in the skin and intestine so that an increased flow of blood reaches the muscles and allows them to cope with the demands of exercise. Epinephrine has been produced synthetically as a drug since 1900. It remains the drug of choice for treatment of anaphylaxis.

Source: Excerpted from "Allergy-Immunology Glossary," © 2005 American College of Allergy, Asthma, and Immunology. All rights reserved. Reprinted with permission.

Chapter 10

You And Your Stuffy Nose

Nasal congestion, stuffiness, or obstruction to nasal breathing is one of man's oldest and most common complaints. While it may be a mere nuisance to some persons, to others it is a source of considerable discomfort, and it detracts from the quality of their lives.

Medical writers have classified the causes of nasal obstruction into four categories, recognizing that overlap exists between these categories and that it is not unusual for a patient to have more than one factor involved in his particular case.

Infection

An average adult suffers a common "cold" two to three times per year, more often in childhood and less often the older he gets as he develops more immunity. The common "cold" is caused by any number of different viruses, some of which are transmitted through the air, but most are transmitted from hand-to-nose contact. Once the virus gets established in the nose, it causes release of the body chemical histamine, which dramatically increases the blood flow to the nose, causing swelling and congestion of nasal tissues, and stimulating the nasal membranes to produce excessive amounts of mucus. Antihistamines and decongestants help relieve the symptoms of a "cold," but time alone cures it.

Table 10.1. Is It a Cold or an Allergy?

Symptoms	Cold	Airborne Allergy
Cough	Common	Sometimes
General Aches, Pains	Slight	Never
Fatigue, Weakness	Sometimes	Sometimes
Itchy Eyes	Rare or Never	Common
Sneezing	Usual	Usual
Sore Throat	Common	Sometimes
Runny Nose	Common	Common
Stuffy Nose	Common	Common
Fever	Common	Never
Duration	3 to 14 days	Weeks (for example, 6 weeks for ragweed or grass pollen seasons)
Treatment	Antihistamines, Decongestants, Nonsteroidal anti-inflammatory medicines	Antihistamines—over the counter or by prescription, Nasal steroids, Decongestants
Prevention	Wash your hands often, Avoid close contact with anyone with a cold	Avoid those things that you are allergic to such as pollen, house dust mites, mold, pet dander, cockroaches
Complications	Sinus infection, Middle ear infection, asthma	Sinus infection, Asthma

Source: U.S. Department of Health and Human Services, National Institutes of Health, National Institute of Allergy and Infectious Diseases (http://www.niaid.nih.gov), April 2005.

During a virus infection, the nose has poor resistance against bacterial infections, which explains why bacterial infections of the nose and sinuses so often follow a "cold." When the nasal mucus turns from clear to yellow or green, it usually means that a bacterial infection has taken over and a physician should be consulted.

Acute sinus infections produce nasal congestion, thick discharge, and pain and tenderness in the cheeks and upper teeth, between and behind the eyes, or above the eyes and in the forehead, depending on which sinuses are involved.

Chronic sinus infections may or may not cause pain, but nasal obstruction and offensive nasal or postnasal discharge is often present. Some persons develop polyps (fleshy growths in the nose) from sinus infections, and the infection can spread down into the lower airways leading to chronic cough, bronchitis, and asthma. Acute sinus infection generally responds to antibiotic treatment; chronic sinusitis usually requires surgery.

Structural Causes

Included in this category are deformities of the nose and the nasal septum, which is the thin, flat cartilage and bone that separates the nostrils and nose into its two sides. These deformities are usually due to an injury at some time in one's life. The injury may have been many years earlier and may even have been in childhood and long since forgotten. It is a fact that seven percent of newborn babies suffer significant nasal injury just from the birth process; and, of course, it is almost impossible to go through life without getting hit on the nose at least once. Therefore, deformities of the nose and the deviated septum should be fairly common problems—and they are. If they create obstruction to breathing, they can be corrected with surgery.

One of the most common causes for nasal obstruction in children is enlargement of the adenoids: tonsil-like tissues that fill the back of the nose up behind the palate. Children with this problem breath noisily at night and even snore. They also are chronic mouth breathers, and they develop a "sad" long face and sometimes dental deformities. Surgery to remove the adenoids and sometimes the tonsils may be advisable.

Other causes in this category include nasal tumors and foreign bodies. Children are prone to inserting various objects such as peas, beans, cherry pits, beads, buttons, safety pins, and bits of plastic toys into their noses. Beware of one-sided foul smelling discharge, which can be caused by a foreign body. A physician should be consulted.

Allergy

Hay fever, rose fever, grass fever, and "summertime colds" are various names for allergic rhinitis. Allergy is an exaggerated inflammatory response to a foreign substance which, in the case of a stuffy nose, is usually a pollen, mold, animal dander, or some element in house dust. Foods sometime play a role. Pollens cause problems in spring (trees) and summer (grasses) or fall (weeds)

♣ It's A Fact!!
What Makes Me Sneeze?

AHHH-CHOO!

If you just sneezed, something was probably irritating or tickling the inside of your nose. Sneezing, also called sternutation, is your body's way of removing an irritation from your nose.

When the inside of your nose gets a tickle, a message is sent to a special part of your brain called the sneeze center. The sneeze center then sends a message to all the muscles that have to work together to create the amazingly complicated process that we call the sneeze.

Some of the muscles involved are the abdominal (belly) muscles, the chest muscles, the diaphragm (the large muscle beneath your lungs that makes you breathe), the muscles that control your vocal cords, and muscles in the back of your throat. Don't forget the eyelid muscles! Did you know that you always close your eyes when you sneeze?

It is the job of the sneeze center to make all these muscles work together, in just the right order, to send that irritation flying out of your nose. And fly it does—sneezing can send tiny particles speeding out of your nose at up to 100 miles per hour!

whereas house dust allergies and mold may be a year-around problem. Ideally the best treatment is avoidance of these substances, but that is impractical in most cases.

In the allergic patient, the release of histamine and similar substances results in congestion and excess production of watery nasal mucus. Antihistamines help relieve the sneezing and runny nose of allergy. Many antihistamines are now available without a prescription. The most familiar brands include Chlor-Trimeton®, Benadryl®, Clarinex®, Claritin®, Allegra®, and Zyrtec® (although most are also available in generic forms). Decongestants, such as Sudafed® (also available in generic forms) shrink congested

Most anything that can irritate the inside of your nose can start a sneeze. Some common things include dust, cold air, or pepper. When you catch a cold in your nose, a virus has made a temporary home there and is causing lots of swelling and irritation. Some people have allergies, and they sneeze when they are exposed to certain things, such as animal dander (which comes from the skin of many common pets) or pollen (which comes from some plants).

Do you know anyone who sneezes when they step outside into the sunshine? About one out of every three people sneezes when exposed to bright light. They are called photic sneezers (photic means light). If you are a photic sneezer, you got it from one of your parents because it is an inherited trait. You could say that it runs in your family. Most people have some sensitivity to light that can trigger a sneeze.

Have you ever had the feeling that you are about to sneeze, but it just gets stuck? Next time that happens, try looking toward a bright light briefly (but don't look right into the sun)—see if that doesn't unstick a stuck sneeze!

Source: This information was provided by KidsHealth, one of the largest resources online for medically reviewed health information written for parents, kids, and teens. For more articles like this one, visit www.KidsHealth.org, or www.TeensHealth.org. © 2003 The Nemours Center for Children's Health Media, a division of The Nemours Foundation.

nasal tissues. Combinations of antihistamines with decongestants are also available; for example, Actifed®, Allegra D®, Chlor-Trimeton D®, Claritin D®. All these preparations have potential side effects, and patients must heed the warnings of the package or prescription insert. This is especially important if the patient suffers from high blood pressure, glaucoma, irregular heart beats, difficulty in urination, or is pregnant.

Allergy shots are the most specific treatment available, and they are highly successful in allergic patients. Skin tests or at times blood tests are used to make up treatment vials of substances to which the patient is allergic. The physician determines the best concentration for initiating the treatment. These treatments are given by injection. They work by forming blocking antibodies in the patient's blood stream, which then interfere with the allergic reaction. Many patients prefer allergy shots over drugs because of the side effects of the drugs.

Vasomotor Rhinitis

"Rhinitis" means inflammation of the nose and nasal membranes. "Vaso-motor" means blood vessel forces. The membranes of the nose have an abundant supply of arteries, veins, and capillaries, which have a great capacity for both expansion and constriction. Normally these blood vessels are in a half-constricted, half-open state. But when a person exercises vigorously, his/her hormones of stimulation (i.e., adrenaline) increase. The adrenaline causes constriction or squeezing of the nasal membranes so that the air passages open up and the person breathes more freely.

The opposite takes place when an allergic attack or a "cold" develops: The blood vessels expand, the membranes become congested (full of excess blood), and the nose becomes stuffy, or blocked.

In addition to allergies and infections, other events can also cause nasal blood vessels to expand, leading to vasomotor rhinitis. These include psychological stress, inadequate thyroid function, pregnancy, certain anti–high blood pressure drugs, and overuse or prolonged use of decongesting nasal sprays and irritants such as perfumes and tobacco smoke.

In the early stages of each of these disorders, the nasal stuffiness is temporary and reversible. That is, it will improve if the primary cause is corrected.

However, if the condition persists for a long enough period, the blood vessels lose their capacity to constrict. They become somewhat like varicose veins. They fill up when the patient lies down and when he/she lies on one side, the lower side becomes congested. The congestion often interferes with sleep. So it is helpful for stuffy patients to sleep with the head of the bed elevated two to four inches accomplish this by placing a brick or two under each castor of the bedposts at the head of the bed. Surgery my offer dramatic and long time relief.

☞ Remember!!

Stuffy nose is one symptom caused by a remarkable array of different disorders, and the physician with special interest in nasal disorders will offer treatments based on the specific causes.

Source: © 2005 American Academy of Otolaryngology–Head and Neck Surgery Foundation.

Chapter 11

Rhinitis

Do you suffer from a runny or stuffy nose much of the time? In the U.S., about 40 million people do. This problem is known as rhinitis. Approximately 40 million people in the U.S. have rhinitis. There are several types of rhinitis.

What are the types of rhinitis?

Allergic Rhinitis: If you sneeze and have a runny or stuffy nose during the spring, summer or fall allergy seasons, you may have seasonal allergic rhinitis or hay fever. Hay fever is the most common type of allergy problem. It mainly affects the eyes and nose. Hay fever symptoms include sneezing, itching, runny or stuffy nose and red, watery eyes.

Rhinitis can be a problem all year or only some of the year. It can be a problem when inside or when outside. Allergy symptoms are caused when someone has a problem when around a certain substance. These substances are called allergens. They can be inside, such as cats or dust. They can be outside such as tree and grass pollen in the spring and weed pollen and molds in the summer and fall. Hay fever is mainly an allergy caused by outdoor allergens.

Non-Allergic Rhinitis: This type of rhinitis is not as well understood. Although not triggered by allergy, the symptoms are often the same as seen with allergic rhinitis. Although the symptoms are similar, allergy skin test results are negative. Nasal polyps may also be seen with this type of rhinitis.

Vasomotor Rhinitis: Common symptoms of vasomotor rhinitis are often nasal congestion and postnasal drip. A person with this type of rhinitis may have symptoms when exposed to temperature and humidity changes. Symptoms may also occur with exposure to smoke, odors, and emotional upsets. Allergy skin test results are negative.

Infectious Rhinitis: This can occur as a cold, which may clear rapidly or continue with symptoms longer than a week. Some people may also develop an acute or chronic bacterial sinus infection. Symptoms include an increased amount of colored (yellow-green) and thickened nasal discharge and nasal congestion.

Rhinitis Medicamentosa: This type of rhinitis is seen with long-term use of decongestant nasal sprays or recreational use of cocaine. Symptoms may include nasal congestion and postnasal drip. Decongestant nasal sprays are intended for short-term use only. Over-use can cause rebound nasal congestion. It is very important for a person with rebound congestion to work closely with a doctor to gradually decrease the nasal spray.

Mechanical Obstruction: This is most often seen with a deviated septum or enlarged adenoids. Symptoms often include nasal obstruction, that may be one sided.

✎ What's It Mean?

Rhinitis: Rhinitis is an inflammation of the mucous membrane that lines the nose, often due to an allergy to pollen, dust or other airborne substances. Seasonal allergic rhinitis also is known as "hay fever," a disorder which causes sneezing, itching, a runny nose and nasal congestion.

Source: Excerpted from "Allergy-Immunology Glossary," © 2005 American College of Allergy, Asthma, and Immunology. All rights reserved. Reprinted with permission.

Hormonal: This type of rhinitis is often seen with changes in the hormones. This often occurs during pregnancy, puberty, menses, or hypothyroidism.

How is rhinitis diagnosed?

Often a person may have more than one types of rhinitis. In making the diagnosis, an evaluation by your doctor may include the following:

- **History:** The doctor will ask questions about your health and your symptoms.

- **Physical exam**

- **Nasal smears**

- **Nasal secretions are examined under a microscope.**

- **Allergy testing:** Skin testing by a board-certified allergist is often recommended for someone with recurrent symptoms. A positive skin test often is seen with allergies. In most cases, an allergic person will react to more than one substance. Your doctor will compare your prick skin test results with your history of symptoms.

> ♣ **It's A Fact!!**
>
> The goal of treatment is to reduce symptoms. This often includes the following:
>
> • Identifying, controlling and/or treating things that make your symptoms worse.
>
> • Using and understanding medications.
>
> Source: © Copyright 2005 National Jewish Medical and Research Center.

- **Sinus X-ray or CT Scan:** Changes in the sinus x-ray or CT scan may indicate sinusitis (inflammation of the sinuses) with or without infection or nasal polyps.

How can you manage symptoms?

The best way to prevent allergic rhinitis is to avoid the things to which you are allergic. Because allergic rhinitis is caused by outdoor allergies this can be hard to do. If you have outdoor allergies there are some things you can do to help:

- Keep your doors and windows shut during pollen season.

- Use an air conditioner to cool your home instead of coolers or fans that bring in outside air.

- Consider pollen counts when planning outdoor activities. It may help to limit your outdoor activities when pollen and mold counts are at their highest.

Pollen and mold counts can vary throughout the day. Peak times are:

- Grass: afternoon and early evening;

- Ragweed: early midday;

- Mold: some types peak during warm, dry, windy afternoons; other types occur at high levels during periods of dampness and rain.

House Dust Mites: If you are allergic to house dust mites and live in a humid area:

- Cover your mattress and box spring in zippered, dust proof encasings.

- Wash your pillows, sheets and blankets weekly in hot water. Dust mites will survive in lukewarm water.

Animals: Dander, urine and saliva from feathered or furry animals is a major year-round allergen. Cats, dogs, birds, hamsters, gerbils and horses are common pets. If you are allergic to an animal:

- Do not keep any furry or feathered pets in your home.

- If you must keep the pet, try to keep it outdoors. If the pet comes indoors, make sure it stays out of your bedroom at all times. After exposure to the pet, wash your hands and change your clothes.

Irritants: Many substances can irritate the nose, throat or airways. Common irritants include smoke such as tobacco smoke from wood-burning stoves, or kerosene stoves and fireplaces, aerosol sprays, strong odors, dust and air pollution. Reducing exposure to irritants can be very helpful.

- It is important that no one smokes in the home or car.

> ### ☞ Remember!!
>
> Rhinitis can be managed so you can have an active, fun life. Talk with your doctor if you think you have rhinitis. Your doctor is your partner in your healthcare.
>
> Source: © Copyright 2005 National Jewish Medical and Research Center.

- Always look for non-smoking sections in public areas.

- Avoid aerosol spray, perfumes, strong cleaning products and other odor sources in the home.

What medications treat rhinitis?

Anti-inflammatory medicines: These control inflammation in the body. This inflammation causes redness and swelling (congestion).

Cromolyn and nedocromil are anti-inflammatory medicines that are not steroids. They may help prevent nasal and eye symptoms.

Nasal steroid sprays: These work well to reduce nasal symptoms of sneezing, itching, runny and stuffy nose. Nasal steroids may also improve eye symptoms. A steroid nasal spray may work after several hours or take several days to work. Nasal steroids work best if you take them daily.

Common nasal steroid sprays include the following:

- Beconase®, Beconase AQ®, Vancenase®, Vancenase AQ® (beclomethasone)

- Rhinocort® (flunisolide)

- Nasarel® (flunisolide)

- Flonase® (fluticasone)

- Nasonex® (mometasone)

- Nasacort®, Nasacort AQ® (triamcinolone)

Nasal wash: A nasal wash with salt water may help clean out your nose. When done routinely, this can also lessen post-nasal drip. If you do a nasal wash, do this before using other nasal medicine.

Antihistamine medicine: Antihistamines can help decrease allergy symptoms. They may be used daily during allergy season or when allergy symptoms occur. There are many different antihistamines. If one doesn't work, another can be tried. Some can make you sleepy and some do not.

Common antihistamines that do not make you sleepy include the following:

- Claritin® (loratadine)
- Clarinex® (desloratadine)
- Allegra® (fexofenadine)
- Zyrtec® (cetirizine) (can cause some people to be sleepy)

Some over-the-counter antihistamines can make you feel sleepy. They may also affect thinking and your reflexes. If you take one of these, use caution when driving or using any kind of machine.

Astelin® (azelastine) is an antihistamine nasal spray. It usually does not make you sleepy.

Decongestant medicine: Decongestants help when your nose is stuffy (congestion). They are available as pills, liquids or nasal sprays. Many are available over the counter. A common over the counter decongestant is Sudafed (pseudoephedrine). Use caution when taking a decongestant nasal spray. Using one longer than four days can have a rebound effect. This causes you to have more nasal congestion.

Atrovent® (ipratropium bromide) is a nasal spray. Atrovent may be helpful for decreasing symptoms of a runny nose. This nasal spray may be helpful for vasomotor rhinitis.

Immunotherapy (allergy shots): Allergy shots may be helpful for specific allergies that aren't controlled with medicine. It is recommended that you see a board certified allergist for allergy testing or allergy shots.

Chapter 12

Sinusitis

You're coughing and sneezing and tired and achy. You think that you might be getting a cold. Later, when the medicines you've been taking to relieve the symptoms of the common cold are not working and you've now got a terrible headache, you finally drag yourself to the doctor. After listening to your history of symptoms, examining your face and forehead, and perhaps doing a sinus x-ray, the doctor says you have sinusitis.

Sinusitis simply means your sinuses are infected or inflamed, but this gives little indication of the misery and pain this condition can cause. Health care experts usually divide sinusitis cases into one of three categories:

- Acute, which last for 3 weeks or less
- Chronic, which usually last for 3 to 8 weeks but can continue for months or even years
- Recurrent, which are several acute attacks within a year

Health care experts estimate that 37 million Americans are affected by sinusitis every year. Health care providers report nearly 32 million cases of chronic sinusitis to the Centers for Disease Control and Prevention annually. Americans spend millions of dollars each year for medications that promise relief from their sinus symptoms.

About This Chapter: From a fact sheet produced by the National Institute of Allergy and Infectious Diseases (NIAID), January 2005.

The Sinuses

Sinuses are hollow air spaces in the human body. When people say, "I'm having a sinus attack," they usually are referring to symptoms in one or more of four pairs of cavities, or sinuses, known as paranasal sinuses. These cavities, located within the skull or bones of the head surrounding the nose, include the following:

- Frontal sinuses over the eyes in the brow area

- Maxillary sinuses inside each cheekbone

- Ethmoid sinuses just behind the bridge of the nose and between the eyes

- Sphenoid sinuses behind the ethmoids in the upper region of the nose and behind the eyes

Each sinus has an opening into the nose for the free exchange of air and mucus, and each is joined with the nasal passages by a continuous mucous membrane lining. Therefore, anything that causes a swelling in the nose— an infection, an allergic reaction, or another type of immune reaction—also can affect the sinuses. Air trapped within a blocked sinus, along with pus or other secretions, may cause pressure on the sinus wall. The result is the sometimes intense pain of a sinus attack. Similarly, when air is prevented from entering a paranasal sinus by a swollen membrane at the opening, a vacuum can be created that also causes pain.

✎ What's It Mean?

Sinuses: The sinuses (paranasal sinuses) are air cavities within the facial bones. They are lined by mucous membranes similar to those in other parts of the airways.

Sinusitis: Sinusitis is inflammation of the membrane lining the facial sinuses, often caused by bacterial or viral infection.

Source: Excerpted from "Allergy-Immunology Glossary," © 2005 American College of Allergy, Asthma, and Immunology. All rights reserved. Reprinted with permission.

Symptoms

The location of your sinus pain depends on which sinus is affected:

- Headache when you wake up in the morning is typical of a sinus problem.

- Pain when your forehead over the frontal sinuses is touched may indicate that your frontal sinuses are inflamed.

- Infection in the maxillary sinuses can cause your upper jaw and teeth to ache and your cheeks to become tender to the touch.

- Since the ethmoid sinuses are near the tear ducts in the corner of the eyes, inflammation of these cavities often causes swelling of the eyelids and tissues around your eyes, and pain between your eyes. Ethmoid inflammation also can cause tenderness when the sides of your nose are touched, a loss of smell, and a stuffy nose.

- Although the sphenoid sinuses are less frequently affected, infection in this area can cause earaches, neck pain, and deep aching at the top of your head.

Most people with sinusitis, however, have pain or tenderness in several locations, and their symptoms usually do not clearly indicate which sinuses are inflamed.

Sinusitis can also produce other symptoms:

- Fever

- Weakness

- Tiredness

- A cough that may be more severe at night

- Runny nose (rhinitis) or nasal congestion

In addition, the drainage of mucus from the sphenoid or other sinuses down the back of your throat (postnasal drip) can cause you to have a sore throat. Mucus drainage also can irritate the membranes lining your larynx (upper windpipe). Not everyone with these symptoms, however, has sinusitis.

Some Causes Of Acute Sinusitis

Most cases of acute sinusitis start with a common cold, which is caused by a virus. These viral colds do not cause symptoms of sinusitis, but they do inflame the sinuses. Both the cold and the sinus inflammation usually go away without treatment in two weeks. The inflammation, however, might explain why having a cold increases your likelihood of developing acute sinusitis. For example, your nose reacts to an invasion by viruses that cause infections such as the common cold or flu by producing mucus and sending white blood cells to the lining of the nose, which congest and swell the nasal passages.

When this swelling involves the adjacent mucous membranes of your sinuses, air and mucus are trapped behind the narrowed openings of the sinuses. When your sinus openings become too narrow, mucus cannot drain properly. This increase in mucus sets up prime conditions for bacteria to multiply.

♣ **It's A Fact!!**
On rare occasions, acute sinusitis can result in brain infection and other serious complications.

Source: NIAID.

Most healthy people harbor bacteria, such as *Streptococcus pneumoniae* and *Haemophilus influenzae*, in their upper respiratory tracts with no problems until the body's defenses are weakened or drainage from the sinuses is blocked by a cold or other viral infection. Thus, bacteria that may have been living harmlessly in your nose or throat can multiply and invade your sinuses, causing an acute sinus infection.

Sometimes, fungal infections can cause acute sinusitis. Although fungi are abundant in the environment, they usually are harmless to healthy people, indicating that the human body has a natural resistance to them. Fungi, such as *Aspergillus*, can cause serious illness in people whose immune systems are not functioning properly. Some people with fungal sinusitis have an allergic-type reaction to the fungi.

Acute sinusitis is much more common in some people than in the general population. For example, sinusitis occurs more often in people who have reduced immune function (such as those with primary immune deficiency diseases or HIV infection) and with abnormality of mucus secretion or mucus movement (such as those with cystic fibrosis).

Causes Of Chronic Sinusitis

It can be difficult to determine the cause of chronic sinusitis. Some investigators think it is an infectious disease but others are not certain. It is an inflammatory disease that often occurs in patients with asthma. If you have asthma, an allergic disease, you may have chronic sinusitis with exacerbations. If you are allergic to airborne allergens, such as dust, mold, and pollen, which trigger allergic rhinitis, you may develop chronic sinusitis. An immune response to antigens in fungi may be responsible for at least some cases of chronic sinusitis. In addition, people who are allergic to fungi can develop a condition called "allergic fungal sinusitis." If you are subject to getting chronic sinusitis, damp weather, especially in northern temperate climates, or pollutants in the air and in buildings also can affect you.

If you have an immune deficiency disease or an abnormality in the way mucus moves through and from your respiratory system (for example, primary immune deficiency, HIV infection, and cystic fibrosis) you might develop chronic sinusitis with frequent flare-ups of acute sinusitis due to infections. In otherwise normal individuals, sinusitis may or may not be infectious. In addition, if you have severe asthma, nasal polyps (small growths in the nose), or a severe asthma attacks caused by aspirin and aspirin-like medicines such as ibuprofen, you might have chronic sinusitis.

Diagnosis

Because your nose can get stuffy when you have a condition like the common cold, you may confuse simple nasal congestion with sinusitis. A cold, however, usually lasts about 7 to 14 days and disappears without treatment. Acute sinusitis often lasts longer and typically causes more symptoms than just a cold.

Your doctor can diagnose sinusitis by listening to your symptoms, doing a physical examination, taking x-rays, and if necessary, an MRI or CT scan (magnetic resonance imaging and computed tomography).

Treatment

After diagnosing sinusitis and identifying a possible cause, a doctor can suggest treatments that will reduce your inflammation and relieve your symptoms.

Acute Sinusitis

If you have acute sinusitis, your doctor may recommend treatments such as these:

- Decongestants to reduce congestion

- Antibiotics to control a bacterial infection, if present

- Pain relievers to reduce any pain

> **✔ Quick Tip**
>
> You should use over-the-counter or prescription decongestant nose drops and sprays for only few days. If you use these medicines for longer periods, they can lead to even more congestion and swelling of your nasal passages.
>
> Source: NIAID.

If bacteria cause your sinusitis, antibiotics used along with a nasal or oral decongestant will usually help. Your doctor can prescribe an antibiotic that fights the type of bacteria most commonly associated with sinusitis.

Many cases of acute sinusitis will end without antibiotics. If you have allergic disease along with sinusitis, however, you may need medicine to relieve your allergy symptoms. If you already have asthma and then get sinusitis, you may experience worsening of your asthma and should be in close touch with your doctor.

In addition, your doctor may prescribe a steroid nasal spray, along with other treatments, to reduce your sinus congestion, swelling, and inflammation.

Chronic Sinusitis

Doctors often find it difficult to treat chronic sinusitis successfully, realizing that symptoms persist even after taking antibiotics for a long period. As discussed below, many doctors treat with steroids such as steroid nasal sprays. Many doctors do treat chronic sinusitis as though it is an infection, by using antibiotics and decongestants. Other doctors use both antibiotics and steroid nasal sprays. Further research is needed to determine what is the best treatment.

Some people with severe asthma are said to have dramatic improvement of their symptoms when their chronic sinusitis is treated with antibiotics.

Doctors commonly prescribe steroid nasal sprays to reduce inflammation in chronic sinusitis. Although doctors occasionally prescribe these sprays to treat people with chronic sinusitis over a long period, doctors don't fully understand the long-term safety of these medications, especially in children. Therefore, doctors will consider whether the benefits outweigh any risks of using steroid nasal sprays.

If you have severe chronic sinusitis, your doctor may prescribe oral steroids, such as prednisone. Because oral steroids are powerful medicines and can have significant side effects, you should take them only when other medicines have not worked.

When medical treatment fails, surgery may be the only alternative for treating chronic sinusitis. Research studies suggest that the vast majority of people who undergo surgery have fewer symptoms and better quality of life.

In children, problems often are eliminated by removal of adenoids obstructing nasal-sinus passages.

Adults who have had allergic and infectious conditions over the years sometimes develop nasal polyps that interfere with

✔ **Quick Tip**

Although home remedies cannot cure sinus infection, they might give you some comfort.

• Inhaling steam from a vaporizer or a hot cup of water can soothe inflamed sinus cavities.

• Saline nasal spray, which you can buy in a drug store, can give relief.

• Gentle heat applied over the inflamed area is comforting.

Source: NIAID.

proper drainage. Removal of these polyps and/or repair of a deviated septum to ensure an open airway often provides considerable relief from sinus symptoms.

The most common surgery done today is functional endoscopic sinus surgery, in which the natural openings from the sinuses are enlarged to allow drainage. This type of surgery is less invasive than conventional sinus surgery, and serious complications are rare.

Prevention

Although you cannot prevent all sinus disorders—any more than you can avoid all colds or bacterial infections—you can do certain things to reduce the number and severity of the attacks and possibly prevent acute sinusitis from becoming chronic.

- You may get some relief from your symptoms with a humidifier, particularly if room air in your home is heated by a dry forced-air system.

- Air conditioners help to provide an even temperature.

- Electrostatic filters attached to heating and air conditioning equipment are helpful in removing allergens from the air.

If you are prone to getting sinus disorders, especially if you have allergies, you should avoid cigarette smoke and other air pollutants. If your allergies inflame your nasal passages, you are more likely to have a strong reaction to all irritants.

If you suspect that your sinus inflammation may be related to dust, mold, pollen, or food—or any of the hundreds of allergens that can trigger an upper respiratory reaction—you should consult your doctor. Your doctor can use various tests to determine whether you have an allergy and its cause. This will help you and your doctor take appropriate steps to reduce or limit your allergy symptoms.

Drinking alcohol also causes nasal and sinus membranes to swell.

If you are prone to sinusitis, it may be uncomfortable for you to swim in pools treated with chlorine, since it irritates the lining of the nose and sinuses.

Divers often get sinus congestion and infection when water is forced into the sinuses from the nasal passages.

You may find that air travel poses a problem if you are suffering from acute or chronic sinusitis. As air pressure in a plane is reduced, pressure can build up in your head blocking your sinuses or eustachian tubes in your ears. Therefore, you might feel discomfort in your sinus or middle ear during the plane's ascent or descent. Some health experts recommend using decongestant nose drops or inhalers before a flight to avoid this problem.

♣ It's A Fact!!

Scientific studies have shown a close relationship between having asthma and sinusitis. As many as 75 percent of people with asthma also get sinusitis. Some studies state that up to 80 percent of adults with chronic sinusitis also had allergic rhinitis. NIAID conducts and supports research on allergic diseases as well as bacteria and fungus that can cause sinusitis. This research is focused on developing better treatments and ways to prevent these diseases.

Source: NIAID.

Research

At least two-thirds of sinusitis cases caused by bacteria are due to two organisms that can also cause otitis media (middle ear infection) in children as well as pneumonia and acute exacerbations of chronic bronchitis. The National Institute of Allergy and Infectious Diseases (NIAID) is supporting multiple studies to better understand the basis for infectivity of these organisms as well as identifying potential candidates for future vaccines strategies that could eliminate these diseases.

A project supported by NIAID is developing an advanced "sinuscope" that will permit improved airway evaluation during a medical examination especially when surgical intervention is contemplated.

Scientists supported by NIAID and other institutions are investigating whether chronic sinusitis has genetic causes. They have found that certain alterations in the gene that causes cystic fibrosis may also increase the likelihood of developing chronic sinusitis. This research will give scientists new insights into the cause of the disease in some people and points to new strategies for diagnosis and treatment.

Another NIAID-supported research study has recently demonstrated that blood cells from patients with chronic sinusitis make chemicals that produce inflammation when exposed to fungal antigens, suggesting that fungi may play a role in many cases of chronic sinusitis. Further research, including clinical trials of antifungal drugs, will help determine whether, and for whom, this new treatment strategy holds promise.

♣ It's A Fact!!

Chronic inflammation of the nasal passages also can lead to sinusitis. If you have allergic rhinitis or hay fever, you can develop episodes of acute sinusitis. Vasomotor rhinitis, caused by humidity, cold air, alcohol, perfumes, and other environmental conditions, also may be complicated by sinus infections.

Source: NIAID.

Chapter 13

Conjunctivitis (Pink Eye)

The conjunctiva is the thin, clear membrane over the white part of the eye; it also lines the eyelids. Inflammation of this membrane is called conjunctivitis. Its common name, pink eye, can refer to all forms of conjunctivitis, or just to its contagious forms.

Pink Eye Symptoms And Signs

The most obvious symptom of pink eye is, of course, a pink eye. The pink or red color is due to inflammation. Your eye may also hurt or itch.

How can you tell what type of pink eye you have? The way your eyes feel will give some clues:

- **Viral conjunctivitis** usually affects only one eye and causes excessive eye watering and a light discharge.

- **Bacterial conjunctivitis** affects both eyes and causes a heavy discharge, sometimes greenish.

- **Allergic conjunctivitis** affects both eyes and causes itching and redness in the eyes and sometimes the nose, as well as excessive tearing.

About This Chapter: This chapter includes text from "Conjunctivitis (Pink Eye)" and "Eye Allergies," both reprinted with permission from http://www.allaboutvision.com. © 2005 Access Media Group, LLC.

- **Giant papillary conjunctivitis (GPC)** usually affects both eyes and causes contact lens intolerance, itching, a heavy discharge, tearing, and red bumps on the underside of the eyelids.

To pinpoint the cause and then choose an appropriate treatment, your doctor will ask some questions, examine your eyes, and possibly collect a sample on a swab to send out for analysis. Give a careful account of the episode, because oftentimes your answers alone with reveal the diagnosis.

Eye Allergies

Similar to processes that occur with other types of allergic responses, the eye may overreact to a substance perceived as harmful even though it may not be. For example, dust that is harmless to most people can cause excessive production of tears and mucus in eyes of overly sensitive, allergic individuals. Eye allergies are often hereditary.

Allergies can trigger other problems, such as conjunctivitis (pink eye) and asthma. Most of the more than 22 million Americans who suffer from allergies also have allergic conjunctivitis, according to the American Academy of Ophthalmology.

✔ **Quick Tip**
Eye Allergies Self-Test

Take this quiz to help determine if you have eye allergies. Always consult your doctor if you suspect you have an eye condition needing care.

1. Do allergies run in your family?

2. Do your eyes often itch, particularly during spring pollen season?

3. Have you ever been diagnosed with "pink eye" (conjunctivitis)?

4. Are you allergic to certain animals such as cats?

5. Do you often need antihistamines and/or decongestants to control sneezing, coughing, and congestion?

6. When pollen is in the air, are your eyes less red and itchy when you stay indoors under an air conditioner?

7. Do your eyes begin tearing when you wear certain cosmetics or lotions, or when you're around certain strong perfumes?

If you answered "yes" to most of these questions, then you may have eye allergies. Make an appointment with an optometrist or ophthalmologist to determine the best course of action.

Source: © 2005 Access Media Group, LLC.

Allergy Symptoms And Signs

Common signs of allergies include: red, swollen, tearing or itchy eyes; runny nose; sneezing; coughing; difficulty breathing; itchy nose, mouth or throat; and headache from sinus congestion.

What Causes Eye Allergies?

Many allergens are in the air, where they come in contact with your eyes and nose. Airborne allergens include pollen, mold, dust and pet dander. Other causes of allergies, such as certain foods or bee stings, do not typically affect the eyes the way airborne allergens do. Adverse reactions to certain cosmetics or drugs such as antibiotic eyedrops also may cause eye allergies.

Eye Allergy Treatment

Avoidance: The most common "treatment" is to avoid what's causing your eye allergy. Itchy eyes? Keep your home free of pet dander and dust, and stay inside with the air conditioner on when a lot of pollen is in the air. Air conditioners filter out allergens, though you must clean the filters from time to time.

Medications: If you're not sure what's causing your eye allergies, or you're not having any luck avoiding them, your next step will probably be medication to alleviate the symptoms.

Over-the-counter and prescription medications each have their advantages; for example, over-the-counter products are often less expensive, while prescription ones are often stronger.

Eyedrops are available as simple eye washes, or they may have one or more active ingredients such as antihistamines, decongestants or mast cell stabilizers. Antihistamines relieve many symptoms caused by airborne allergens, such as itchy, watery eyes, runny nose and sneezing.

Decongestants clear up redness. They contain vasoconstrictors, which simply make the blood vessels in your eyes smaller, lessening the apparent redness. They treat the symptom, not the cause.

In fact, with extended use, the blood vessels can become dependent on the vasoconstrictor to stay small. When you discontinue the eyedrops, the

✔ Quick Tip

National Jewish pediatrician Dan Atkins, M.D., recommends several steps that people can take to reduce pollen's irritating effect on their eyes.

Wash your hands: During high allergy season, pollen is everywhere. You get it on your hands opening a car door, running your hands through your hair, or touching other outdoor surfaces. If you rub your eyes with those pollen-coated hands, they will only get more irritated. Washing your hands frequently can reduce the amount of pollen that gets in your eyes.

Use saline rinses or artificial tears: These can provide significant relief by removing or diluting the pollen grains in the eye.

Wear sunglasses: Sunglasses can reduce the amount of pollen that gets in the eyes by deflecting the wind carrying it toward you.

Close the windows and use the air conditioner: This can reduce pollen floating in the air both in the house and in the car.

Apply cold compresses: A bag of frozen peas or a moist washcloth that has been place briefly in the freezer can reduce both itching and swelling when put on the eyes.

Medications: Several medications can also help people whose eyes bear the brunt of their seasonal allergies. For people with mild symptoms oral antihistamines can prevent irritation of both the eye and the nose. For those with more severe allergic conjunctivitis, physicians can prescribe a number of medications that can be applied directly to the eye. These include topical antihistamines, vasoconstrictors, mast-cell stabilizers, topical non-steroidal anti-inflammatory medications, and topical corticosteroids. Patients should consult their own physicians to learn what would work best for them.

Patients should also remember to take these medications continuously throughout the pollen season rather than intermittently because most of them work best if taken before the allergen exposure, rather than after the eyes have already become irritated.

Source: © Copyright 2005 National Jewish Medical and Research Center. All rights reserved. For additional information, visit http://asthma .nationaljewish.org/ or call 1-800-222 LUNG.

vessels actually get bigger than they were to begin with. This process is called rebound hyperemia, and the result is that your red eyes get worse over time.

Some products have ingredients that act as mast cell stabilizers, which alleviate redness and swelling. Mast cell stabilizers are similar to antihistamines, but while antihistamines are known for their immediate relief, mast cell stabilizers are known for their long-lasting relief.

Antihistamines, decongestants and mast cell stabilizers are available in pill form, but pills don't work as quickly as eyedrops or gels to bring eye relief.

Nonsteroidal anti-inflammatory drug (NSAID) eyedrops may be prescribed to decrease swelling, inflammation, and other symptoms associated with seasonal allergic conjunctivitis, otherwise known as hay fever. Prescription corticosteroid eyedrops also may provide similar, quick relief. However, steroids have been associated with side effects such as increased inner eye pressure (intraocular pressure) leading to glaucoma, which can damage the optic nerve. Steroids also have been known to cause the eye's natural lens to become cloudy, producing cataracts.

Check the product label or insert for a list of side effects of over-the-counter medications. For prescription medication, ask your doctor. In some cases, combinations of medications may be used.

Immunotherapy: You may benefit from immunotherapy, in which an allergy specialist injects you with small amounts of the allergen to help you gradually build up immunity.

Eye Allergies And Contact Lenses

Even if you are generally a successful contact lens wearer, allergy season can make your contacts uncomfortable. Airborne allergens can get on your lenses, causing discomfort. Allergens can also stimulate the excessive production of natural substances in your eyes, which bind to your contacts and also become uncomfortable.

Ask your eye doctor about eyedrops that can help relieve your symptoms and keep your contact lenses clean: certain drops can discolor or damage certain lenses, so it makes sense to ask first before trying out a new brand.

Another alternative is daily disposable contact lenses, which are discarded nightly. Because you replace them so frequently, these types of lenses are unlikely to develop irritating deposits that can build up over time and cause or heighten allergy-related discomfort.

♣ It's A Fact!!
Watery Eyes

Two common causes of excessively watery eyes are allergies and dry eye syndrome, two very different problems. With allergies, your body's release of histamine causes your eyes to water, just as it may cause your nose to run.

Although it may not initially make sense that watery eyes would result from dry eye syndrome, this is sometimes the case, because the excessive dryness works to overstimulate production of the watery component of your eye's tears.

Source: © 2005 Access Media Group, LLC.

Chapter 14

Rashes: The Itchy Truth

Question: What is red and itchy, but can also be bumpy, lumpy, or scaly?

Answer: If you said a rash, you're right!

Types Of Rashes

A rash can also be called dermatitis (say: dur-muh-tye-tus), which is any swelling (puffiness) or irritation of the skin. It can be red, dry, scaly, and itchy. Rashes also can include lumps, bumps, blisters, and even pimples. Most people have had a rash or two. When you were a baby, you probably had diaper rash.

But some rashes, especially combined with a fever, can be signs of serious illnesses. Hives, also called urticaria (say: ur-tuh-kar-ee-ah), also can be serious because they can be a sign of an allergic reaction and the person may need immediate medical attention.

Hives, which are reddish or pale swellings, appear on a person's body when a chemical called histamine (say: his-tuh-meen) is released in response

About This Chapter: This information was provided by KidsHealth, one of the largest resources online for medically reviewed health information written for parents, kids, and teens. For more articles like this one, visit www.KidsHealth.org, or www.TeensHealth.org. © 2004 The Nemours Center for Children's Health Media, a division of The Nemours Foundation.

to an allergen. The trigger could be a certain food, medicine, or insect bite. A virus also can cause hives.

Here are some other common types of rashes:

- **Eczema** (say: ek-zuh-muh), also called atopic dermatitis, is a common rash for kids. Eczema can cause dry, chapped, bumpy areas around the elbows and knees or more serious cases of red, scaly, and swollen skin all over the body.

- **Irritant contact dermatitis** is caused by contact with something irritating, such as a chemical, soap, or detergent. It can be red, swollen, and itchy. Even sunburn can be a kind of irritant dermatitis because it's red and may itch while it's healing.

✔ Quick Tip

Rash Prevention

Prevention is also the name of the game when it comes to other kinds of rashes.

- If a poison plant is your problem, learn what the plant looks like and avoid it. It also may help to wear long sleeves and pants when you're camping or hiking in the woods.

- If bugs bug you, have a parent help you apply some insect repellent when you'll be going outside.

- For allergic dermatitis or irritant contact dermatitis, try to avoid that substance. If you are allergic to nickel, wear only nickel-free jewelry. Or if you discover that bubble bath bothers your skin, don't use it.

- With eczema, stay away from harsh soaps that may dry out your skin. Also, make an effort to moisturize your skin with creams or lotions. Short, cool showers are a good idea, too, because hot showers and baths can further dry out your skin.

- When it comes to sun, you should always wear sunscreen to avoid a red and itchy sunburn.

- **Allergic contact dermatitis** is a rash caused by contact with an allergen (say: ah-lur-jun). An allergen is something you are allergic to, such as rubber, hair dye, or nickel, a metal found in some jewelry. If you have nickel allergy, you might get a red, scaly, crusty rash wherever the jewelry touched the skin, like around your finger if you were wearing a ring. Urushiol (say: yoo-roo-shee-ol), an oil or resin contained in poison ivy, oak, and sumac, also can cause this kind of rash.

What To Do If You Get A Rash

Some rashes form right away and others can take several days to occur. When a rash appears, you usually know it because it will start to bother you. If you develop a rash, tell a parent or another adult as soon as you can. For instance, you might want to see the school nurse if you are at school.

Try not to scratch. If you do, the rash may take longer to heal and you'll be more likely to develop an infection or scar.

A visit to the doctor is a good idea if you have a rash. Although all rashes may look alike to you, a skin doctor called a dermatologist (say: dur-muh-tah-luh-jist) knows the difference. And knowing which kind of rash you have can help the dermatologist choose the best treatment to heal your rash.

For eczema, the doctor may suggest special moisturizers called emollients (say: ih-mal-yunts). Emollients retain the water in your skin, keeping it soft and smooth while soothing the itchy feeling.

With poison ivy, the doctor may prescribe cool showers and calamine lotion. In more severe cases, a liquid or pill medicine called an antihistamine may be needed. It decreases itching and redness.

For rashes that are caused by an allergen, including hives, the doctor will probably want more information. He or she will want to find out which food, substance, medicine, or insect caused your rash or hives. He or she may recommend a medical test to determine which allergens are causing you trouble. It's important to find this out because the best way to prevent rashes and hives caused by allergens is to avoid the problem food, substance, medicine, or insect.

Remember!!

Being a kid means getting a few rashes. But now you know what to do if you get that awful itchy feeling.

Chapter 15

Eczema

All About Eczema

Three midterms, extra household chores because his mom was on a business trip, and inventory at his part-time job had left Rick exhausted by the end of the week. But he wasn't just tired—the skin on the back of his neck and upper chest was beginning to get red and itchy, too. Not again, he thought—not another eczema flare!

Eczema is a common teen skin problem. If you have eczema, keep reading to find out more about it and how you can deal with the skin stress.

What Is Eczema?

Eczema is a group of skin conditions that cause skin to become irritated. Teens who have it may develop rashes more easily and more frequently than others. There are many forms of eczema, but atopic eczema is the most common form. Doctors don't know exactly what causes atopic eczema, also called atopic dermatitis, but they think it's caused by a difference in the way a

About This Chapter: This chapter begins with text from "All About Eczema"; this information was provided by TeensHealth, one of the largest resources online for medically reviewed health information written for parents, kids, and teens. For more articles like this one, visit www.TeensHealth.org, or www.KidsHealth.org. © 2003 The Nemours Center for Children's Health Media, a division of The Nemours Foundation. Text under the heading "Hand Eczema" is reprinted with permission from the American Academy of Dermatology. All rights reserved. © 2004.

person's immune system reacts to things. Skin allergies may be involved in some forms of eczema.

If you have eczema, you're probably not the only one you know who has it. Eczema isn't contagious like a cold or mono, but most people with eczema have family members with the same condition, so researchers think it's inherited or passed through the genes. In general, it's fairly common—about 3% of all the people in the United States have eczema.

People with eczema also may have asthma and certain allergies, such as hay fever. In some people with eczema, food allergies (such as allergies to cow's milk, soy, eggs, fish, or wheat) may bring on or worsen eczema. Allergies to animal dander, rough fabrics, and dust may also trigger the condition in some teens.

Signs And Symptoms

It can be difficult to avoid all the triggers, or irritants, that may cause your eczema to flare or become worse. In teens and young adults, the itchy patches of eczema usually break out where the elbow bends; on the backs of the knees, ankles, and wrists; and on the face, neck, and upper chest—although any part of the body can be affected.

If you have eczema, at first your skin may feel hot and itchy. Then, if you scratch, your skin may become red, inflamed, or blistered. Some teens who have eczema scratch their skin so much it becomes almost leathery in texture. Other teens find that their skin becomes extremely dry and scaly. Even though a lot of teens experience eczema, the symptoms quite a bit from person to person.

What Do Doctors Do?

If you think you have eczema, your best bet is to visit your doctor. He or she may refer you to a dermatologist, a doctor who specializes in treating skin conditions. Diagnosing atopic eczema can be difficult because it may be confused with other skin conditions such as contact dermatitis, which occurs when your skin comes in contact with an irritating substance like the perfume in a certain detergent.

In addition to doing a physical examination, the doctor will ask you about any concerns and symptoms you have, your past health, your family's health, any medications you're taking, any allergies you may have, and other issues. This is called the medical history. Your doctor will also help you identify things in your environment that may be contributing to your skin irritation. For example, if you started using a new shower gel or body lotion before the symptoms appeared, mention this to your doctor because a substance in the cream or lotion might be irritating your skin.

Emotional stress can lead to eczema flares, so your doctor might also ask you about any stress you're feeling at home, school, or work.

✎ What's It Mean?

Eczema: An inflammation of the skin, usually causing itching and sometimes accompanied by crusting, scaling, or blisters. A type of eczema often made worse by allergen exposure is termed *atopic dermatitis*.

Source: Excerpted from "Allergy-Immunology Glossary," © 2005 American College of Allergy, Asthma, and Immunology. All rights reserved. Reprinted with permission.

Once your doctor has diagnosed the condition, he or she may suggest avoiding the things that may be triggers for your eczema. The doctor may also prescribe medications to soothe the redness and irritation of eczema. External creams or ointments that contain corticosteroids are frequently prescribed to help control itching. Your doctor might also recommend medications you take internally, such as antihistamines or corticosteroids. In teens who have severe eczema, ultraviolet light therapy may help clear up their condition and make them more comfortable. Newer medications that change the way the skin's immune system reacts are also prescribed in some cases.

Allergy testing is sometimes used to help people who have eczema that doesn't respond to normal treatment, especially if a teen has asthma or seasonal allergies.

If a person is tested for food allergies, he or she may be given certain foods (such as eggs, milk, soy, or nuts) and observed to see if the food causes an eczema flare. Food allergy testing can also be done by pricking the person's skin with an extract of the food substance and observing the reaction. But sometimes allergy testing can be misleading because the person may have an allergic reaction to a food that is not causing the eczema flare.

If a person is tested for allergy to dyes or fragrances, a patch of the substance will be placed against the person's skin and he or she will be monitored to see if skin irritation develops.

✔ Quick Tip

If you have eczema and can't wear certain types of makeup, find brands that are free of fragrances and dyes. Your dermatologist may be able to recommend some brands that will help keep you looking great and are less likely to irritate your skin.

Source: © 2003 The Nemours Center for Children's Health Media, a division of The Nemours Foundation.

Can I Prevent Eczema?

Eczema can't be cured, but there are plenty of things you can do to prevent a flare. For facial eczema, wash gently with a nondrying facial cleanser or soap substitute, use a facial moisturizer that says noncomedogenic/oil-free, and apply only hypoallergenic makeup and sunscreens. In addition, the following tips may help:

- **Avoid triggers and substances that stress skin.** Besides your known triggers, some things you may want to avoid include household cleaners, detergents, lotions, and harsh soaps.

- **H_2O is a no-no.** Too much exposure to water can dry out your skin, so take short warm, not hot, showers and baths and wear gloves if your hands will be in water for long periods of time.

- **Say yes to cotton.** Clothes made of scratchy fabric like wool can irritate your skin. Cotton clothes are a better bet.

- **Moisturize!** An unfragranced moisturizer such as petroleum jelly will prevent your skin from becoming irritated and cracked.

- **Don't scratch that itch.** Even though it's difficult to resist, scratching your itch can worsen eczema and make it more difficult for the skin to heal because you can break the skin and bacteria can get in, causing an infection.

- **Keep it cool.** Sudden changes in temperature, sweating, and becoming overheated may cause your eczema to kick into action.

- **Take your meds.** Follow your doctor's or dermatologist's directions and take your medication as directed.

- **Chill out.** Stress can aggravate eczema, so try to relax.

Dealing With Eczema

There's good news if you have eczema—usually eczema will go away before the age of 25. Until it clears up, you'll have to deal with it, even though at best it's annoying and at worst it can make you want to stay in your room and hide.

Your self-esteem doesn't have to suffer just because you have eczema, and neither does your social life! Getting involved in your school and extracurricular activities can be a great way to get your mind off the itch. If certain activities will aggravate your eczema, such as swimming in a heavily chlorinated pool, suggest activities to your friends that won't harm your skin.

Even if sweat tends to aggravate your skin, it's still a good idea to exercise. Exercise is a great way to blow off stress—just try walking, bike riding, or another sport that keeps your skin cool and dry while you work out.

Hand Eczema

What causes a hand rash?

A hand rash, also called hand dermatitis or hand eczema, may be caused by many things.

Hand rashes are extremely common. Many people start with dry, chapped hands that later become patchy, red, scaly, and inflamed. Numerous items can irritate skin. These include overexposure to water, too much dry air, soaps, detergents, solvents, cleaning agents, chemicals, rubber gloves, and even ingredients in skin and personal care products. Once skin becomes red and dry, even so-called "harmless" things like water and baby products can irritate the rash, making it worse. Your doctor will try to find out what substance in your everyday routine could be causing or contributing to the problem. Often your skin will get better by changing products or avoiding an ingredient completely.

A tendency to get skin reactions is often inherited. People with these tendencies may have a history of hay fever and/or asthma. They may also have food allergies and a skin condition called atopic dermatitis or eczema. Their skin can turn red, and itch, indicating an allergy, after contact with many substances that might not bother other people's skin.

How do I find the culprit?

Your dermatologist will work with you to uncover and identify the possible causes of a hand rash. Could it be irritation? Could it be an allergy? Like a detective, your dermatologist will ask many questions. These may include information about previous rashes, whether you have any history of hay fever or asthma, or any other medical problems. The dermatologist will also want to know what kinds of things your hands are exposed to all day long, what creams or lotions you apply to your skin, and whether or not you wear gloves. The doctor may examine your hands, feet, and the rest of your skin to determine what's causing the rash. Your doctor may order special tests to see if you have a skin infection or other problems. Your dermatologist may do a skin scraping and a microscope exam while you wait in the office. Most of the causes usually fall into one of the three types: an externally triggered "contact" rash, an internally generated skin reaction, or a fungal infection.

If your doctor suspects the rash is due to an allergy to some external substance, a patch test may be done. This involves testing the skin on your arms or back to see what specific ingredients might be causing your skin to react. If so, you will receive a list of products that contain those ingredients.

How are hand rashes treated?

Your dermatologist may offer a combination of methods to heal your skin. It is possible you may need an oral antibiotic if an infection is present. Medicated ointment or cream may also be prescribed. Be certain not to use this in combination with other hand creams unless your doctor approves. If the prescribed cream doesn't seem to be helping, tell your doctor right away. You can speed up the healing process by keeping your hands away from other irritants. Discuss with your doctor what to avoid while your skin is healing.

Is hand protection really important?

It may take months for your hands to be normal. Regardless of the cause of your rash, you'll want your hand to heal and to stay healthy. There are ways to pamper them now, and in the future, to lessen the chance of getting a rash again:

- Protect hands against soaps, cleansers, and other chemicals by wearing vinyl gloves—available at local grocery stores and pharmacies. Have four or five pairs and keep them in the kitchen, bathroom, nursery, and laundry areas. Have other pairs for non-wet housework and gardening.

Avoid rubber/latex gloves since many people are sensitive to them. Always replace any gloves that develop holes. Dry out gloves between cleaning jobs. Wear your gloves even when folding laundry, peeling vegetables, or handling citrus fruits or tomatoes.

Remember!!

Hand eczema is not contagious. Although some fungal infections may look like eczema, it is important to have your rash checked by a dermatologist who can do the appropriate testing. Hand rashes sometimes temporarily look worse while they are healing—and sometimes rashes just come back. Try to remember which substance or what activity triggered the recent "flare-up." Let your doctor know about it. Since many hand rashes can be stubborn, it's important to keep up with your medication, stay in contact with your doctor, and not get discouraged.

Source: © 2004 American Academy of Dermatology.

- Use an automatic dishwasher as much as possible. Avoid hand washing dishes or clothes as much as you can.

- When you wash your hands, use lukewarm water and very little soap. Remove rings whenever washing or working with your hands because they trap soap and moisture next to the skin.

- When outdoors in cool weather, wear unlined leather gloves to prevent dry and chapped skin. Always use a dermatologist recommended product to keep your hands soft and supple. Apply it as many times a day as you need it.

- If the type of work you do is affecting your hands, talk to your supervisor about ways that you and other employees can better protect your skin.

Chapter 16

Contact Dermatitis

Allergic contact dermatitis is caused by your body's reaction to something that directly contacts the skin. Many different substances can cause allergic contact dermatitis, which are called 'allergens'. Usually these substances cause no trouble for most people, and may not even be noticed the first time the person is exposed. But once the skin becomes sensitive or allergic to the substance, any exposure will produce a rash. The rash usually doesn't start until a day or two later, but can start a soon as hours or as late as a week.

Allergic contact dermatitis is not usually caused by things like acid, alkali, solvent, strong soap or detergent. These harsh compounds, which can produce a reaction on anyone's skin, are known as 'irritants'. Although some chemicals are both irritants and allergens, allergic contact dermatitis results from brief contact with substances that don't usually provoke a reaction in most people.

The dermatitis usually shows redness, swelling and water blisters, from tiny to large. The blisters may break, forming crusts and scales. Untreated, the skin may darken and become leathery and cracked. Allergic contact dermatitis can be difficult to distinguish from other rashes, especially after it been present for a while.

About This Chapter: "Allergic Contact Dermatitis," reprinted with permission from the American Osteopathic College of Dermatology (AOCD), © 2004. All rights reserved. For additional information, visit the AOCD website at www.aocd.org.

The dermatologist and patient will discuss the materials that touch the person's skin at work and home, and try to identify the allergen. The dermatologist may also perform patch tests. Patch testing is a safe and quick way to diagnose contact allergies. A small amount of the suspected allergen is applied to the skin for a fixed time, usually two days. Some things like nickel, rubber, dyes, and poison ivy, poison oak and related plants are fairly common allergens.

Nickel

Nickel, part of certain metals, is found in many products. Many chrome-plated objects contain enough nickel to produce a reaction in sensitive people. Stainless steel also contains nickel, but it is bound in such a way that makes stainless steel safe for most nickel-sensitive individuals.

Earrings containing nickel can cause earlobe dermatitis, a very common problem in people allergic to nickel. Needles used to pierce ears, and earrings may trigger this. Only sterile stainless needles should be used for piercing. After piercing wear only nickel-free earrings for at least the first three weeks.

Clothing accessories made of nickel buckles, zippers, buttons and metal clips can cause dermatitis. Nickel-sensitive people can substitute nylon accessories.

Sweating increases dermatitis in nickel-sensitive people. In the summer, items containing nickel can cause an itchy, prickly sensation within 15 to 20

✎ What's It Mean?

Contact dermatitis: Contact dermatitis is an inflammation of the skin or a rash caused by contact with various substances of a chemical, animal or vegetable nature. The reaction may be an immunologic response or a direct toxic effect of the substance. Among the more common causes of a contact dermatitis reaction are detergents left on washed clothes, nickel (in watch straps, bracelets and necklaces, and the fastenings on underclothes), chemicals in rubber gloves and condoms, certain cosmetics, plants such as poison ivy, and topical medications.

Source: Excerpted from "Allergy-Immunology Glossary," © 2005 American College of Allergy, Asthma, and Immunology. All rights reserved. Reprinted with permission.

minutes of touching perspiring skin. A rash may appear within a day or two. These same items can be worn for several hours without any symptoms, if perspiration is not present.

Latex

Rubber products (latex) often cause allergic contact dermatitis. Rubber can also cause immediate allergic reactions, including itching or burning and hives (welts) under the rubber object. Some people experience itching and tearing eyes and, occasionally, shortness of breath. This is more common in people who wear tight fitting rubber gloves, such as medical workers. Rubber gloves may also cause dermatitis on the skin of the hands under the glove. Vinyl or other synthetic gloves may be substituted.

Many women with rubber allergy can wear foundation garments of non-sensitizing spandex if they do not have rubber-backed fasteners or edges. Some manufacturers market girdles and bras containing no rubber.

Ingredients in the rubber used in the shoe's construction cause most cases of allergic contact dermatitis from footwear. Adhesives, both rubber and non-rubber, can also cause problems. Even leather shoes may contain these. Shoes without rubber should be substituted.

Paraphenylenediamine

Paraphenylenediamine (PPDA) is an ingredient found in permanent hair dyes. This ingredient is mixed with an oxidizing agent, such as peroxide, before application. People allergic to PPDA should not use any permanent hair dyes. About one fourth of the people allergic to PPDA are also allergic to ingredients in semi-permanent dyes. Follow the package instructions for a patch test before using any hair dye. Most PPDA allergic people can use temporary dyes or rinses, to blend in gray and brighten hair. A few people, however, will react to these dyes also.

A final option to color hair is henna (vegetable dyes). However, henna doesn't work on all hair. Metallic or progressive dyes are also called hair-color restorers are safe to use if the scalp is not irritated.

While PPDA dyes are rarely used in clothing, other dyes that may cross-react with PPDA are in clothing. As a result, some PPDA-sensitive patients cannot wear dark clothing, but can wear fabrics dyed in lighter shades. About 25% of PPDA sensitivity people are allergic to certain widely used local anesthetics that are chemical relatives of PPDA. Substitutes may be used.

Chromates

Chromates, compounds containing chromium, are commonly responsible for allergic contact dermatitis from contact with cement, leather, some matches, paints and anti-rust compounds. Occupational exposure to chromium is common in jobs in the automobile, welding, foundry, cement, railroad and building repair industries.

Chromates are used to tan leather for shoes and clothing. 'Shoe dermatitis' may result from leather containing chromates. Vegetable-tanned footwear can be substituted.

Some matches contain chromates. Touching unlit matches can contaminate fingers. Fumes from a lit match and the charred match head also contain traces of chromates. Placing used matches in a pocket will contaminate the pocket lining, as will book matches.

Plants

Poison ivy and its relatives include poison ivy, poison oak and poison sumac. In the U.S. these plants produce many cases of allergic contact dermatitis. The reaction looks the same whether caused by poison ivy, oak or sumac. Often patients develop lines of small blisters on the skin where the plant brushed against them.

People sensitive to poison ivy, oak and sumac are often allergic to oils from plants from other countries. A furniture lacquer obtained from the Japanese lacquer tree contains such oil, as do mango rinds and cashew shells.

☞ **Remember!!**

People with allergic contact dermatitis should:

1. Avoid the allergen that causes the reaction, and materials that cross-react with it. Your dermatologist can help you identify items to avoid.

2. Substitute products made of materials that do not cause reactions.

Patch testing by a dermatologist can alert patients to which substances to avoid.

Source: © 2004 American Osteopathic College of Dermatology (AOCD).

Chapter 17

Urticaria (Hives) And Angioedema

Hives Explained

Hives (urticaria) is a type of rash characterized by circular wheals of reddened and itching skin. The wheals can vary in size, from relatively small to as large as a dinner plate. The condition can afflict any part of the body, but is common to the trunk, throat, arms, and legs. The wheals generally rise in clusters, with one cluster waxing as another wanes. This type of skin rash is an allergy, which means the immune system reacts to a substance as if it were toxic. Hives can be triggered by a number of different factors, including medications, insect bites, and certain foods. Underlying conditions (such as systemic lupus erythematosus, rubella, hepatitis, and infections) can also bring on an attack of hives in susceptible people. It is thought that around one in every six people will experience at least one attack of hives at some point in their lives.

Symptoms

Symptoms of hives include:

• Raised circular wheals that look like mosquito bites;

About This Chapter: This chapter begins with "Hives Explained"; this information was provided by the Better Health Channel. Material on the Better Health Channel is regularly updated. For the latest version of this information please visit: www.betterhealth .vic.gov.au. Text under the heading "Angioedema," is © 2005 A.D.A.M., Inc.; reprinted with permission.

- The wheals are red on the outer rim and white in the center;

- Localized itching;

- An individual wheal has a lifespan of around 24 hours;

- The wheals appear in batches or clusters;

- One batch fades away as a new batch appears;

- The rash may last for days or weeks, depending on the individual.

✎ What's It Mean?

Histamine: Histamine is a chemical present in cells throughout the body that is released during an allergic reaction. Histamine is one of the substances responsible for the symptoms of inflammation and is the major reason for running of the nose, sneezing, and itching in allergic rhinitis. It also stimulates production of acid by the stomach and narrows the bronchi or airways in the lungs.

Mast cell: Mast cells play an important role in the body's allergic response. Mast cells are present in most body tissues, but are particularly numerous in connective tissue, such as the dermis (innermost layer) of skin. In an allergic response, an allergen stimulates the release of antibodies, which attach themselves to mast cells. Following subsequent allergen exposure, the mast cells release substances such as histamine (a chemical responsible for allergic symptoms) into the tissue.

Urticaria: Urticaria is a skin condition, common known as hives, characterized by the development of itchy, raised white lumps surrounded by an area of red inflammation.

Source: Excerpted from "Allergy-Immunology Glossary," © 2005 American College of Allergy, Asthma, and Immunology. All rights reserved. Reprinted with permission.

Mast Cells And Histamines

The lining of the deepest layer of the skin, the dermis, houses 'mast cells' that form part of the immune system. Mast cells contain chemicals, including histamine, that are designed to kill micro-organisms and other foreign invaders. The immune system of a person with hives will react to certain substances, such as particular foods, by producing antibodies. These specialized proteins trigger a variety of immune system responses, including the release of mast cell chemicals—notably histamine. In small amounts, these chemicals cause itching and reddening of the local area. In large amounts, the nearby blood vessels become dilated and the area swells due to the accumulation of fluid.

Allergens That Commonly Cause Hives

In around one third of cases, the cause of hives is unknown. For the remaining two thirds, some type of allergen is the culprit. An allergen is any substance that prompts an allergic reaction. Some of the allergens and other factors that commonly cause hives include:

- Medications: such as antibiotics, aspirin, and codeine.
- Foods: such as shellfish, eggs, nuts, chocolate, cheese, tomatoes, soy products, and strawberries.
- Some food additives.
- Infections: including bacterial, viral, or parasitic.
- Certain underlying conditions: such as systemic lupus erythematosus, rubella, and hepatitis.
- Emotional stress.
- Certain plants.
- Sunshine and heat.
- Cold temperatures.
- Exercise and sweating.
- Bee and wasp stings.

Anaphylactic Shock Is A Medical Emergency

In most cases, the skin rash is unpleasant but harmless. However, complications may include a more serious allergic reaction known as anaphylactic shock. This is a medical emergency and an ambulance should be called immediately. Symptoms of anaphylactic shock include:

- Hives;

- Swelling of the tongue and throat;

- Breathing difficulties;

- Choking;

- Collapse.

People who have experienced anaphylactic reactions are sometimes advised to have ready access to adrenaline. They may also choose to wear a Medi-alert pendant or bracelet, to indicate to others which substance may cause them to have an allergic reaction.

Diagnosis Methods

Hives can be commonly mistaken for insect bites or some other types of skin rashes. Diagnosis methods can include:

- Medical history;

- Physical examination;

- Allergy tests, such as skin prick tests;

- Elimination diet, under medical supervision—to identify the allergen, if certain foods are suspected.

Treatment Options

For most people, each attack of hives will build in severity and intensity, if their sensitive immune system is repeatedly exposed to the same trigger. Avoiding the known trigger is an important management technique. Treatment for severe or recurring hives may include:

- Checking that the rash isn't caused by an underlying disorder.

- Medications, such as antihistamines and corticosteroids, to reduce the immune system response.

- Avoidance of known triggers.

- Avoidance of factors that exacerbate the condition—such as sunshine, heat, and hot showers.

Where To Get Help

- Your doctor

- Dermatologist

Things To Remember

- Hives is a skin rash characterized by reddened and raised circular wheals.

- This type of skin rash is an allergic reaction, which means the immune system responds to a substance as if it were toxic.

- Treatment options include avoidance of known triggers, and medications—such as antihistamines and corticosteroids.

Angioedema

Alternative names: Angioneurotic edema; Swelling—eyes

Definition: Angioedema is the development of large welts below the surface of the skin, especially around the eyes and lips. The welts may also affect the hands, feet, and throat. The condition can be associated with allergies and histamine release.

Causes, Incidence, And Risk Factors

Angioedema is a swelling similar to urticaria (hives), but the swelling is beneath the skin rather than on the surface. There seems to be a hereditary tendency toward the development of both angioedema and hives (see hereditary angioedema). Angioedema is associated with the release of histamine and other chemicals into the bloodstream, which is part of the allergic response.

Common allergens include:

- medications;
- foods (such as berries, shellfish, fish, nuts, eggs, milk, and others);
- pollen;
- animal dander (scales of shed skin);
- insect bites;
- exposure to water, sunlight, cold or heat;
- emotional stress.

Hives and angioedema may also occur after infections or illness (including autoimmune disorders, leukemia, and others).

Symptoms

- sudden development of wheals or welts
- usually located on the eyes and mouth, but may also occur on the hands and feet or in the throat
- red
- itching or painful
- blanch and swell if irritated
- deep
- localized edema (eyes and mouth appear swollen)
- abdominal cramping
- difficulty breathing
- chemosis (swollen conjunctiva)

Signs And Tests

The diagnosis is primarily based on the appearance of the skin and a history of exposure to an irritant/allergen. There may be stridor (crowing sound when inhaling) if the throat is affected. Rarely, allergy testing may be performed to determine the causative allergen.

Treatment

Mild symptoms may not need treatment. Moderate to severe symptoms may need treatment. Difficulty breathing or stridor indicates an emergency condition.

Self-care includes cool compresses or soaks to the area to provide pain relief and reduce symptoms.

Medications to reduce the allergic response and associated symptoms include antihistamines, adrenaline (epinephrine), terbutaline, cimetidine, corticosteroids, sedatives, and tranquilizers.

For an emergency condition, protect the airway. At the hospital, there may be a need for intubation (placement of a tube in the throat to keep the airway open).

To prevent recurrence of angioedema avoid irritating the affected area, avoid known allergens, and avoid temperature extremes.

Expectations (Prognosis)

Angioedema that does not affect the breathing may be uncomfortable, but it generally is harmless and resolves itself in a few days.

Complications

- Life-threatening airway obstruction (if swelling occurs in the throat)
- Anaphylactic reaction

Calling Your Health Care Provider

Call your health care provider if angioedema is severe and does not respond to treatment.

Go to the emergency room or call the local emergency number (such as 911) if difficulty breathing, wheezing, stridor, or fainting occurs with an episode of angioedema.

Prevention

Avoid known allergens and don't take medications that are not prescribed for you.

♣ It's A Fact!!
Urticaria Can Be Acute Or Chronic

Acute urticaria lasts from a few hours to six weeks and is more common in children and young adults. The cause or trigger often can be determined because hives typically develop a few minutes to a few hours after exposure.

Chronic urticaria lasts more than six weeks, may come and go for months or years and disappear on its own and is more common in middle-aged women. The trigger is identified only about 20 percent of the time.

Urticaria Is Classified As
Allergic Or Non-Allergic

Allergic urticaria: is caused by the immune system's overreaction to a trigger; is more common in children than adults; and can be caused by foods (especially eggs, nuts, and shellfish), medication (especially penicillin and sulfa drugs), infection, insect stings, blood transfusions or other substances.

Non-allergic urticaria: is the label given when an allergic source can't be found; is more prevalent than allergic urticaria; and is caused by many things, including cold temperatures, food dyes, and additives, medication, exercise, anxiety, constricting clothing (such as a belt or bra strap), the sun, and stroking the skin with a firm object.

Source: Excerpted from "Urticaria (Hives), © 2005 American College of Allergy, Asthma, and Immunology (ACAAI). Reprinted with permission. The ACAAI has more information that can help you get your allergies and asthma under control. Call its toll-free number 800-842-7777 or visit www.acaai.org.

Chapter 18

Headaches May Be Caused By Allergies

Headache is one of the top health complaints of Americans. We're bombarded with advertisements and we pay many millions of dollars for pain relievers. Headache also is one of the most common reasons people see physicians.

Everybody gets headaches. How do you know when you should see your doctor about them?

Because each of us is different in how we handle pain, you must decide yourself. However, here are some conditions that might call for a visit with your physician:

- The recent onset of frequent, moderate to severe headaches, associated with other symptoms such as nausea or vomiting.

- Headaches that occur on a daily or weekly basis.

- Headaches that make it impossible for you to think, do your work, go to school, or enjoy life.

- Headaches that respond only to a great deal of over-the-counter pain-relief medication.

- Headaches with fever that last more than a day or two.

About This Chapter: Text in this chapter is from "Headaches," © 2005 American College of Allergy, Asthma, and Immunology (ACAAI). Reprinted with permission. The ACAAI has more information that can help you get your allergies under control. Call its toll-free number 800-842-7777 or visit www.acaai.org.

How are headaches diagnosed?

Your doctor will ask you to describe how severe your pain is, where it's strongest, how you obtain relief, if other symptoms accompany your headaches, and if you've found that some things make your headache worse. A physical examination will reveal the causes of some headaches. If necessary, your doctor will order laboratory tests, x-rays, and brain-wave tests. Often these tests are ordered after consultation with a neurologist, a physician who specializes in nerve and brain problems.

Some types of headaches have an allergic basis, but most do not. Before you see an allergist-immunologist for evaluation and treatment of your headaches, you should first visit your primary care physician first to rule out the other more common causes of your headaches.

In some cases, a careful evaluation allergy evaluation may pinpoint the allergen (allergy-causing substance) causing a headache.

What kinds of headaches may be caused by allergies?

Three types of headaches may possibly be related to allergic disease—"sinus headaches" (facial pain), migraines, and cluster headaches.

What are the symptoms of "sinus headache"?

The four groups of sinus cavities in the head are hollow air spaces with openings into the nose for exchange of air and mucus. They're located inside each cheekbone, behind the eyes, behind the bridge of the nose, and in the forehead. Secretions from the sinus cavities normally drain into the nose.

Sinus headaches and pain occur when the sinuses are swollen and their openings into the nasal passages are obstructed, stopping normal drainage and causing pressure to build up. Often the pain is localized over the affected sinus, perhaps causing facial pain rather than a headache. For example, if the maxillary sinus in the cheeks is obstructed, your cheeks may be tender to the touch and pain may radiate to your jaw and teeth. Other sinuses can cause pain on the top of your head, or elsewhere. Sinus pain can be dull to intense, often begins in the morning and becomes less intense after you move from a lying down to an upright position.

Similar pain can also be caused by severe nasal congestion, particularly if you have a septal deviation or septal "spur" from a previous nasal injury. Such "headaches" or facial pain can involve one side only.

Oral or nasal spray decongestants often help relieve symptoms of facial pain or headaches due to nasal or sinus blockage. Antihistamines are generally less helpful. Obstructed sinuses can get infected, requiring more intensive treatment, including antibiotics.

One hint that allergy might play a role in your sinus headaches or facial pain is if you have other upper airway symptoms such as the itching, sneezing, and runny nose of seasonal allergic rhinitis (hay fever). Allergy is not usually a direct cause of these types of headaches when the other allergic rhinitis symptoms are not present. Allergic reactions to things like airborne pollens, dust, animal dander, molds, as well as foods, can lead to sinus obstruction. Treatment of the underlying allergic cause of sinus pain can result in long-term relief. Medications used to treat allergies include antihistamines, decongestants, intranasal steroids, and cromolyn. In some cases, allergen immunotherapy (allergy shots), may be recommended. When possible, of course, avoid the allergen if an avoidable substance causes your allergy.

What are migraines?

Migraine headaches vary from very intense and disabling to mild. Migraines tend to be throbbing, usually one-sided headaches, that often are aggravated by sunlight and are frequently accompanied by nausea. Migraine headaches can run in families. There are two general types of migraine: classic and common (plus many variations). If you are having these types of headaches, you should schedule an appointment with your doctor for evaluation because certain new medications are very effective in preventing and stopping migraines in their tracks.

What is the role of allergy in these types of headaches?

Years of published data and clinical experience suggest that food allergy may be a trigger of recurrent, persistent migraine headaches in a few, but by no means all patients. In such cases, only a few foods trigger migraines and, by limiting or avoiding them, you can experience complete or marked relief

> ✎ **What's It Mean?**
>
> *Classic migraine* attacks tend to be severe and of long duration. They are preceded by aura, a sensation that signals the start of a headache. The aura may be a funny smell, partial vision loss, or a strange sound.
>
> *Common migraine* is more prevalent than classic migraine. Attacks are generally milder and shorter. There is no aura. However, because the attacks may occur more frequently, common migraine also can be quite disabling.
>
> Source: From "Headaches," © 2005 American College of Allergy, Asthma, and Immunology (ACAAI). Reprinted with permission.

without medication. If you have a firm diagnosis of migraine made by a physician expert in the diagnosis and treatment of migraine headaches, you may want to keep a diary of foods eaten and their relation to your headaches, and then request consultation with an allergist for evaluation and possible allergy testing. On a nonallergic basis, some migraines are provoked by food additives or naturally occurring food chemicals such as monosodium glutamate (often added to oriental food and packaged foods), tyramine (found in many cheeses), phenylethylamine (found in chocolate), or alcohol. The artificial sweetener aspartame has also been reported as a trigger migraine in some people.

Chapter 19

Allergic Diseases And Cognitive Impairment

Sneezing, wheezing, watery eyes, and runny nose aren't the only symptoms of allergic diseases. Many people with allergic rhinitis also report feeling "slower" and drowsy. When their allergies are acting up, they have trouble concentrating and remembering.

Many parents of children with allergic rhinitis observe increased bad moods and irritability in their child's behavior during the allergy season. Since children cannot always express their uncomfortable or painful symptoms verbally, they may express their discomfort by acting up at school and at home. In addition, some kids feel that having an allergic disease is a stigma that separates them from other kids.

It is important that the irritability or other symptoms caused by ear, nose, or throat trouble are not mistaken for attention deficit disorder. With proper treatment, symptoms can be kept under control and disruptions in learning and behavior can be avoided.

About This Chapter: Text in this chapter is from "Allergic Diseases and Cognitive Impairment," © 2005 American College of Allergy, Asthma, and Immunology (ACAAI). Reprinted with permission. The ACAAI has more information that can help you get your allergies under control. Call its toll-free number 800-842-7777 or visit www.acaai.org.

Causes

Experts believe the top two culprits contributing to cognitive impairment of people with allergic rhinitis are sleep interruptions and over the counter (OTC) medications.

Secondary factors, such as blockage of the eustachian tube (ear canal), also can cause hearing problems that have a negative impact on learning and comprehension. Constant nose blowing and coughing can interrupt concentration and the learning process, and allergy-related absences can cause people to miss school or work and subsequently fall behind.

Sleep Disruption

Chronic nasal congestion can cause difficulty in breathing, especially at night. Waking is a hard-wired reflex to make you start breathing again. If you have bad allergic rhinitis, you may waken a dozen times a night. Falling back asleep can be difficult, cutting your total number of sleep hours short.

The average person needs about eight hours of sleep per night to function normally the next day. Losing just a few hours of sleep can lead to a significant decrease in your ability to function. Prolonged loss of sleep can cause difficulty in concentration, inability to remember things, and can contribute to automotive accidents. Night after night of interrupted sleep can cause serious decreases in learning ability and performance in school or on the job.

> ## ♣ It's A Fact!!
>
> Allergic rhinitis can be associated with the following symptoms:
>
> - Decreased ability to concentrate and function
> - Activity limitation
> - Decreased decision-making capacity
> - Impaired hand-eye coordination
> - Problems remembering things
> - Irritability
> - Sleep disorders
> - Fatigue
> - Missed days at work or school
> - More motor vehicle accidents
> - More school or work injuries
>
> Source: © 2005 American College of Allergy, Asthma, and Immunology (ACAAI).

Over-The-Counter Medications

Most allergy therapies don't take into account the effects of allergic rhinitis on mental functioning—they treat the more obvious physical symptoms. Some allergy therapies may even cause some cognitive or mental impairment.

In a recent poll in which allergy sufferers were asked how they treat their symptoms, about 50 percent responded that they use over-the-counter (OTC) medications. The most commonly used OTC medications for allergy symptoms are decongestants and antihistamines—both of which can cause sleep disturbances.

Decongestants

Decongestants constrict small blood vessels in the nose. This opens the nasal passageways and lets you breathe easier. Some decongestants are available over-the-counter, while higher strength formulas are available with a prescription. In some people, oral decongestants can cause problems with getting to sleep, appetite loss, and irritability, which can contribute to allergy problems. If you have any of these symptoms, discuss them with your doctor.

Antihistamines

Antihistamines block the effects of histamine, a chemical produced by the body in response to allergens. Histamine is responsible for the symptoms of allergic rhinitis, including an itchy runny nose, sneezing, and itchy eyes. OTC antihistamines are an inexpensive choice when it comes to treating the symptoms of an allergy—but all OTC antihistamines available in the United States also can cause drowsiness. Regularly taking OTC antihistamines can lead to a feeling of constant sluggishness, affecting learning, memory, and performance.

Non-sedating antihistamines, such as Allegra® (fexofenadine) and Claritin® (loratadine), are available with a prescription. These antihistamines are designed to minimize drowsiness while still blocking the effects of histamine.

Solutions

With all the allergic diseases, the best way to control your symptoms is to avoid coming into contact with your triggers—the substances that cause you to have an allergic reaction. This is often easier said than done. Sometimes it is impossible to avoid the substances that cause symptoms, especially when you are not in control of your environment.

If your allergens can't be avoided, your doctor can help you to create an allergy treatment plan. People who are allergic to indoor things like dust mites or animal dander may need medication on a daily basis, while people who have seasonal symptoms may only need treatment at certain times during the year. An allergist-immunologist can help you determine to which substances you are allergic.

Several types of non-sedating medications are available to help control allergies. One nonsedating nasal spray, Nasalcrom® (cromolyn), is available without a prescription. In addition to the newer antihistamines discussed above, your doctor may also prescribe nasal steroid sprays to treat nasal inflammation. Nasal steroid sprays are highly effective in treating allergy symptoms. The most common side effect associated with nasal sprays is headache.

If medications are not effective or cause unwanted side effects, your doctor may suggest immunotherapy, or "allergy shots". Immunotherapy is used to treat allergy to pollen, ragweed, dust mites, animal dander and other allergens. This process gradually desensitizes you to these substances by changing the way that your body's immune system responds to them. For example, if you are allergic to ragweed, immunotherapy treatments would involve injecting a tiny amount of ragweed pollen extract under your skin every week. Immunotherapy treatments usually last three to five years or longer. Once your body is able to tolerate the substance without producing the symptoms of an allergy, immunotherapy can be stopped, and the need for oral medications should be gone or greatly reduced.

☞ Remember!!

If allergies are affecting your ability to concentrate or function, several treatment options may be beneficial. Getting allergy symptoms under control can help you sleep at night and function during the day.

If you suspect that you or a family member may have an allergic disorder, make an appointment with your doctor for proper diagnosis. Treating allergies sooner rather than later can help prevent disruptions in learning and behavior.

Source: © 2005 American College of Allergy, Asthma, and Immunology (ACAAI).

Part 3

Food Allergies And Intolerances

Chapter 20

Food Allergy: An Overview

Introduction

If you have an unpleasant reaction to something you have eaten, you might wonder if you have a food allergy. One out of three people either believe they have a food allergy or modify their or their family's diet. Thus, while food allergy is commonly suspected, health care providers diagnose it less frequently than most people believe.

This chapter describes allergic reactions to foods and their possible causes as well as the best ways to diagnose and treat allergic reactions to food. It also describes other reactions to foods, known as food intolerances, which can be confused with food allergy, and describes some unproven and controversial food allergy theories.

How Allergic Reactions Work

An immediate allergic reaction involves two actions of your immune system.

- Your immune system produces immunoglobulin E (IgE), a type of protein that works against a specific food. This protein is called a food-specific antibody, and it circulates through the blood.

About This Chapter: Text in this chapter is from "Food Allergy: An Overview," National Institute of Allergy and Infectious Diseases, NIH Pub. No. 04-5518, July 2004.

- The food-specific IgE then attaches to mast cells, cells found in all body tissues. They are more often found in areas of your body that are typical sites of allergic reactions. Those sites include your nose, throat, lungs, skin, and gastrointestinal (GI) tract.

Generally, your immune system will form IgE against a food if you come from a family in which allergies are common—not necessarily food allergies but perhaps other allergic diseases such as hay fever or asthma. If you have two allergic parents, you are more likely to develop food allergy than someone with one allergic parent.

If your immune system is inclined to form IgE to certain foods, you must be exposed to the food before you can have an allergic reaction.

- As this food is digested, it triggers certain cells in your body to produce a food-specific IgE in large amounts. The food-specific IgE is then released and attaches to the surfaces of mast cells.

- The next time you eat that food, it interacts with food-specific IgE on the surface of the mast cells and triggers the cells to release chemicals such as histamine.

♣ **It's A Fact!!**
What Is Food Allergy?

Food allergy is an abnormal response to a food triggered by the body's immune system.

Allergic reactions to food can cause serious illness and, in some cases, death. Therefore, if you have a food allergy, it is extremely important for you to work with your health care provider to find out what food(s) causes your allergic reaction. Sometimes, a reaction to food is not an allergy at all but another type of reaction called "food intolerance." Food intolerance is more common than food allergy. The immune system does not cause the symptoms of a food intolerance, though these symptoms can look and feel like those of a food allergy.

Source: NIAID, 2004.

- Depending upon the tissue in which they are released, these chemicals will cause you to have various symptoms of food allergy.

Food allergens are proteins within the food that enter your bloodstream after the food is digested. From there, they go to target organs, such as your skin or nose, and cause allergic reactions.

An allergic reaction to food can take place within a few minutes to an hour. The process of eating and digesting food affects the timing and the location of a reaction.

- If you are allergic to a particular food, you may first feel itching in your mouth as you start to eat the food.

- After the food is digested in your stomach, you may have GI symptoms such as vomiting, diarrhea, or pain.

- When the food allergens enter and travel through your bloodstream, they may cause your blood pressure to drop.

- As the allergens reach your skin, they can cause hives or eczema.

- When the allergens reach your lungs, they may cause asthma.

♣ It's A Fact!! Cross-Reactivity

If you have a life-threatening reaction to a certain food, your health care provider will show you how to avoid similar foods that might trigger this reaction. For example, if you have a history of allergy to shrimp, testing will usually show that you are not only allergic to shrimp but also to crab, lobster, and crayfish. This is called "cross-reactivity."

Another interesting example of cross-reactivity occurs in people who are highly sensitive to ragweed. During ragweed pollen season, they sometimes find that when they try to eat melons, particularly cantaloupe, they experience itching in their mouths and simply cannot eat the melon. Similarly, people who have severe birch pollen allergy also may react to apple peels. This is called the "oral allergy syndrome."

Source: NIAID, 2004.

Food Allergy Vs. Intolerance

If you go to your health care provider and say, "I think I have a food allergy," your provider has to consider other possibilities that may cause symptoms and could be confused with food allergy, such as food intolerance. To find out the difference between food allergy and food intolerance, your provider will go through a list of possible causes for your symptoms. This is called a "differential diagnosis." This type of diagnosis helps confirm that you do indeed have a food allergy rather than a food intolerance or other illness.

Types Of Food Intolerance

Food Poisoning: One possible cause of symptoms like those of food allergy is foods contaminated with microbes, such as bacteria, and bacterial products, such as toxins. Contaminated meat and dairy products sometimes cause symptoms, including GI discomfort, that resemble a food allergy when it is really a type of food poisoning.

Histamine Toxicity: There are substances, such as histamine present in certain foods, that cause a reaction like an allergic reaction. For example, histamine can reach high levels in cheese, some wines, and certain kinds of fish such as tuna and mackerel.

In fish, histamine is believed to come from contamination by bacteria, particularly in fish that are not refrigerated properly. If you eat one of these foods with a high level of histamine, you could have a reaction that strongly resembles an allergic reaction to food. This reaction is called "histamine toxicity."

Lactose Intolerance: Another cause of food intolerance confused with a food allergy is lactose intolerance or lactase deficiency. This common food intolerance affects at least one out of ten people.

- Lactase is an enzyme that is in the lining of the gut.
- Lactase breaks down lactose, a sugar found in milk and most milk products.
- There is not enough lactase in the gut to digest lactose.
- Lactose, instead, is used by bacteria to form gas which causes bloating, abdominal pain, and sometimes diarrhea.

There are tests your health care provider can use to find out whether your body can digest lactose.

Food Additives: Another type of food intolerance is a reaction to certain products that are added to food to enhance taste, provide color, or protect against the growth of microbes. Several compounds, such as MSG (monosodium glutamate) and sulfites, are tied to reactions that can be confused with food allergy.

MSG

MSG is a flavor enhancer, and, when taken in large amounts, can cause some of the following signs.

- Flushing
- Sensations of warmth
- Headache
- Chest discomfort
- Feelings of detachment

These passing reactions occur rapidly after eating large amounts of food to which MSG has been added.

Sulfites

Sulfites occur naturally in foods or may be added to increase crispness or prevent mold growth. Sulfites in high concentrations sometimes pose problems for people with severe asthma. Sulfites can give off a gas called sulfur dioxide that the asthmatic inhales while eating the sulfited food. This irritates the lungs and can send an asthmatic into severe bronchospasm, a tightening of the lungs.

♣ It's A Fact!! Common Food Allergies

In adults, the foods that most often cause allergic reactions include:

- Shellfish such as shrimp, crayfish, lobster, and crab;
- Peanuts;
- Tree nuts such as walnuts;
- Fish;
- Eggs.

The most common foods that cause problems in children are:

- Eggs;
- Milk;
- Peanuts.

Tree nuts and peanuts are the leading causes of deadly food allergy reactions called anaphylaxis.

Adults usually keep their allergies for life, but children sometimes outgrow them. Children are more likely to outgrow allergies to milk or soy, however, than allergies to peanuts or shrimp. The foods to which adults or children usually react are those foods they eat often. In Japan, for example, rice allergy is more frequent. In Scandinavia, codfish allergy is more common.

Source: NIAID, 2004.

The Food and Drug Administration (FDA) has banned sulfites as spray-on preservatives in fresh fruits and vegetables. Sulfites are still used in some foods, however, and occur naturally during the fermentation of wine.

Gluten Intolerance: Gluten intolerance is associated with the disease called gluten-sensitive enteropathy" or "celiac disease." It happens if your immune system responds abnormally to gluten, which is a part of wheat and some other grains.

Psychological Causes: Some people may have a food intolerance that has a psychological trigger. If your food intolerance is caused by this type of trigger, a careful psychiatric evaluation may identify an unpleasant event in your life, often during childhood, tied to eating a particular food. Eating that food years later, even as an adult, is associated with a rush of unpleasant sensations.

Other Causes: There are several other conditions, including ulcers and cancers of the GI tract, that cause some of the same symptoms as food allergy. These problems include vomiting, diarrhea, and cramping abdominal pain made worse by eating.

Diagnosis

After ruling out food intolerances and other health problems, your health care provider will use several steps to find out if you have an allergy to specific foods.

Detailed History

This technique is the most valuable. Your provider will ask you several questions and listen to your history of food reactions to decide if the facts go with a food allergy.

- What was the timing of your reaction?

- Did your reaction come on quickly, usually within an hour after eating the food?

- Did allergy medicines help? Antihistamines should relieve hives, for example.

- Is your reaction always associated with a certain food?

- Did anyone else who ate the same food get sick? For example, if you ate fish contaminated with histamine, everyone who ate the fish should be sick.

- How much did you eat before you had a reaction? The severity of a reaction is sometimes related to the amount of food eaten.

- How was the food prepared? Some people will have a violent allergic reaction only to raw or undercooked fish. Complete cooking of the fish may destroy the allergen, and they can then eat it with no allergic reaction.

- Did you eat other foods at the same time you had the reaction? Some foods may delay digestion and thus delay the start of the allergic reaction.

Elimination Diet

The next step some health care providers use is an elimination diet. Under your provider's direction:

- You don't eat a food suspected of causing the allergy, such as eggs;

- You then substitute another food—in the case of eggs, another source of protein;

- Your provider can almost always make a diagnosis if the symptoms go away after you remove the food from your diet.

♣ It's A Fact!!
Diet Diary

Sometimes your health care provider can't make a diagnosis solely on the basis of your history. In that case, you may be asked to keep a record of the contents of each meal you eat and whether you have a reaction. This gives more detail from which you and your provider can see if there is a consistent pattern in your reactions.

Source: NIAID, 2004.

The diagnosis is confirmed if you then eat the food and the symptoms come back. You should do this only when the reactions are not significant and under health care provider direction.

Your provider can't use this technique, however, if your reactions are severe or don't happen often. If you have a severe reaction, you should not eat the food again.

Skin Test

If your history, diet diary, or elimination diet suggests a specific food allergy is likely, your health care provider will then use tests to confirm the diagnosis.

One of these is a scratch skin test, during which an extract of the food is placed on the skin of your lower arm. Your provider will then scratch this portion of your skin with a needle and look for swelling or redness which would be a sign of a local allergic reaction. If the scratch test is positive, it means that there is IgE on the skin's mast cells that is specific to the food being tested. Skin tests are rapid, simple, and relatively safe.

You can have a positive skin test to a food allergen, however, without having an allergic reaction to that food. A health care provider diagnoses a food allergy only when someone has a positive skin test to a specific allergen and the history of reactions suggests an allergy to the same food.

Blood Test

If you are extremely allergic and have severe anaphylactic reactions, your health care provider cannot use skin testing because causing an allergic reaction could be dangerous. Skin testing also cannot be done if you have eczema over a large portion of your body.

In those cases, a health care provider may use blood tests such as the RAST (radioallergosorbent test) or the ELISA (enzyme-linked immunosorbent assay). These tests measure the presence of food-specific IgE in your blood. As with skin testing, positive tests do not necessarily mean you have a food allergy.

Double-Blind Food Challenge

The final method health care providers use to diagnose food allergy is double-blind food challenge. This testing has come to be the "gold standard" of allergy testing.

- Your health care provider will give you individual opaque capsules containing various foods, some of which are suspected of starting an allergic reaction.

- You swallow a capsule and are watched to see if a reaction occurs. This process is repeated until you have swallowed all the capsules.

♣ **It's A Fact!!**

Can foods trigger asthma?

Only a few. For years it has been suspected that foods or food ingredients may cause or exacerbate symptoms in those with asthma. After many years of scientific and clinical investigation, there are very few confirmed food triggers of asthma. Sulfites and sulfiting agents in foods (found in dried fruits, prepared potatoes, wine, bottled lemon or lime juice, and shrimp), and diagnosed food allergens (such as milk, eggs, peanuts, tree nuts, soy, wheat, fish, and shellfish) have been found to trigger asthma. Many food ingredients such as food dyes and colors, food preservatives like BHA and BHT, monosodium glutamate, aspartame, and nitrite, have not been conclusively linked to asthma.

What can individuals with asthma do to prevent a food-triggered asthma attack?

The best way to avoid food-induced asthma is to eliminate or avoid the offending food or food ingredient from the diet or from the environment. Reading ingredient information on food labels and knowing where food triggers of asthma are found are the best defenses against a food-induced asthma attack. The main objectives of an asthmatic's care and treatment are to stay healthy, to remain symptom free, to enjoy food, to exercise, to use medications properly, and to follow the care plan developed between the physician and patient.

Source: Excerpted from "Food Allergies and Asthma," reprinted from the International Food Information Council Foundation, © 2004.

In a true double-blind test, your health care provider is also "blinded" (the capsules having been made up by another medical person). In that case your provider does not know which capsule contains the allergen. The advantage of such a challenge is that if you react only to suspected foods and not to other foods tested, it confirms the diagnosis. You cannot be tested this way if you have a history of severe allergic reactions.

In addition, this testing is difficult because it takes a lot of time to perform and many food allergies are difficult to evaluate with this procedure. Consequently, health care providers seldom do double-blind food challenges.

♣ **It's A Fact!!**
Exercise-Induced
Food Allergy

At least one situation may require more than simply eating food with allergens to start a reaction: exercise-induced food allergy. People who have this reaction only experience it after eating a specific food before exercising. As exercise increases and body temperature rises, itching and lightheadedness start and allergic reactions such as hives may appear and even anaphylaxis may develop.

The cure for exercised-induced food allergy is simple—avoid eating for a couple of hours before exercising.

Source: NIAID, 2004.

This type of testing is most commonly used if your health care provider thinks the reaction you describe is not due to a specific food and wishes to obtain evidence to support this. If your provider finds that your reaction is not due to a specific food, then additional efforts may be used to find the real cause of the reaction.

Treatment

Food allergy is treated by avoiding the foods that trigger the reaction. Once you and your health care provider have identified the food(s) to which you are sensitive, you must remove them from your diet. To do this, you must read the detailed ingredient lists on each food you are considering eating.

Many allergy-producing foods such as peanuts, eggs, and milk, appear in foods one normally would not associate them with. Peanuts, for example, are often used as a protein source, and eggs are used in some salad dressings.

The U.S. Food and Drug Administration (FDA) requires ingredients in a packaged food to appear on its label. You can avoid most of the things to which you are sensitive if you read food labels carefully and avoid restaurant-prepared foods that might have ingredients to which you are allergic.

If you are highly allergic, even the tiniest amounts of a food allergen (for example, a small portion of a peanut kernel) can prompt an allergic reaction.

If you have severe food allergies, you must be prepared to treat unintentional exposure. Even people who know a lot about what they are sensitive to occasionally make a mistake. To protect yourself if you have had allergic reactions to a food, you should:

- Wear a medical alert bracelet or necklace stating that you have a food allergy and are subject to severe reactions;

- Carry a syringe of adrenaline (epinephrine), obtained by prescription from your health care provider, and be prepared to give it to yourself if you think you are getting a food allergic reaction;

- Seek medical help immediately by either calling the rescue squad or by getting transported to an emergency room.

Anaphylactic allergic reactions can be fatal even when they start off with mild symptoms such as a tingling in the mouth and throat or GI discomfort. Schools and day care centers must have plans in place to address any food allergy emergency. Parents and caregivers should take special care with children and learn how to:

- protect children from foods to which they are allergic;

- manage children if they eat a food to which they are allergic;

- give children epinephrine.

There are several medicines that you can take to relieve food allergy symptoms that are not part of an anaphylactic reaction. These include:

- antihistamines to relieve GI symptoms, hives, or sneezing and a runny nose;

- bronchodilators to relieve asthma symptoms.

You should take these medicines if you have accidentally eaten a food to which you are allergic. They do not prevent an allergic reaction when taken before eating the food. No medicine in any form will reliably prevent an allergic reaction to that food before eating it.

Food Allergy In Infants And Children

Allergy to cow's milk is particularly common in infants and young children. In addition to causing hives and asthma, it can lead to colic and sleeplessness, and perhaps blood in the stool or poor growth. Infants are thought to be particularly susceptible to this allergic syndrome because their immune and digestive systems are immature. Milk allergy can develop within days to months of birth.

If a baby is on cow's milk formula, a healthcare provider may suggest a change to soy formula or an elemental formula if possible. Elemental formulas are produced from processed proteins with supplements added (basically sugars and amino acids). There are few if any allergens within these materials.

Health care providers sometimes prescribe glucocorticosteroid drugs to treat infants with very severe GI reactions to milk formulas. Fortunately, this food allergy tends to go away within the first few years of life.

Breast feeding often helps babies avoid feeding problems related to allergic reactions. Therefore, health experts often suggest that a mother feed her baby only breast milk for the first 6 to 12 months of life to avoid milk allergy from developing within that time frame.

Some babies are very sensitive to a certain food. If the mother is nursing and eats that food, sufficient amounts can enter her breast milk to cause a food reaction in her baby. To keep possible food allergens out of the breast milk, a mother might try not eating those foods that could cause an allergic reaction in her baby, such as peanuts.

There is no conclusive evidence that breast feeding prevents allergies from developing later in the child's life. It does, however, delay the start of food allergies by delaying the infant's exposure to those foods that can prompt allergies. Plus, it may avoid altogether food allergy problems sometimes seen in infants.

By delaying the introduction of solid foods until a baby is six months old or older, the baby's allergy-free period is prolonged. In addition, the American Academy of Pediatrics recommends delaying adding eggs to a child's diet until he or she is two years old and peanuts, tree nuts, and fish until he or she is three years old.

Some Controversial And Unproven Theories

There are several disorders that are popularly thought by some to be caused by food allergies. There is not enough scientific evidence, or evidence that does exist goes against such claims.

Migraine Headaches: There is controversy about whether migraine headaches can be caused by food allergy. Studies show people who are prone to migraines can have their headaches brought on by histamines and other substances in foods. The more difficult issue is whether food allergies actually cause migraines in such people.

Arthritis: There is virtually no evidence that most rheumatoid arthritis or osteoarthritis can be made worse by foods, despite claims to the contrary.

Allergic Tension Fatigue Syndrome: There is no evidence that food allergies can cause a disorder called the allergic tension fatigue syndrome, in which people are tired, nervous, and may have problems concentrating, or have headaches.

Cerebral Allergy: Cerebral allergy is a term that has been given to people who have trouble concentrating and have headaches as well as other complaints. These symptoms are sometimes blamed on mast cells activated in the brain but no other place in the body. Researchers have found no evidence that such a scenario can happen. Most health experts do not recognize cerebral allergy as a disorder.

Environmental Illness: In a seemingly pristine environment, some people have many non-specific complaints such as problems concentrating or depression. Sometimes this is blamed on small amounts of allergens or toxins in the environment. There is no evidence that such problems are due to food allergies.

Childhood Hyperactivity: Some people believe hyperactivity in children is caused by food allergies. But researchers have found that this behavioral disorder in children is only occasionally associated with food additives, and then only when such additives are consumed in large amounts. There is no evidence that a true food allergy can affect a child's activity except for the possibility that if a child itches and sneezes and wheezes a lot, the child may be uncomfortable and therefore more difficult to guide. Also, children who are on antiallergy medicines that cause drowsiness may get sleepy in school or at home.

Controversial And Unproven Diagnostic Methods

Cytotoxicity Testing: One controversial diagnostic technique is cytotoxicity testing, in which a food allergen is added to your blood sample. A technician then examines the sample under the microscope to see if white cells in the blood "die." Scientists have evaluated this technique in several studies and have found it does not effectively diagnose food allergy.

Provocative Challenge: Another controversial approach is called sublingual (placed under the tongue) or subcutaneous (injected under the skin) provocative challenge. In this procedure, diluted food allergen is put under your tongue if you feel that your arthritis, for instance, is due to foods. The technician then asks you if the food allergen has made your arthritis symptoms worse. In clinical studies, researchers have not shown that this procedure can effectively diagnose food allergy.

Immune Complex Assay: An immune complex assay is sometimes done on people suspected of having food allergies to see if groups, or complexes, of certain antibodies connect to the food allergen in the bloodstream. Some think that these immune groups link with food allergies. But the formation of such immune complexes is a normal offshoot of food digestion, and everyone, if tested with a sensitive enough measurement, has them. To date, no one has conclusively shown that this test links with allergies to foods.

IgG Subclass Assay: Another test is the IgG subclass assay, which looks specifically for certain kinds of IgG antibody. Again, there is no evidence that this diagnoses food allergy.

Controversial And Unproven Treatments

Controversial treatments include putting a diluted solution of a particular food under your tongue about a half hour before you eat the food suspected of causing an allergic reaction. This is an attempt to "neutralize" the subsequent exposure to the food that you believe is harmful. The results of a carefully conducted clinical study show this procedure does not prevent an allergic reaction.

Allergy Shots: Another unproven treatment involves getting shots (immunotherapy) containing small quantities of the food extracts to which you are allergic. These shots are given regularly for a long period of time with the aim of "desensitizing" you to the food allergen. Researchers have not yet proven that allergy shots reliably relieve food allergies.

Research

The National Institute of Allergy and Infectious Diseases does research on food allergy and other allergic diseases. This research is focused on understanding what happens to the body during the allergic process—the sequence of events leading to the allergic response and the factors responsible for allergic diseases. This understanding will lead to better methods of diagnosing, preventing, and treating allergic diseases. Researchers also are looking at better ways to study allergic reactions to foods.

One study by the Johns Hopkins Children's Center showed that simply washing your hands with soap and water will remove peanut allergens. Also, most household cleaners will remove them from surfaces such as food preparation areas at home as well as day care facilities and schools. These easy-to-do measures will help prevent peanut allergy reactions in children and adults.

Educating people, including patients, health care providers, school teachers, and day care workers, about the importance of food allergy is also an important research focus. The more people know about the disorder, the better equipped they will be to control food allergies.

✔ Quick Tip

How Can I Help My Friend Who Has A Food Allergy?

Here are a few guidelines to help your friend stay safe.

Do

- Learn what food or foods your friend must avoid.
- Ask about symptoms of a food allergy reaction.
- Find out what medications your friend uses to treat a reaction and how you can help in the event of an allergic emergency.
- Remind your friend to read labels.
- Wash your hands after eating.

Don't

- Pressure your friend to try a food.
- Ignore the symptoms of a reaction.
- Exclude your friend because of food allergy.
- Allow others to make fun of your friend.

Source: © 2005 The Food Allergy & Anaphylaxis Network. All Rights Reserved. Reprinted with permission. For additional information, visit http://www.foodallergy.org or http://www.fankids.org.

Chapter 21

Problem Foods: Is It An Allergy Or Intolerance?

What is a food allergy?

A food allergy is an immune system response. It occurs when the body mistakes an ingredient in food—usually a protein—as harmful and creates a defense system (antibodies) to fight it. Allergy symptoms develop when the antibodies are battling the "invading" food. The most common food allergies in adults are peanuts, tree nuts (such as walnuts, pecans and almonds), fish, and shellfish. The most common food allergies in children are milk, eggs, soy products, peanuts, tree nuts, wheat, fish, and shellfish.

What is food intolerance?

Food intolerance is a digestive system response rather than an immune system response. It occurs when something in a food irritates a person's digestive system or when a person is unable to properly digest or breakdown, the food. Intolerance to lactose, which is found in milk and other dairy products, is the most common food intolerance.

About This Chapter: "Problem Foods: Is It An Allergy Or Intolerance?" © 2005 The Cleveland Clinic Foundation, 9500 Euclid Avenue, Cleveland, OH 44195, www.clevelandclinic.org. Additional information is available from the Cleveland Clinic Health Information Center, 216-444-3771, tollfree 800-223-2273 extension 43771, or at http://www.clevelandclinic.or g/health.

What are the symptoms of food allergy?

Symptoms of a food allergy can range from mild to severe, and the amount of food necessary to trigger a reaction varies from person to person. Symptoms of food allergy may include the following:

- Rash or hives

- Nausea

- Stomach pain

- Diarrhea

- Itchy skin

- Shortness of breath

- Chest pain

- Swelling of the airways to the lungs

- Anaphylaxis

♣ **It's A Fact!!**
Food allergies often run in families, suggesting that the condition can be inherited.

Source: © 2005 The Cleveland Clinic Foundation.

What are the symptoms of food intolerance?

Symptoms of food intolerance include the following:

- Nausea

- Stomach pain

- Gas, cramps, or bloating

- Vomiting

- Heartburn

- Diarrhea

- Headaches

- Irritability or nervousness

What causes food allergies and intolerances?

Food allergies arise from sensitivity to chemical compounds (proteins) in food. They develop after you are exposed to a food protein that your body thinks is harmful. The first time you eat the food containing the protein, your immune system responds by creating specific disease-fighting antibodies (called immunoglobulin E or IgE). When you eat the food again, it triggers the release of IgE antibodies and other chemicals, including histamine, in an effort to expel the protein "invader" from your body. Histamine is a powerful chemical that can affect the respiratory system, gastrointestinal tract, skin, or cardiovascular system.

As a result of this response, allergy symptoms occur. The allergy symptoms you have depend on where in the body the histamine is released. If it is released in the ears, nose, and throat, you may have an itchy nose and mouth, or trouble breathing or swallowing. If histamine is released in the skin, you may develop hives or a rash. If histamine is released in the gastrointestinal tract, you likely will develop stomach pains, cramps, or diarrhea. Many people experience a combination of symptoms as the food is eaten and digested.

There are many factors that may contribute to food intolerance. In some cases, as with lactose intolerance, the person lacks the chemicals, called enzymes, necessary to properly digest certain proteins found in food. Also common are intolerances to some chemical ingredients added to food to provide color, enhance taste, and protect against the growth of bacteria. These ingredients include various dyes and monosodium glutamate (MSG), a flavor enhancer.

Substances called sulfites are also a source of intolerance for some people. They may occur naturally, as in red wines, or may be added to prevent the growth of mold.

♣ **It's A Fact!!**

How common are food allergies and intolerances?

Food allergies affect about 1% of adults and 7% of children, although some children outgrow their allergies. Food intolerances are much more common. In fact, nearly everyone at one time has had an unpleasant reaction to something they ate. Some people have specific food intolerances. Lactose intolerance, the most common food intolerance, affects about 10% of Americans.

Source: © 2005 The Cleveland Clinic Foundation.

Salicylates are a group of plant chemicals found naturally in many fruits, vegetables, nuts, coffee, juices, beer, and wine. Aspirin also is a compound of the salicylate family. Foods containing salicylates may trigger symptoms in people who are sensitive to aspirin. Of course, any food consumed in excessive quantities can cause digestive symptoms.

How can you tell the difference between a food allergy and intolerance?

Food allergies can be triggered by even a small amount of the food and occur every time the food is consumed. People with food allergies are generally advised to avoid the offending foods completely. On the other hand, food intolerances often are dose related.

People with food intolerance may not have symptoms unless they eat a large portion of the food or eat the food frequently. For example, a person with lactose intolerance may be able to drink milk in coffee or a single glass of milk, but becomes sick if he or she drinks several glasses of milk.

Food allergies and intolerances also are different from food poisoning, which generally results from spoiled or tainted food and affects more than one person eating the food. Your healthcare provider can help determine if you have an allergy or intolerance, and establish a plan to help control your symptoms.

How are food intolerances diagnosed?

Most food intolerances are found through trial and error to determine which food or foods cause symptoms. You may be asked to keep a food diary to record what you eat and when you get symptoms, and then look for common factors.

Another way to identify problem foods is to go on an elimination diet. This involves completely eliminating any suspect foods from your diet until you are symptom-free. You then begin to reintroduce the foods, one at a time. This can help you pinpoint which foods cause symptoms. Seek the advice of your healthcare provider or a registered dietitian before beginning an elimination diet to be sure your diet provides adequate nutrition.

Can food intolerances be prevented?

Taking a few simple steps can help you prevent the symptoms associated with food intolerance.

- Learn which foods in which amounts cause you to have symptoms and limit your intake to amounts you can handle.

- When you dine out, ask your server about how your meal will be prepared. Some meals may contain foods you cannot tolerate and that may not be evident from the description on the menu.

- Learn to read food labels and check the ingredients for problem foods. Don't forget to check condiments and seasonings. They may contain MSG or another additive that can lead to symptoms.

☞ Remember!!
How are food intolerances treated?

Treatment is based on avoiding or reducing your intake of problem foods and treating symptoms when they arise.

Source: © 2005 The Cleveland Clinic Foundation.

Chapter 22

Food Challenges Identify True Food Allergies

Food challenges play a vital role in the evaluation and management of patients with histories suggestive of food allergy. The necessity of food challenges is supported by studies revealing that more than 50% of patients presenting with a history of an adverse reaction to a food fail to react during blinded challenges to the suspected food. There are a number of reasonable explanations for this.

Sometimes the wrong food is suspected as the cause of symptoms. For example, a child reacting in a restaurant to a French fry cooked in peanut oil might be suspected of having a reaction to peanut, when the actual cause was contamination of the French fry with fish protein from fish fried in the same oil.

Sometimes the reaction is caused by a nonfood contaminant as exemplified by reactions to latex proteins deposited on foods by food handlers wearing latex gloves or reactions to dust mites in mite-contaminated baked goods.

Sometimes the reactions are not related to food ingestion at all, but are precipitated by medications, toxins, parasites, allergen exposures by inhalation or contact, viral illness, exercise or panic, to list just a few potential causes.

About This Chapter: "Food Challenges: Why Bother?" by Dan Atkins, M.D., © Copyright 2005 National Jewish Medical and Research Center. All rights reserved. For additional information, visit http://asthma.nationaljewish.org/ or call 800-222 LUNG.

Skin testing can identify foods that may have caused symptoms, but the positive predictive accuracy of a properly performed food prick skin test is only about 50%. Thus, there are patients with reasonable histories of food allergy and a positive skin test to the suspected food who do not react during food challenge.

♣ **It's A Fact!!**

What is a food challenge?

A food challenge consists of having a patient eat a food suspected of previously causing symptoms in a controlled fashion under medical supervision. The basic structure of a food challenge involves feeding gradually increasing doses of the suspected food at predetermined time intervals until symptoms occur or a normal portion of the food ingested openly is tolerated.

The history of previous suspected reactions to the food is reviewed and an interval history is taken to insure that the patient is stable. Performing a food challenge in a patient whose asthma is not well controlled is contraindicated. Obviously, a food challenge should be postponed if the child is thought to be coming down with another illness to avoid confusing results or the potential for an accelerated reaction. Vital signs, spirometry and a physical examination are performed before starting the challenge and prior to subsequent doses or whenever the patient complains of symptoms.

Food challenges come in a variety of flavors and are categorized into open, single-blind placebo-controlled or double-blind placebo-controlled depending upon who knows what the patient is receiving in each dose during the challenge.

In an open food challenge (OFC), both the patient and medical staff are aware that the patient is eating the suspected food. For example, a child receiving an OFC to egg might be given increasing doses of scrambled egg every 30 minutes until a whole egg is ingested.

In a single-blind placebo-controlled food challenge (SBPCFC) the medical staff is aware of what the patient is being fed, but the patient is not. A child receiving a SBPCFC to egg receives egg masked by concealing it in another

The CAP System FEIA (CAP FEIA) is a quantitative antibody fluorescent-enzyme immunoassay that measures the amount of circulating allergen-specific IgE in the serum in kilounits of antibody (allergen-specific IgE) per liter (kUA/L). For several foods, such as milk, egg, peanut, soy, wheat, and

food. The medical staff knows if and how much egg is contained in each challenge dose, but the patient and the patient's family do not. Each dose could either contain concealed egg or be a placebo. However, the final dose of any food challenge is the open ingestion of a normal portion of the suspected food. SBPCFCs are performed to eliminate bias on the part of the patient and/or the patient's family. In a double-blind placebo-controlled food challenge (DBPCFC) neither the patient nor the medical team involved in administering the challenge is aware of what the patient is being fed.

The DBPCFC is performed to eliminate both patient and observer bias. For the safety of the patient at least one physician not directly involved in the challenge must be aware of the challenge contents even in a DBPCFC. Again, the final dose of the DBPCFC is a normal portion of the suspected food ingested openly.

A food challenge is completed when the patient has an obvious reaction to the food or when a normal portion of the food has been ingested openly without symptoms. The length of time a patient is kept for observation after completion of the challenge depends upon several factors including the timing and severity of previous reactions and any concern about biphasic anaphylaxis. The results of the challenge should be thoroughly reviewed with the patient and his or her family and all questions should be addressed in light of the findings of the challenge.

Source: "What Is a Food Challenge?" by Dan Atkins, M.D., © Copyright 2005 National Jewish Medical and Research Center. All rights reserved. For additional information, visit http://asthma.nationaljewish.org/ or call 1-800-222 LUNG.

fish, threshold CAP FEIA levels have been calculated. Patients with CAP FEIA values higher than the threshold values have a 95% likelihood of reacting after ingestion of the food. However, individual CAP FEIA results may fall in the gray zone below the threshold or threshold values may not have been established for the suspected food. As a result of these and other nuances, food challenges are often necessary to document the association between the ingestion of the suspected food and the onset of symptoms.

Performing food challenges in patients with suspected food allergies is often anxiety producing for patients and their families. At first glance having someone eat a food that might make him or her ill seems contrary to that basic premise of medicine (and parenthood) "first do no harm." However, there are a number of situations where the information to be gained is worth the risk. It is also important to remember that in experienced hands with appropriate attention to detail and sound clinical judgment, food challenges can be safely performed.

Food challenges are performed to address a variety of clinical questions. Sometimes the food responsible for the reaction is not apparent from the history or after attempts to document sensitization. For example, the patient may have a positive skin test to several foods ingested before a reaction and food challenges may be necessary to determine which, if any, of the suspected foods is the culprit. Determining which food actually caused the reaction is necessary to aid in preventing future reactions and to avoid needlessly eliminating foods from the diet.

Documenting the degree of sensitivity is another reason for performing food challenges. Some patients or their families become concerned that exposure to even miniscule amounts of a food might cause a reaction. Others are worried that any exposure would result in a life-threatening reaction. These concerns occasionally inhibit participation in normal activities and can lead to social isolation. Although some patients are indeed exquisitely sensitive, others find that a larger exposure to the food than was expected can be tolerated without a severe reaction. This can be liberating for patients who have markedly curtailed activities out of concern about the possibility of exquisite sensitivity. Some patients, despite large positive skin tests and histories suggestive of contact reactions, do not develop systemic symptoms after the ingestion of significant amounts of the suspected food. Alternatively, some patients are found to be more sensitive than was previously suspected and the importance of strict avoidance as well as being thoroughly prepared to treat severe reactions is reinforced.

Some food challenges are performed to prove that a food is not the cause of symptoms. An example is the patient who has been inaccurately labeled as allergic to one or more foods despite an unconvincing history or suspicious skin test results. A food challenge is indicated to find out if ingestion of the food causes symptoms.

Some patients outgrow their food allergies. The majority of infants and young children allergic to milk, egg, or soy outgrow their food allergies by their third birthday. Studies over the past few years have even suggested that approximately 20% of children with allergic reactions to peanut in the first years of life outgrow their sensitivity. CAP FEIA results can help in making a decision about when to challenge these children. Skin tests often remain positive even when the food allergy has been outgrown. The careful performance of food challenges can safely document when the food can be returned to the diet or if continued avoidance is necessary.

Food challenges should be performed in a medical setting with the necessary medications and equipment as well as personnel experienced in the treatment of anaphylaxis. Decisions about who should be challenged are reached only after a thorough evaluation and discussion of the risks and benefits with the patient or his or her family. However, few procedures in medicine answer a posed clinical question as directly as a properly performed food challenge and the information obtained can be life altering.

Chapter 23

Egg Allergy

For as long as you can remember, you've had to deal with being allergic to eggs. Sometimes it's a pain—you get tired of checking labels to make sure foods don't have eggs in them, and you may even think about skipping a meal completely to avoid all the hassle. But that's never a good idea. Instead, use these pointers for making life with an egg allergy easier.

What Is An Egg Allergy?

First, let's learn a bit about the allergy itself. When a person is allergic to eggs, the body's immune system overreacts to proteins in the egg. It thinks that these proteins are harmful invaders and produces antibodies called immunoglobulin E (IgE) to fight them off. Whenever a person who has an egg allergy eats something that contains egg proteins, the body sends out antibodies and histamines (chemicals released from the body's cells during most allergic reactions). This reaction makes the person feel sick.

Most people who are allergic react to the proteins in egg whites, but some can't tolerate proteins in the yolk. The allergy usually first appears when kids are very young, but most outgrow it by the time they're five years old.

About This Chapter: This information was provided by TeensHealth, one of the largest resources online for medically reviewed health information written for parents, kids, and teens. For more articles like this one, visit www.TeensHealth.org, or www.KidsHealth.org. © 2003 The Nemours Center for Children's Health Media, a division of The Nemours Foundation.

Because vaccines are an important part of children's medical care, some people have been concerned about kids who are allergic to eggs receiving flu and measles/mumps/rubella (MMR) vaccines. The vaccines are grown in cultures from egg cells and may contain a small amount of egg protein. Experts say the MMR vaccine is safe for people who are allergic to eggs but advise you to ask your doctor about getting a flu shot.

Signs And Symptoms

People who are allergic to eggs may either feel sick just a few minutes after consuming egg proteins or a couple of hours later. Most reactions last less than a day and may affect any of three body systems:

- **The skin:** in the form of red, bumpy rashes (hives), eczema, or redness and swelling around the mouth

- **The gastrointestinal tract:** in the form of belly cramps, diarrhea, nausea, or vomiting

- **The respiratory tract:** symptoms can range from a runny nose, itchy, watery eyes, and sneezing to the triggering of asthma with coughing and wheezing

> ✔ **Quick Tip**
> *Good Enough To Eat*
>
> Be careful of shiny snacks and baked goods. Egg yolks are sometimes used to glaze pretzels, bagels, and other baked items. Eggs also may be used as a foaming agent in beer, lattes, or cappuccinos. Even some makeup, shampoos, and medicines contain egg proteins.
>
> Source: © 2003 The Nemours Center for Children's Health Media, a division of The Nemours Foundation.

People who have a serious egg allergy may suffer anaphylaxis (pronounced: ah-nuh-fuh-lak-sis). This severe allergic reaction causes swelling of the mouth, throat, and airways leading to the lungs, resulting in an inability to breathe. In addition, there is a dangerous drop in blood pressure, which can make someone dizzy or pass out, and may quickly lead to shock. For people who are especially sensitive to eggs, even egg fumes or getting egg on the skin can cause an anaphylactic reaction, so eggs should be kept out of the house completely.

How Is It Diagnosed?

Determining if someone has an egg allergy isn't always simple. If a person has the same reaction every time he or she eats eggs, the diagnosis may be easier to make. But most people who are allergic to eggs react to egg proteins that are found in lots of foods, and this makes pinpointing the allergy harder.

As part of the diagnosis, your doctor or a doctor who specializes in allergies will probably do skin testing. The doctor will scratch a bit of skin on your forearm or back and place a weak extract of egg on the spot. If the area swells or becomes red, this is considered an allergic reaction. Blood tests can also be used to measure the amount of antibodies to egg proteins in the body.

Doctors often put patients on an elimination diet to help diagnose an allergy to eggs. If you are placed on such a diet, you will be told to not eat eggs or anything made with eggs for a certain period of time—usually about a week. If your symptoms go away during this time, it supports the diagnosis of an allergy. If the symptoms return when you eat eggs again, it's a pretty sure bet you have an egg allergy.

How Is It Treated?

If you have an egg allergy, you need to avoid eggs as well as anything that is made from eggs. If you have a serious allergy, you might want to wear a medical alert bracelet or necklace so other people will know you're at risk.

If you have a severe egg allergy—or any kind of serious allergy—you should probably keep a shot of epinephrine (pronounced: eh-puh-neh-frin) in an easy-to-carry container that looks like a pen with you in case of an emergency. If you accidentally eat something with egg in it and start having serious allergic symptoms, like swelling inside your mouth, chest pain, or difficulty breathing, you can give yourself the shot right away to counteract the reaction while you're waiting for medical help. (Always call for emergency help [911] when using epinephrine.) You should make sure your school and even good friends' houses have injectable epinephrine on hand, too.

Living With An Egg Allergy

Keeping epinephrine on hand at all times should be just part of your action plan for living with an egg allergy. You may also want to keep antihistamines at home and in a traveling first-aid kit.

To make sure the foods you eat are egg free, you'll need to be on the lookout for any ingredients that might come from eggs. That means asking

✔ **Quick Tip**

Tips For Managing An Egg Allergy

Baking: For each egg, substitute one of the following in recipes:

- 1 tsp. baking powder, 1 T. liquid, 1 T. vinegar
- 1 tsp. yeast dissolved in ¼ cup warm water
- 1½ T. water, 1½ T. oil, 1 tsp. baking powder
- 1 packet gelatin, 2 T. warm water. Do not mix until ready to use.

These substitutes work well when baking from scratch and substituting 1 to 3 eggs.

Some Hidden Sources Of Egg

- Eggs have been used as to create the foam or milk topping on specialty coffee drinks and are used in some bar drinks.
- Some commercial brands of egg substitutes contain egg whites.
- Most commercially processed cooked pastas (including those used in prepared foods such as soup) contain egg or are processed on equipment shared with egg-containing pastas. Boxed, dry pastas are usually egg-free. Fresh pasta is sometimes egg-free, too. Read the label or ask about ingredients before eating pasta.

Source: Excerpted from "Common Food Allergens," © 2005 The Food Allergy & Anaphylaxis Network. All Rights Reserved. Reprinted with permission. For additional information, visit http://www.foodallergy.org or http://www.fankids.org.

questions when eating out at restaurants or at a friend's home and carefully reading food labels. Besides obvious ingredients like egg whites and powdered egg, you should also watch out for:

- albumin;
- globulin;
- livetin;
- lysozyme;
- ovalbumin;
- ovoglobulin;
- ovomucin;

- ovomucoid;
- ovotransferrin;
- ovovitella;
- ovovitellin;
- silici albuminate;
- Simplesse;
- vitellin.

Sometimes you might want to bring your own food when hanging out with friends or sleeping away from home just to be sure what you're eating is safe. Many fast foods are made with eggs, including burgers, cheese sticks, chicken nuggets, fries, and pizza dough.

When cooking at home, always carefully scrub the utensils you're using in case they have been used on egg products. It's also a good idea to talk to a nutritionist or registered dietitian about your diet. That person can help you plan healthy, tasty alternatives to foods made with eggs. Before long, you'll realize that living with an egg allergy isn't as hard as you thought.

Chapter 24

Milk Allergy

You're allergic to milk. Maybe you're wondering what that really means. Is it like your friend who's lactose intolerant? And is it really a big deal? After all, it's not like you're a little kid who needs milk to grow, right?

A milk allergy can be a big deal because milk is in lots of foods. Some are obvious, like pizza, and others may not be so obvious, like baked goods. If someone who has a milk allergy eats any of these foods, they can make the person sick. Plus, teens do need calcium and vitamin D, which milk has lots of, because their bones are still growing. So how can a person who's allergic to milk deal with the allergy? Read on to find out.

What Is A Milk Allergy?

People who are allergic to cow's milk react to one or more of the proteins in it. Curd, the substance that forms chunks in sour milk, contains 80% of milk's proteins, including several called caseins (pronounced: kay-seenz). Whey (pronounced: way), the watery part of milk, holds the other 20%. A person may be allergic to proteins in either or both parts of milk, but whey is responsible for most problems.

About This Chapter: This information was provided by TeensHealth, one of the largest resources online for medically reviewed health information written for parents, kids, and teens. For more articles like this one, visit www.TeensHealth.org, or www.KidsHealth.org. © 2003 The Nemours Center for Children's Health Media, a division of The Nemours Foundation.

When a person who is allergic to milk ingests milk or a food that contains milk products, the body's immune system mistakenly sees the milk proteins as dangerous "invaders" and tries to fight them off. It starts an allergic reaction that involves the release of chemicals called histamines (pronounced: his-tuh-meenz) from some of the body's cells and the production of immunoglobulin E (IgE) antibodies to fight the proteins. This reaction can make a person feel sick.

A milk allergy usually starts when an infant is given formula and has a reaction. Up to 7% of babies and toddlers are allergic to milk, but most outgrow the allergy within the first six years of life. Some kids never outgrow it, however.

Signs And Symptoms

The symptoms of milk allergy can occur within minutes (this is called a fast-onset type of milk allergy) or several hours or more after eating or drinking something containing milk protein. Symptoms can include runny nose, hives (itchy bumps on the skin), facial swelling, wheezing and other breathing problems, irritability, vomiting, diarrhea, and eczema (an itchy, scaly rash).

People often confuse milk allergy with lactose intolerance because the two can share some symptoms. But the conditions are not related. Milk allergy is a problem involving the immune system, whereas lactose intolerance involves the digestive system. When someone is lactose intolerant, it means that his digestive system doesn't produce enough of the enzyme needed to break down the sugar in milk. The sugar ends up fermenting in the small intestine, which can lead to nausea, cramps, bloating of the abdomen, gas, and diarrhea.

How Is An Allergy To Milk Diagnosed?

People who have the fast-onset type of milk allergy, in which the body reacts almost immediately, often can be diagnosed with a blood or skin test that detects IgE antibodies to milk protein. The skin test involves placing bits of milk protein on the forearm, scratching the skin, and waiting to see if a reddish, raised spot forms, indicating an allergic reaction. For the blood test, a sample of blood will be analyzed in a laboratory to look for the antibodies.

But for people who have the slower-developing form of milk allergy, skin and blood tests are not as helpful. In these cases doctors try to make a diagnosis based on dietary elimination. The person is told not to eat or drink anything made with milk for a period of time. If the person is symptom free during this trial, the doctor can diagnose a milk allergy fairly confidently. And if the person has a reaction when he begins eating products containing milk again, the diagnosis is confirmed.

✔ Quick Tip
Tips For Managing A Milk Allergy

Baking

- Fortunately, milk is one of the easiest ingredients to substitute in baking and cooking. It can be substituted, in equal amounts, with water or fruit juice. (For example, substitute 1 cup milk with 1 cup water.)

Some Hidden Sources Of Milk

- Deli meat slicers are frequently used for both meat and cheese products.

- Some brands of canned tuna fish contain casein, a milk protein.

- Many non-dairy products contain casein (a milk derivative), listed on the ingredient labels. (The Food Allergy and Anaphylaxis Network is currently working with the U.S. Food and Drug Administration to have the term "non-dairy"" eliminated on products that contain milk derivatives.

- Some meats may contain casein as a binder. Check all labels carefully.

- Many restaurants put butter on steaks after they have been grilled to add extra flavor. The butter is not visible after it melts.

Source: Excerpted from "Common Food Allergens," © 2005 The Food Allergy & Anaphylaxis Network. All Rights Reserved. Reprinted with permission. For additional information, visit http://www.foodallergy.org or http://www.fankids.org.

How Is It Treated?

To treat a milk allergy, the person who's allergic needs to completely avoid any foods that contain milk or milk products. Babies diagnosed with the allergy can be switched to a soy or hypoallergenic formula relatively easily. For older kids and teens, though, cutting out favorite treats like ice cream, pizza, and many sweets can be a drag. But avoiding milk involves more than just leaving the cheese off your cheese fries. If you are allergic to milk, you need to read food labels carefully and not eat anything that's questionable. It may sound hard, but there are many milk substitutes available as well as foods that can give you plenty of calcium and vitamin D.

Some people who are allergic to milk can have a severe reaction to even the smallest exposure to milk proteins. For them, just inhaling the powder in powdered milk might be dangerous enough to bring on an anaphylactic (pronounced: ah-nuh-fuh-lak-tik) reaction. Anaphylaxis can cause a person's blood pressure to drop, airways to narrow, and tongue to swell, resulting in serious breathing difficulty and, in some cases, death.

If you're one of these people, you should probably keep a shot of epinephrine (pronounced: eh-puh-ne-frin) in an easy-to-carry container that looks like a pen with you in case of an emergency. If you accidentally ingest milk protein and have an anaphylactic reaction, you can give yourself the shot to help counteract it. Make sure your school and close friends' houses each have injectable epinephrine on hand, too.

Living With A Milk Allergy

It may be challenging to eliminate milk from your diet, but it's not impossible. Because most people don't get enough calcium in their diets even if they do drink milk, many other foods are now enriched with calcium, such as juices, cereals, and rice and soy beverages. These are good substitutes for dairy foods, and they're tasty, too. But before you eat or drink anything calcium enriched, make sure it's also dairy free.

Milk and milk products can lurk in strange places. For instance, be sure to check the labels of processed meats and "non-dairy" products. And for anything made with chocolate, be sure to check if it contains dairy products.

Look for these ingredients on food labels and avoid them. In some cases, you may need to check with the product's manufacturer to be sure:

- ammonium caseinate
- artificial butter flavor
- butter
- butter fat
- butter solids/fat
- butter oil
- buttermilk
- calcium caseinate
- caramel color
- caramel flavoring
- casein
- caseinate
- cheese
- condensed milk
- cottage cheese
- cream
- cream curds
- custard
- delactosed whey
- demineralized whey
- dry milk
- dry milk solids
- evaporated milk
- flavoring (this may contain milk products, so make sure it is dairy free)
- ghee
- goat's milk
- half-and-half
- high protein flour
- hydrolysates
- hydrolyzed casein
- hydrolyzed milk protein
- iron caseinate
- lactalbumin
- lactalbumin phosphate
- lactate
- lactic acid
- lactoferrin
- lactoglobulin
- lactose
- lactulose
- low-fat milk
- magnesium caseinate
- malted milk
- margarine (this may contain milk products so make sure it is dairy free)
- milk
- milk derivative
- milk fat
- milk powder
- milk protein
- milk solids
- natural flavoring
- nonfat milk
- nougat
- opta
- potassium caseinate
- powdered milk
- protein (this ingredient could be milk protein so check to be sure)
- rennet casein
- Simplesse
- skimmed milk
- sodium caseinate
- sour cream
- sour cream solids
- sour milk solids
- whey
- whey powder
- whey protein concentrate
- whey protein hydrolysate
- whole milk
- yogurt
- zinc caseinate

After looking at this list, you may wonder what someone who's allergic to milk can eat. To help answer that question, it's important to talk with a registered dietitian. He or she will help you substitute other foods for dairy products to make sure you get all the nutrition you need and still enjoy your meals and snacks.

♣ **It's A Fact!!**

Milk Allergy Diet: Foods That Might Contain Milk

Butter	Goat's milk	milk fat, milk powder, milk protein, milk solids, malted milk, and powdered milk)
Canned fish	Half-and-half	
Cheese	"High-energy" foods with high-protein flour or added protein	Processed meats
Chocolate		
Cottage cheese		Seasoned and ranch-style potato and tortilla chips
Cream and cream curds	Ice cream	
Custard	Margarine	Seasoned French fries
Foods marked with "D" or "DE" kosher labels	Milk in all forms (including condensed milk, dry milk, dry milk solids, evaporated milk, low-fat milk, nonfat or skim milk, milk derivative,	Sour cream, sour cream solids, and sour milk solids
Frozen yogurt		Yogurt
Ghee (clarified butter)		

Examine food labels for these milk-based ingredients:

Artificial butter flavor	Coconut cream flavoring	Hydrolysates
Bavarian cream flavoring	Delactosed whey	Hydrolyzed cosein
Binding agents	Demineralized whey	Milk protein
Brown sugar flavoring	Lactalbumin	Natural butter flavor
Butter fat	Lactalbumin phosphate	Natural egg flavor
Buttermilk	Lactate	Opta
Butter oil	Lactic acid	Simplesse
Butter solids	Lactoferrin	Whey
Caramel color	Lactoglobulin	Whey powder
Caramel flavoring	Lactose	Whey protein concentrate
Caseinates	Lactulose	Whey protein hydrolysate
Casein products	High-protein flour	

Source: This information was provided by TeensHealth, one of the largest resources online for medically reviewed health information written for parents, kids, and teens. For more articles like this one, visit www.TeensHealth.org, or www.KidsHealth.org. © 2003 The Nemours Center for Children's Health Media, a division of The Nemours Foundation.

Chapter 25

Lactose Intolerance

Jessie was so embarrassed! About an hour after chowing down on pizza and ice cream with a group of friends, her stomach suddenly started rumbling, and she began farting over and over. Then Jessie's stomach began to ache and she had to run to the restroom every few minutes. In the excitement of an afternoon hanging out at the mall, Jessie had forgotten to watch her dairy intake. Jessie has lactose intolerance and her symptoms flare up when she eats more dairy than her body can handle.

What Is Lactose Intolerance And What Causes It?

Lactose intolerance is the inability to digest a sugar called lactose that is present in milk and dairy products. Normally when you eat something containing lactose, the body produces an enzyme called lactase in the small intestine. Lactase breaks down lactose into simpler sugar forms called glucose and galactose, which are then easily absorbed into the bloodstream and turned into energy—fuel for our bodies.

People with lactose intolerance do not produce enough of the lactase enzyme to break down lactose. Instead undigested lactose sits in the gut

About This Chapter: This information was provided by TeensHealth, one of the largest resources online for medically reviewed health information written for parents, kids, and teens. For more articles like this one, visit www.TeensHealth.org, or www.KidsHealth.org. © 2004 The Nemours Center for Children's Health Media, a division of The Nemours Foundation.

causing gas, bloating, and stomach cramps, and then usually diarrhea because the intestine cannot absorb the lactose-containing foods.

The American Dietetic Association estimates that between 30 and 50 million Americans are lactose intolerant. Lactose intolerance seems to affect guys and girls equally. But certain ethnic groups are more likely to be affected. About 90% of Asian Americans are lactose intolerant, and up to 75% of African Americans, Hispanic Americans, and Native Americans also have symptoms of lactose intolerance.

Most people eventually become lactose intolerant in adulthood—some while they are still in their teen years. Many health care providers view lactose intolerance as a normal human condition likely to occur in the majority of people in the world (especially as they get older), and therefore don't really consider lactose intolerance a true disease.

Who Gets Lactose Intolerance?

There are different reasons why a person may be or may become lactose intolerant:

- People who are of Asian, African, Native American, and Hispanic backgrounds are more likely to develop lactose intolerance at a younger age.

- People with irritable bowel syndrome or Crohn disease have a reduced level of the lactase enzyme.

- Certain antibiotics can trigger temporary lactose intolerance by interfering with the intestine's ability to produce the lactase enzyme.

- After a bout of infectious diarrhea, some kids can develop a temporary lactose intolerance that usually improves after a few days or weeks.

- As people get older, their bodies usually stop producing the lactase enzyme, and most people will naturally become lactose intolerant over time.

What Happens To People With Lactose Intolerance?

Depending on how much dairy or how many milk-containing foods you eat and how little lactase you produce, you could have a variety of symptoms.

Usually within 30 minutes to two hours after eating, someone with lactose intolerance will experience nausea, stomach cramps, bloating, gas, and diarrhea. This can be unpleasant and embarrassing if you're at school or out with friends.

Because many people may think they're lactose intolerant when they really aren't, it's important to watch what you eat to figure out if dairy products really are the problem. It can also help to see a doctor who can diagnose the condition correctly and advise you on steps you can take to manage it.

How Do Doctors Diagnose It?

The most common test for lactose intolerance is the hydrogen breath test. This is a simple test that can be performed by your doctor. Normally very little hydrogen gas is detectable in the breath. However, undigested lactose in the colon ferments (breaks down) and produces various gases, including hydrogen.

For the hydrogen breath test, your doctor will ask you to blow into a tube for a beginning sample. You'll then swallow a drink with lactose in it or eat lactose-containing food, wait 30 minutes, and breathe into the tube again. The hydrogen level of the sample is then checked.

Doctors can also find out if you are able to digest lactose by testing for the presence of lactase during a procedure called endoscopy. During this procedure, doctors view the inside of the intestines by inserting a long tube with a light and a tiny camera on the end into the mouth or rectum. They can then take tissue samples and pictures of the inside of your gut and look for clues as to why you've been having problems with what you're eating.

In addition to doing a physical examination, the doctor will ask you about any concerns and symptoms you have, your past health, your family's health, any medications you're taking, any allergies you may have, and other issues. This is called the medical history.

Living With Lactose Intolerance

A person's body doesn't need lactose to be healthy. After early childhood, milk is a good source of nutrition but it's not absolutely necessary in the diet. (Calcium is very important, though, especially in teens, for good health and bone growth.)

✔ Quick Tip

Here are some other tips for dealing with lactose intolerance:

- Choose lactose-reduced or lactose-free milk.

- Take a lactase enzyme supplement (such as Lactaid) just before you eat dairy products. These can be taken in drops or tablets and even added directly to milk (they tend to make milk taste a bit sweeter if left for a long time).

- When you do drink milk or eat lactose-containing foods, eat other non-lactose foods at the same meal to slow digestion and avoid problems. (For example, if you are going to have a milkshake, don't drink it by itself. Have something else with it—like a healthy sandwich.)

- Drink juices that are fortified with calcium.

- Eat a variety of dairy-free foods that are rich in calcium, such as leafy greens (like spinach, brussels sprouts, or broccoli).

- Consider hard (aged) cheeses such as cheddar, which are lower in lactose.

- Try tofu or soy milk. These foods are high in calcium and can be prepared in dozens of different ways.

- Yogurts that contain active cultures are easier to digest and much less likely to cause lactose problems.

- Eliminating dairy can also reduce a person's intake of vitamin D. But several minutes in the sun two or three times a week should allow your body to produce enough vitamin D on its own.

- Learn to read food labels. Lactose is added to some boxed, canned, frozen, and prepared foods like bread, cereal, lunch meats, salad dressings, mixes for cakes and cookies, and coffee creamers. Be aware of certain words that may mean the food has lactose in it: butter, cheese, cream, dried milk, milk solids, powdered milk, and whey, for example.

Source: © 2004 The Nemours Center for Children's Health Media, a division of The Nemours Foundation.

Lactose intolerance is a very individual condition and it's often easy to manage if you're in tune with your body. Most people with lactose intolerance are able to eat a small amount of dairy, but the trick is to remember to always eat the dairy in combination with other foods that don't contain lactose and not go overboard. But because each case is different, there's no one simple way of dealing with it. Each person needs to learn the strategies that work best for him or her depending upon the symptoms and how much, if any, lactase the body produces.

Teens with the most severe symptoms of lactose intolerance must avoid all dairy products. Others can control problems by keeping a food diary and learning what they can and can't tolerate.

Because growing teens need about 1,200 milligrams (mg) of calcium each day, it's extremely important that teens who have to eliminate dairy products from their diets find other good calcium sources. It's probably a good idea to seek help from a registered dietitian. Dietitians are trained in nutrition and they can help people who are lactose intolerant come up with eating alternatives and develop a well-balanced diet that provides lots of calcium for developing strong bones.

Chapter 26

Nut And Peanut Allergies

Nut And Peanut Allergy Diet

When you're allergic to nuts or peanuts, any food—even the chocolate rabbit the Easter bunny brought or the burrito you had after school—is fair game for an exhaustive content analysis. But you don't have to be a chemist to distinguish an allergy-free food from one that could cause a potentially dangerous allergic reaction. You can keep yourself safe simply by reading labels on prepackaged foods and being open about your allergies with people who are preparing foods for you.

What Is A Nut And Peanut Allergy?

An allergic reaction is when the immune system mistakenly believes that a harmless substance, in this case a nut or peanut, is actually harmful to your body. Your immune system will create specific antibodies to that food; these trigger the release of certain chemicals (such as histamine) in an attempt to protect your body. So, when a person with a nut or peanut allergy eats a nut, peanut, or a food that contains nuts or peanuts, the immune system unleashes this army of chemicals to protect the body. These chemicals can affect the

About This Chapter: This information was provided by TeensHealth, one of the largest resources online for medically reviewed health information written for parents, kids, and teens. For more articles like this one, visit www.TeensHealth.org, or www.KidsHealth.org. © 2003 The Nemours Center for Children's Health Media, a division of The Nemours Foundation.

✔ Quick Tip
Tips For Managing A Peanut Allergy

Some Hidden Sources Of Peanuts

- Artificial nuts can be peanuts that have been deflavored and reflavored with a nut, such as pecan or walnut. Mandelonas are peanuts soaked in almond flavoring.

- Arachis oil is peanut oil.

- It is advised that peanut-allergic patients avoid chocolate candies unless they are absolutely certain there is no risk of cross-contact during manufacturing procedures.

- African, Chinese, Indonesian, Mexican, Thai, and Vietnamese dishes often contain peanuts, or are contaminated with peanuts during preparation of these types of meals. Additionally, foods sold in bakeries and ice cream shops are often in contact with peanuts. It is recommended that peanut-allergic individuals avoid these types of foods and restaurants.

- Many brands of sunflower seeds are produced on equipment shared with peanuts.

Keep In Mind

- Studies show that most allergic individuals can safely eat peanut oil (not cold pressed, expelled, or extruded peanut oil—sometimes represented as gourmet oils). Patients should ask their doctors whether or not to avoid peanut oil.

- Most experts recommend peanut-allergic patients avoid tree nuts as well.

- Peanuts can be found in many foods. Check all labels carefully. Contact the manufacturer if you have questions.

- Peanuts can cause severe allergic reactions. If prescribed, carry epinephrine at all times.

Source: Excerpted from "Common Food Allergies," © 2005 The Food Allergy & Anaphylaxis Network. All Rights Reserved. Reprinted with permission. For additional information, visit http://www.foodallergy.org or http://www.fankids.org.

♣ It's A Fact!!

Public awareness about all types of food allergies is increasing. Some companies have even changed their practices to accommodate customers. For example, several airlines have stopped serving peanuts altogether because some people are so severely allergic to them that even being around peanuts causes a reaction.

Source: © 2003 The Nemours Center for Children's Health Media, a division of The Nemours Foundation.

respiratory system, gastrointestinal tract, skin, or cardiovascular system— causing allergy symptoms such as wheezing, nausea, itchy hives and, in some people, a dangerous reaction called anaphylaxis (pronounced: ah-nuh-fuh-lak-sis).

About 7 million people in the United States have food allergies and, of these, 3 million are allergic to nuts and peanuts. Nut and peanut allergies can be so severe that every year up to 100 people die from eating nuts or peanuts in the United States. Although many kids outgrow allergies to milk, wheat, and eggs, only about 20% of the people with allergies to nuts and peanuts outgrow their allergies.

Although peanuts aren't true nuts, but groundnuts or legumes (in the same family as peas and lentils), the reaction in people allergic to them is similar to the reaction in people who are allergic to tree nuts, such as walnuts, cashews, and pecans.

What Are The Signs And Symptoms Of A Nut And Peanut Allergy And What Should I do?

People have different allergic reactions to nuts and peanuts. Some people may not even recognize an allergic reaction—in fact, people sometimes confuse an allergy with a cold. Other people experience the drastic (even life-threatening) changes associated with anaphylaxis, such as difficulty breathing, swelling of the throat, a drop in blood pressure, and sometimes a loss of consciousness.

Symptoms usually appear within seconds to a couple of hours after eating a nut or peanut. The first signs of an allergic reaction could be a runny nose, an itchy skin rash all over the body, or a tingly tongue. Other possible symptoms include vomiting, abdominal cramps, and diarrhea.

In some highly allergic people, symptoms can quickly become serious. In case of an emergency, doctors recommend that people with severe nut or peanut allergies keep a shot of epinephrine (pronounced: eh-puh-neh-frin) with them in an easy-to-carry container that looks like a pen. That way, if they accidentally eat nuts or peanuts and have an anaphylactic reaction, they can give themselves the epinephrine shot to help counteract it.

If you're one of these highly allergic people, you should remember to keep the pen on you at all times (you may want to have several—one for home, one for school, etc.) and make sure that the expiration date hasn't passed. Your doctor should give you instructions on how to use and store the epinephrine injection pen. (If you're taking the epinephrine pen to school, talk to your principal and school nurse: State laws about carrying medication in school vary from state to state.)

✔ Quick Tip
Nutty Nut Names

Some nuts, like walnuts, are easy to figure out—they're called nuts and they are nuts. Other nuts like pistachios, filberts, and cashews are nuts, even though they're not called nuts. Nutmeg has the word "nut" in it, but it's actually a spice—so it won't harm people with nut allergies.

Source: © 2003 The Nemours Center for Children's Health Media, a division of The Nemours Foundation.

If you've had to take an epinephrine shot, go immediately to a medical facility or hospital emergency room where you can get additional treatment, if needed. Up to one third of anaphylactic reactions can have a second wave of symptoms several hours following the initial attack.

Reading Food Labels

If you know you have a nut or peanut allergy, you must read every label on every item, and then teach others—including your parents and other people who prepare food for you—to do the same.

Most manufacturers are good about labeling every ingredient in their products. However, peanuts and peanut by-products may go by different names, such as arachis.

Peanuts are used in many foods as flavorings or oils—they're even found in non-food products like cosmetics. The Food and Drug Administration requires food manufacturers to list every ingredient in a product with a few exceptions: Flavors, colors, spices, and ingredients that appear in insignificant (or trace) amounts don't have to be listed on food labels.

It's also possible that a food that doesn't contain peanut ingredients may have come into contact with nuts or peanuts if it's produced in a factory that also processes these ingredients (this is called cross contamination). This is because some factories may use the same equipment to process nuts or peanuts as they do for products that don't contain them, so tiny amounts of nuts or peanuts could be transferred to other foods. You may have seen warnings on some food labels that a food may contain trace amounts of nuts or peanuts, but these warnings are entirely up to the manufacturer. Fortunately, as awareness surrounding allergies grows, companies are taking steps to protect consumers.

Living With A Nut and Peanut Allergy

There's no cure for food allergies. The only way to stay healthy and avoid reactions is to stay away from nuts and peanuts. Foods like peanut butter or mixed nuts are obvious, but avoiding nuts isn't always that easy. Stay away from any food you're not sure about, such as baked goods, desserts, or other products that you didn't prepare yourself or for which you don't know the ingredients. You may also come across ingredient names that mean nuts or peanuts but don't have the word "nut" anywhere in sight. Here are a few ingredients to look out for and avoid:

- lecithins or food additive 322

- arachis (an alternative term for peanut)

- hydrolyzed vegetable protein (which may be found in some cereals)

- ingredients that are "emulsified" or "satay" (these could mean a food or sauce has been thickened with peanuts)

Doctors also advise peanut-allergic patients to avoid chocolate candies unless they're absolutely certain there's no risk of cross contamination during manufacturing. Many candy companies are very aware of nut and peanut allergy issues. Some even make sure they manufacture candies that contain nuts separately from those that don't so people with nut allergies can still enjoy their products. To be sure a candy is nut and peanut free, log on to the manufacturer's website or call the toll-free number listed on the package. Most companies have customer service representatives that can answer nut and peanut allergy questions accurately.

African, Chinese, Indonesian, Mexican, Thai, and Vietnamese dishes often contain peanuts, or they may be prepared in a kitchen where the foods come into contact with nuts or peanuts. Bakeries and ice cream shops often keep peanuts on hand. And foods can be produced on equipment that's also used to process peanuts.

Nuts are used in many foods, including some you'd least expect, like chili. Other foods to avoid include:

- ice cream

- certain sauces and condiments, such as barbecue sauce, bouillon, and Worcestershire sauce

- nut and peanut oils

- Asian foods (for example, satay, pad thai, and eggrolls)

- pesto (an Italian sauce made with nuts)

- marzipan (a paste made from ground almonds and sugar)

- mandelonas (peanuts soaked in almond flavoring)

- health food bars

- all cakes and pastries with unknown ingredients, particularly carrot cake, pumpkin cake or pie, and fruit and nut rolls

- praline and nougat

- artificial nuts (they could be peanuts that have been deflavored and reflavored with a nut flavoring, such as pecan or walnut)

- muesli and fruited breakfast cereals

- baking mixes

- certain vegetarian dishes

- prepared salads and salad dressings

- gravy

♣ **It's A Fact!!**
Some Hidden Sources Of Tree Nuts

- Artificial nuts can be peanuts that have been deflavored and reflavored with a nut, such as pecan or walnut. Mandelonas are peanuts soaked in almond flavoring.

- Mortadella may contain pistachios.

- Natural and artificial flavoring may contain tree nuts.

- Tree nuts have been used in many foods including barbecue sauce, cereals, crackers, and ice cream.

- Kick sacks, or hacky sacks, bean bags, and draftdodgers are sometimes filled with crushed nut shells.

Source: Excerpted from "Common Food Allergies," © 2005 The Food Allergy & Anaphylaxis Network. All Rights Reserved. Reprinted with permission. For additional information, visit http://www.foodallergy.org or http://www.fankids.org.

At home, be on the watch for cross contamination with knives or toasters. Make sure the knife used for making peanut butter sandwiches is not used to butter your bread and that nut breads are not toasted in the same toaster you use. Better yet, make sure your home is a nut-free zone.

It's also important for nut- and peanut-allergic people to be cautious when eating out. Here are some tips:

- Avoid Chinese or other ethnic foods and buffet restaurants where spoons go in and out of various bowls that may contain nuts or seeds.

- Tell everyone who handles the food you eat—from waiters and waitresses to chefs and bakers—that you have a nut allergy. If the manager or owner of a restaurant is uncomfortable about your request for peanut- or nut-free food preparation, don't eat there.

- Make your own snacks to take to other people's houses, parties, school, and on field trips so you have some safe food.

- Be sure everyone at school—from the principal and staff to your friends and classmates—knows about your food allergy. Ask for a nut-free table in the lunchroom if your school doesn't already have one.

- Keep an epinephrine pen handy at all times—that means in your backpack or bookbag, not the glove compartment of your car. When it comes to anaphylaxis, seconds count. Talk to your school nurse to ensure that you can keep your medication easily available.

- See your doctor or an allergist regularly.

☞ Remember!!

If you have a nut or peanut allergy, just be sure you know what you're eating no matter where you dine—whether it's while vegging out on the couch or at a restaurant with your Saturday night date.

Source: © 2003 The Nemours Center for Children's Health Media, a division of The Nemours Foundation.

Chapter 27

Seafood Allergies

Seafood, a high-protein, low-fat food, offers many choices for grilling, frying, baking, and fresh food dining. Unfortunately, for a percentage of people, different types of fish and shellfish, no matter how it's cooked, can trigger dangerous allergic reactions.

"Fish and shellfish are among the most common foods that trigger severe allergic reactions," says Dan Atkins, M.D., a National Jewish physician who treats people with food allergies.

For someone with extreme sensitivity, anaphylaxis may occur, resulting in a sudden drop in blood pressure and swelling of the bronchial tissues, causing severe breathing difficulty. These reactions can arise in seconds and can be deadly. Severe anaphylactic shock is fatal if not treated immediately.

General allergic symptoms—occurring within a few minutes to a few hours of eating shellfish—include tingling and swelling in the mouth and throat; runny nose, sneezing, nausea, vomiting, diarrhea, swelling, hives, and difficulty breathing.

✔ Quick Tip

Tips For Managing A Fish And/Or Shellfish Allergy

Allergic reactions to fish and shellfish are commonly reported in both adults and children. It is generally recommended that individuals who have had an allergic reaction to one species of fish or positive skin tests to fish avoid all fish. The same rule applies to shellfish. If you have a fish allergy but would like to have fish in your diet, speak with your allergist about the possibility of being challenged with various types of fish.

Keep In Mind

Fish-allergic individuals should be cautious when eating away from home. They should avoid fish and seafood restaurants because of the risk of contamination in the food-preparation area of their "non-fish" meal from a counter, spatula, cooking oil, fryer, or grill exposed to fish. In addition, fish protein can become airborne during cooking and cause an allergic reaction. Some individuals have had reactions from walking through a fish market.

Allergic reactions to fish and shellfish can be severe and are often a cause of anaphylaxis.

Some Hidden Sources Of Fish

• Caponata, a traditional sweet-and-sour Sicilian relish, can contain anchovies.

• Caesar salad dressings and steak or Worcestershire sauce often contain anchovies.

• Surimi (imitation crabmeat) contains fish.

Source: © 2005 The Food Allergy & Anaphylaxis Network. All Rights Reserved. Reprinted with permission. For additional information, visit http://www.foodallergy.org or http://www.fankids.org.

♣ **It's A Fact!!**

Should carrageenan be avoided by a fish- or shellfish-allergic individual?

Carrageenan is not fish. Carrageenan, or Irish moss, is a red marine algae. This food product is used in a wide variety of foods, particularly dairy foods, as an emulsifier, stabilizer, and thickener. It appears safe for most individuals with food allergies. Carrageenan is not related to fish or shellfish and does not need to be avoided by those with food allergies.

Should iodine be avoided by a fish- or shellfish-allergic individual?

Allergy to iodine, allergy to radiocontrast material (used in some lab procedures), and allergy to fish or shellfish are not related. If you have an allergy to fish or shellfish, you do not need to worry about cross reactions with radiocontrast material or iodine.

Source: © 2005 The Food Allergy & Anaphylaxis Network. All Rights Reserved. Reprinted with permission. For additional information, visit http://www.foodallergy .org or http://www.fan kids.org.

"If someone has a life-threatening reaction to one crustacean, such as shrimp, testing will usually show that other crustaceans—crab, lobster, and crayfish—will also cause a reaction," Dr. Atkins says. "This relationship is known as cross-reactivity."

Raw or cooked, fish can still cause allergies. "For most sufferers it doesn't matter how fish is prepared," he says, "since the allergenic proteins in cod, shrimp, lobster, or any other fish that causes allergic reactions are not destroyed by cooking."

Minimal exposure to seafood can cause symptoms for some people. "Handling fish, or inhaling fish vapors while walking through a fish market or in a restaurant can cause a reaction in extremely sensitive individuals," Dr. Atkins says. Exposure can occur by eating another food cooked on the same surface as fish or absorbing fish protein through a cut.

The good news about food allergies is that only 1 to 2 percent of adults has a true food allergy of any kind. If you suspect you're among this group, meet with your personal physician and, if necessary, devise a treatment plan. Precautions can be taken to avoid triggering a reaction: avoid contact with the food, inform those around you about your food allergy, and wear a medical alert bracelet. Have a plan for treatment of reactions. Know the medicines used to treat reactions and carry them at all times.

"Food allergies may be misdiagnosed without a careful patient history and an appropriate evaluation," Dr. Atkins notes. "If you had just eaten shrimp before a reaction, the assumption might be made that shrimp is the cause of the reaction. It may be, but other potential causes such as another food or ingredients in sauces eaten at the same time need to be considered. Testing is necessary to determine the source of the problem.

Chapter 28

Wheat Allergy Or Gluten Intolerance?

Adverse reactions to wheat, as to any food, can be allergic (wheat or gluten allergy), intolerance (in this case, wheat intolerance, gluten intolerance, and celiac disease), or due to other naturally occurring constituents.

The body's different mechanisms of defense involved in each type of adverse reaction to wheat cause symptoms which may be quite different from or confusingly similar to each other. The severity of symptoms can vary considerably within each type of adverse reaction, but the patterns are distinct. An allergy can cause very mild to quite severe reactions (such as life-threatening anaphylaxis), compared to wheat intolerance, which can cause significant discomfort, but is never dangerous. Celiac disease (CD) can lead to serious long-term complications if left untreated (discussed below).

Wheat allergy may be present in the absence of a family history, but CD is probably always inherited. However, as CD can be silent or latent, a family history is not always reliable.

About This Chapter: "Wheat, Gluten Allergy, Gluten Intolerance and Gluten Enteropathy," by Dr. Harris Steinman. This article was originally published in the December 2001 issue of *Science in Africa*, http://www.scienceinafrica.co.za, updated 2005. © Science in Africa. Reprinted with permission.

About The Proteins/Allergens In Wheat

Wheat, like all other foods, contains a number of proteins (more than 100), including albumin, globulin, gliadin and glutenin (gliadin and glutenin together form gluten). A person can be allergic to one or more of these proteins. The majority of allergies to wheat involve the albumin and globulin fractions, but gluten may also, rarely, cause allergic reactions.

Gluten is composed of two protein groups, namely gliadins, which give wheat dough its flow characteristics, and glutenins, which provide the elasticity in finished wheat products. Gliadin is a type of prolamin (a group of proteins with similar protein structures). Other grains such as rye and barley each contain their own prolamins, which cause the same intestinal damage in CD that gliadin causes. This is due to the similarity in protein structure. By definition, gluten is found only in wheat, although the term is commonly used to refer to any similar prolamin protein in any grain that is harmful to a person with CD.

Because the type and proportion of prolamin proteins in grains vary, the kind of reaction (if any) they are likely to cause also varies. Corn, rice, other cereal grains such as sorghum, millet, teff, ragi and Job's tears as well as buckwheat, quinoa and amaranth can safely be ingested by a person with CD. Wheat, barley, rye, spelt and kamut, however, should be avoided in CD.

The safety of the ingestion of oats has been controversial for a while, but the consumption of oats has recently been proven to be safe. However, it should be considered that most commercial oat products contain wheat flour or gluten. Contamination

> ♣ **It's A Fact!!**
> **Wheat Intolerance**
> Intolerance does not involve the immune system, and the mechanisms responsible for wheat intolerance may be because of an enzyme deficiency or undigested food (as a result of one of many reasons), which result in bacterial fermentation in the colon, causing specific symptoms.

of oats with wheat may occur due to the sharing of equipment in grain processing and the rotation of crops (wheat may be grown on the same field as oats were). Therefore, contamination may be the cause of adverse reactions to oats often reported by gluten-sensitive individuals.

Wheat Allergy

What is wheat allergy?

A wheat allergy involves an immune reaction in response to an allergen (usually a protein in wheat) that the body is exposed to. A person can be allergic to one or more of the proteins in wheat. If inflammatory mediators are released or their levels enhanced by mechanisms that are independent of the immune system, the reaction is due to an intolerance.

Allergic reactions to wheat may be caused by ingestion of wheat-containing foods or by inhalation of flour containing wheat (Baker's asthma).

How common is wheat allergy?

Clinical experience suggests that wheat allergy is a relatively common allergy, but there are no accurate figures for prevalence. It is, however, more prevalent in certain groups: for example, wheat allergy is responsible for occupational asthma in up to 30% of individuals in the baking industry.

Wheat allergy is most common in young children, of which the majority will outgrow it within five years. This occurs more quickly if the wheat-containing food is completely avoided. Those who develop the allergy later in life will probably retain it.

What are the symptoms of wheat allergy?

Allergic reactions to wheat can be acute or delayed, occurring within minutes or a few hours after eating or inhaling wheat. The symptoms can involve the skin (urticaria, eczema, angioedema, atopic dermatitis), the gastrointestinal tract (abdominal cramps, nausea and vomiting) and the respiratory tract (asthma or allergic rhinitis). Wheat can cause Baker's asthma and has also been associated with wheat-dependent exercise-induced reactions (see below).

Baker's Asthma: Contact with or inhalation of wheat flour proteins is one of the causes of baker's asthma (an occupational allergy), but allergens other than the wheat itself (for example, storage mites, yeast and baking additives) may also be causes. Symptoms that may present include rhinitis, skin itching/rash, ocular symptoms (including tearing, itching, and conjunctival injection), respiratory symptoms (including coughing, wheezing, shortness of breath, and sputum production) and grain fever.

Wheat-Dependent Exercise-Induced Reactions: Exercise within 3 hours of wheat consumption can induce an adverse reaction in susceptible individuals. In some cases, this can also occur when wheat is consumed directly after exercise. Typical symptoms experienced include asthma, urticaria, angioedema, dyspnea, syncope, and anaphylaxis.

How is wheat-allergy diagnosed?

The diagnosis may be easy if a person has the same reaction repeatedly after eating wheat-containing food. More often the diagnosis is difficult because wheat is usually consumed with other food. Diagnosis usually entails clinical evaluation (medical history, family history, food history) supported by appropriate laboratory tests (CAP® RAST [RadioAllergoSorbent Test] blood tests, skin prick-testing). An elimination-challenge test may be employed to make the diagnosis.

How is wheat allergy treated?

Medication is ineffective in treating this condition. Avoidance of wheat and wheat-containing foods is the only treatment. This may be difficult to maintain, particularly as wheat protein may be "hidden" in other foods. Rice or maize may be substituted as alternative cereals. A dietitian must supervise treatment. Wheat-allergic patients who have sensitivity to gluten should avoid other gluten-containing cereals.

> ### ♣ It's A Fact!!
>
> Wheat allergy can produce any of the following symptoms:
>
> - urticaria (hives)
> - eczema
> - angioedema
> - atopic dermatitis
> - abdominal cramps
> - nausea
> - vomiting
> - asthma

Celiac Disease (Gluten-Sensitive Enteropathy)

What is celiac disease?

CD is a hereditary disorder of the immune system. The ingestion of gluten leads to damage of the mucosa (lining) of the small intestine. This results in malabsorption of nutrients and vitamins such as proteins, carbohydrates, fats, vitamins, minerals, and, in some cases, water and bile salts. CD is the result of IgA and IgG antibody responses to gluten. It is important to differentiate between CD, mediated by IgA and IgG antibodies, and wheat allergy, which is mediated by IgE antibodies.

The disease is permanent, and damage to the small intestine will occur every time gluten is consumed, regardless whether symptoms are present or not. It has been reported that as little as 0.1 grams of ingested gluten can trigger symptoms.

The onset of noticeable symptoms of CD seems to be dependent on the following: exposure to wheat, as when an infant is weaned (introduction of solids); predisposition through family history; and some kind of "trigger" mechanism. Little is known about this "trigger" but suspected factors include physical or emotional stress, trauma such as surgery or pregnancy, overexposure to wheat, viral infection, other diseases, and even antibiotics.

How common is celiac disease?

CD is one of the most common life-long disorders in certain countries. CD is frequently under-diagnosed, particularly in adults, who may present with only subtle symptoms. In some countries the incidence is as high as 1 in 200 (Sweden).

As CD can be silent or latent, a family history is not always reliable. It primarily affects Caucasians of northwestern European decent and rarely affects Africans, people of Mediterranean extraction, or Asians. It affects twice as many females as males.

CD usually develops in childhood but can begin at any age. Typically the disease presents at the age of 6–24 months, after wheat has been introduced into the diet, and in early adult life (30s and 40s).

What are the symptoms of celiac disease?

There is no typical set of symptoms. However, there are "classic" symptoms (diarrhea, bloating, weight loss, anemia, chronic fatigue, bone pain, and muscle cramps), but CD frequently presents with other symptoms. In some cases only one symptom may be experienced (for example, anemia, a run-down feeling, or behavioral problems) or the symptoms may occur intermittently.

In Infants And Young Children: Symptoms usually arise after weaning and with the introduction of cereals into the diet. In children, gastrointestinal problems are more evident; they include abnormal stools (ranging from diarrhea, to soft, bulky, clay-colored, foul-smelling stools, to constipation), abdominal distension, abdominal pain, flatulence, nausea, vomiting, and intestinal malabsorption. Children also present with irritability, apathy, loss of appetite, weight loss, poor weight gain, short stature, muscle wasting, hypotonia, general failure to thrive, poor school performance, bone and joint pains, and occasionally rickets.

It is not uncommon for symptoms experienced during infancy to disappear during later childhood or adolescence, and then to reappear later in life. The disease does not disappear; the small intestine damage still occurs during these years even though no symptoms are experienced.

In Older Children And Adults: The symptoms may be quite varied, from severe weight loss, diarrhea and bulky, offensive stools to less severe symptoms that may lead to a missed diagnosis. Subtle complaints of abdominal bloating, cramping, flatulence, and constipation are often mistakenly attributed to irritable bowel syndrome. Symptoms such as recurrent mouth ulceration, miscarriages, or failure to conceive may lead to further investigations with an eventual diagnosis.

> **♣ It's A Fact!!**
>
> Celiac disease may produce symptoms such as the following:
>
> - diarrhea
> - bloating
> - weight loss
> - anemia
> - chronic fatigue
> - bone pain
> - muscle cramps
> - anemia
> - behavioral problems

Some individuals present with only anemia-related fatigue and have no gastrointestinal symptoms. Other manifestations of the disease include osteopenic bone disease, infertility, tetany, ataxia, and neurologic disorders.

How is celiac disease diagnosed?

Doctors must have a low threshold of suspicion when seeing patients with symptoms such as those described above. There are various blood tests that can be used to support the diagnosis of CD:

1. The anti-gliadin antibody (AGA) assay, which measures the amount of IgA and IgG antibody produced against the gliadin component of cereals

2. The anti-reticulin antibody (ARA) test, in which IgG antibodies are viewed in an immuno-fluorescent microscope examination

3. The anti-endomysial antibody (AEA) assay, which identifies IgA antibodies against the endomysium tissue

These tests offer simple and fast tools to investigate patients with suspected CD. They are particularly recommended for screening relatives of CD patients or patients who are affected by a related disease such as malabsorption or diabetes mellitus, and for monitoring the compliance to a gluten-free diet.

None of these tests has shown 100% accuracy, and a small-intestinal mucosal biopsy remains the cornerstone for diagnosis. Any provisional diagnosis of CD must be confirmed by this biopsy. The procedure is safe and usually performed at the time of gastrointestinal endoscopy. However, it must be kept in mind that if the patient is on a gluten-free diet, the results of these tests are likely to be negative.

What is dermatitis herpetiformis?

Dermatitis herpetiformis is a form of CD. It is a skin reaction to gluten (granular IgA is deposited under the skin). Dermatitis herpetiformis manifests as a blistering, burning, itchy rash on the extensor surfaces of the body (mainly the back, sacrum, face, trunk, elbows, knees, and buttocks, but also inside the mouth) in strikingly symmetrical patterns. In most of these individuals,

intestinal biopsies are characteristic of CD regardless of whether gastrointestinal symptoms are present. The treatment is the same as for CD, but it may
take two or more years after the initiation of the diet before the rash clears.

How is celiac disease treated?

Medication is ineffective in treating this condition. The only treatment
available is the complete removal of gluten from the diet. This usually entails
life-long avoidance of all cereals containing gluten, including wheat, rye, and
barley. Individuals on any avoidance diet are at risk of developing deficien-
cies of micro-nutrients (for example, thiamine, riboflavin, niacin, iron, sele-
nium, chromium, magnesium, folate, phosphorus and molybdenum). It is
therefore essential that patients be managed in collaboration with a dietitian. Information on gluten-free diets is becoming increasingly available
worldwide. Gluten-free products are also becoming more abundant and more
easily available.

Chapter 29

Learning To Take Control Of Your Food Allergies

"My parents are constantly bugging me about my food allergy. How can I get them off my back?"

"My parents are too strict. They won't let me go to a lot of places by myself, or with my friends, because of my food allergies."

If this sounds like you, step back and take a careful look at your situation. Your parents aren't staying up until the wee hours of the morning devising ways to ruin your fun. They probably feel you are not ready to handle the full responsibility of your food allergy yet.

If you feel that you are, start by talking calmly to your parents. Tell them you would like to be more involved in managing your food allergies. Agree to shift the control of your food allergy slowly; as they see that you are able to handle small responsibilities, they will be more comfortable allowing you to handle the big ones.

Preparing yourself to take on the responsibility of your food allergy is one of the first steps to gaining independence. The following tips may help:

Do your homework: Pay attention to ways your parents help manage your food allergies both at home and in public. For example, note the questions they ask servers in restaurants; keep your own "How to Read a Label" card rather than relying on your mom or dad to have one. Take the lead in asking about ingredients and food preparation the next time you and your family eat in a restaurant.

Actions speak louder than words: Demonstrate that you are willing and able to take responsibility for your food allergy. One way to do this is to show your parents that you have your medications with you when you are going to leave the house—before they ask.

Know who to talk to: Responsibly managing your food allergies doesn't mean doing it by yourself; it means knowing who to consult about which aspects of your allergy.

- Keep your parents in the loop. Tell them about situations you've encountered and how you've handled them. Ask them what they would have done in the same situations.

- Make your doctor your new best friend. Clear communication with your doctor is important. Answer your doctor's questions honestly; if you have questions about your medications or about whether certain situations are safe, ask. If you don't understand something your doctor tells you, say so.

- Let others know how they can help. Teach a few friends about your allergy in detail. Tell them the symptoms of an allergic reaction, and go over what they should do if you have a reaction when you're with them. This will not only give you and your parents peace of mind (and help your parents be more comfortable when you go out without them), but will also give you a safety net of people who can help keep you safe.

Plan ahead: By figuring out how you will handle big events like a school dance or football camp, and small ones like hanging out at the pizza place or going to parties, you'll be able to enjoy the events themselves instead of stressing about your food allergy.

Admit your mistakes: Everyone makes mistakes. If you have a reaction, analyze what happened and how you can prevent it from happening again. Discussing what you've learned from your reaction shows your parents that you are mature enough to use your past mistakes to build future successes.

✔ Quick Tip

Tips For Managing Food Allergies At School

By now you've probably gotten used to your new class schedule, memorized your locker combination, and have joined clubs or teams for after school. Making sure you manage your food allergies with all these activities, though, might not be a piece of cake yet. Here are some tips to keep you safe and fed during the long school days.

- **Enlist The Help Of Your Friends:** Tell your friends about your allergy, what you do to avoid a reaction, and what they should do to help you if you have a reaction. You don't have to tell the whole school, but it is a good idea to tell the people you hang out with most.

- **Update Your Teachers And Coaches:** If you joined an after-school club or sports team, remind teachers and coaches about your food allergy from time to time, particularly if they serve food or snacks so that you know you'll be able to eat with your friends.

- **Keep A Stash In Your Locker:** Sports, clubs, and other activities can keep you at school late in the day—past dinnertime even. Keep a stash of snacks (such as crackers, popcorn, or fruit snacks) in your locker so you always have a "safe" snack available.

Most important, have fun, learn, and don't let food allergies hold you back.

Source: © 2005 The Food Allergy & Anaphylaxis Network. All Rights Reserved. Reprinted with permission. For additional information, visit http://www.foodallergy.org or http://www.fankids.org.

Finally, remember that gaining independence is a process: Celebrate small victories (like the first time you leave the house and your parents don't ask if you have your medications—because they already know you do), and use them as encouragement to keep after the big ones (like going to camp, going to college, or traveling by yourself). By taking the lead in managing your food allergies on a day-to-day basis, you will be preparing yourself to handle unfamiliar situations in the future. Good luck!

Chapter 30

Decoding Food Labels

Background

True food allergies are immune-mediated systemic allergic reactions to certain foods. According to the FDA, true food allergies affect less than 2% of the adult population and 2–8% of children. However, the impact of true allergies can be quite severe. Most childhood food allergies are found in young infants and children under three years old. Food allergies have a genetic component and may be more common among those with asthma.

Reactions to a food allergen can range from uncomfortable skin irritations to gastrointestinal distress to respiratory involvement to life threatening anaphylaxis—a systemic allergic reaction that generally involves several of these areas as well as the cardiovascular system. The number of people with food allergies appears to be increasing, especially among children. To keep pace with this trend, there is an increasing need for preemptive food selection strategies.

Currently, an individual with a food allergy must learn to read labels carefully and critically. This is because a food allergen may take on an unfamiliar

✔ Quick Tip

Currently, the only way to treat food allergies is to avoid the foods that trigger reactions. Even the most diligent label-readers and ingredient-checkers likely will be inadvertently exposed to proteins that elicit an allergic response at some point. That's why people with food allergies severe enough to cause anaphylactic reactions should wear medical alert bracelets or necklaces and carry a syringe of adrenaline (epinephrine) obtained by prescription from their physicians.

Source: From "Food Allergies: When Food Becomes the Enemy," by Ray Formanek, Jr. U.S. Food and Drug Administration (FDA), *FDA Consumer*, July-August 2001, revised April 2004.

name when used for processing purposes. For example, if eggs, one of the most allergenic foods, are used as a binder to retain water in a food product, the term binder rather than egg will appear on the food label. Similarly, soy protein may be used for flavoring and listed on the label as natural flavoring.

New legislation, The Food Allergen Labeling and Consumer Protection Act (FALCPA), would require food manufacturers to use common names to identify major allergens. If approved by the House of Representatives, the FALCPA should provide consistent ingredient information, understandable at-a-glance to the average consumer, by January 2006. Until that time, understanding current labeling information is vital to allergic individuals.

The goal of this chapter is to provide information to help consumers understand ingredient statements on food packages, so they can avoid foods and food-products that might contain specific allergens. It also differentiates between allergies and intolerances, and discusses the potential for cross-contamination of foods both in and away from the home.

Food Allergy Vs. Food Intolerances Vs. Histamine Sensitivity

Most people experience an adverse reaction to some food at some point in their life. This does not necessarily mean that the individual is allergic to that food. Food intolerances, including sensitivity to elevated levels of histamine in foods, can produce a response similar to an allergic reaction. Adverse reactions and suspected allergens can be identified through a detailed history and specific allergy testing by a physician or qualified specialist, to exclude other causes.

The difference between food allergies and food intolerance is how the body handles the offending food. In the case of an allergy, the immune system recognizes a chemical in the food (usually a protein) as an allergen, and produces antibodies against it.

A response to an allergen may manifest as:

- Swelling of the lips
- Stomach cramps, vomiting, diarrhea
- Hives, rashes, eczema
- Wheezing or breathing problems
- Severely reduced blood pressure

Most common allergens are found in the following food groups:

1. Cow's milk (especially among children)
2. Wheat (especially among children)
3. Soy (especially among children)
4. Eggs
5. Peanuts
6. Tree nuts
7. Fish and/or shellfish
8. Food additives (not true allergens, but capable of causing reaction or illness specific to a given person)

In most cases, children will outgrow their allergies to milk, wheat, soy, and eggs, but not to peanuts. Adults do not usually grow out of or loose their allergies.

Food intolerance is more common than a true allergy and does not involve the immune system. Intolerance is a metabolic problem in which the body cannot adequately digest the offending food. This is usually because of a chemical deficiency (i.e., an enzyme deficiency).

An individual with food intolerance can generally consume a small amount of the offending food without becoming symptomatic. However, that specific amount may be different for each individual. Intolerances, unlike allergies, seem to intensify with age.

Histamine sensitivity may be considered a type of food intolerance. Because histamine is a primary mediator of an allergic response in the body, consumption of histamine can elicit a similar response. Histamine toxicity is most frequently associated with the consumption of spoiled fish, but has also been associated with aged cheeses and red wines. Elevated levels of histamine occur naturally in these foods.

Decoding Allergens In Foods

Eggs

If you are allergic to egg protein, you should avoid any product with the word egg on the label. You should also avoid products with the following terms on their label:

- Albumin
- Binder
- Coagulant
- Emulsifier
- Globulin/ ovoglobulin
- Lecithin
- Livetin
- Lysozyme
- Ovalbumin
- Ovomucin
- Ovomucoid
- Ovovitellin
- Vitellin
- Simplesse*

* Simplesse™ is a fat substitute made from egg white and milk protein.

Types of foods that likely contain egg protein include:

- Baked goods and packaged mixes
- Creamy fillings and sauces
- Breakfast cereals
- Malted drinks and mixes
- Pancakes and waffles
- Marzipan*
- Custard
- Marshmallows
- Processed meat products
- Pastas/egg noodles
- Salad dressings/ mayonnaise
- Soups
- Meringue
- Pudding

* Marzipan might be made with egg whites.

Milk

Milk and milk proteins are also found in a variety of processed foods. Individuals with milk protein allergies should avoid all types of milk, ice cream, yogurt and cheese, including vegetarian cheese.

Allergic individuals should avoid foods with the terms butter, cream, casein, caseinate, whey, or emulsifier on the label. Additional labeling terms indicating the presence of milk proteins in a food product include:

- Caramel color or flavoring
- High protein flavor
- Lactalbumin/ lactalbumin phosphate
- Lactoglobulin
- Lactose
- Natural flavoring
- Solids
- Simplesse*

* Simplesse™ is a fat substitute made from egg white and milk protein

Types of foods that likely contain milk protein include:

- Battered foods
- Baked goods and mixes
- Breakfast cereals
- Chocolate
- Cream sauces, soups and mixes
- Gravies and mixes
- Ghee*
- Custard, puddings, sherbet
- Imitation sour cream
- Instant mashed potatoes
- Margarine
- Sausages
- Sweets/candies

*Ghee is clarified butter frequently used in Indian cuisine.

Wheat

Individuals who are allergic to wheat proteins should avoid any product that contains the term wheat, bulgur, couscous, bran, gluten, bread crumbs, or hydrolyzed wheat proteins on the label. Wheat has binding properties that are very useful in the food processing industry, and has been extended to use in the pharmaceutical industry. Individuals with wheat allergies should discuss the composition of prescription or over-the-counter medications with a pharmacist prior to use. The presence of wheat protein in a food product may be indicated by the following label terms:

- Flour—bleached, unbleached, white, whole wheat, all-purpose, enriched, graham, durum, high gluten, high protein
- Cornstarch
- Farina
- Semolina
- Hydrolyzed vegetable protein
- Modified food starch
- Miso**
- MSG (monosodium glutamate)
- Vegetable starch/gum
- Gelatinized starch
- Spelt*
- Kamut*
- Triticale*

*Spelt and Kamut are both relatives of wheat; Triticale is a wheat/rye hybrid. These grains are gaining popularity as wheat substitutes. Spelt, Kamut, and Triticale containing products are marketed primarily through health/natural food stores.

** Fermented soy product with up to 50% wheat.

Types of foods that likely contain wheat proteins include:

- Ale/beer/wine/bourbon/whiskey
- Baked goods and mixes—including barely products
- Battered or breaded foods
- Breakfast cereals
- Candy/chocolate
- Processed meats
- Coffee substitutes
- Gravy
- Ice cream and cones
- Malts and flavorings
- Pasta/egg noodles
- Soup and soup mixes
- Soy sauce
- Pretzels, chips, crackers

Soy

Soy can be consumed as a whole bean, a nut, or a cow-milk alternative. Soy can be processed into foods such as tofu, soy curd, yuba (soy film), and soy flour. Soy can be fermented into products such as tempeh, natto, miso, and soy sauce. Soy has a variety of supportive uses in the food industry as well. It can be a thickener, stabilizer, emulsifier, and a protein extender. Allergic individuals should avoid products with these terms on the label in addition to products containing the terms soy and soybean.

Soybean oil should be protein free, but this is not always the case and some allergic individuals must avoid soybean oil and products made with soybean oil (margarine and products made with margarine, salad dressings, and baby foods). The presence of the following terms on the product label may also indicate the presence of soy protein:

- Guar gum
- Bulking agent
- Carob
- Gum Arabic
- Hydrolyzed vegetable protein (HVP)/Hydrolyzed soy protein
- Lecithin
- Miso*
- Monosodium glutamate (MSG)
- Protein
- Starch
- Textured vegetable protein (TVP)
- Vegetable broth/gum/starch

*Miso is a paste made from fermented soybeans, used as a flavoring agent in Japanese cuisine.

Types of foods that likely contain soy protein include:

- Baked goods
- Some breakfast cereals
- Hamburger patties
- Butter substitutes/shortening
- Chocolates/candy
- Canned meat/fish in sauces
- Canned/packaged soups
- Canned tuna
- Crackers
- Gravies/mixes
- Oriental foods
- Processed meats
- Ice cream
- Liquid/powdered meal replacers
- Seasoning sauces
- Seasoned salt
- Snack bars
- Bouillon cubes
- TV dinners
- Tamari*

*Tamari is a dark sauce, similar to but thicker than soy sauce.

Peanuts And Tree Nuts

Peanuts are one of the most severely allergenic foods available in the market place. Peanuts are frequently used as a flavoring/seasoning agent in a variety of products. Peanuts and peanut oil are commonly used in oriental cooking. As with soy oil, peanut oil (occasionally referred to as arachic oil) may very well contain an amount of peanut protein sufficient to elicit an allergic reaction. The terms peanut, peanut butter, ground-nut, flavoring, extract, and oriental sauce on a product label generally indicates the presence of peanut protein.

Types of foods that may contain peanut protein include:

- Baked goods/ mixes
- Battered foods
- Some breakfast cereals
- Cereal-based products
- Candy/candy bars/sweets (read label)
- Ice cream
- Margarine/ vegetable oil/ vegetable fat
- Some grain breads
- Snack foods
- Barbecue/ Worcestershire sauce
- Sunflower seeds*
- Chili
- Soups
- Marzipan**
- Satay sauce***
- Milk formula
- Chinese dishes/ egg roll
- Asian dishes (e.g., Thai/ Indonesian)
- African dishes
- Energy bars
- Meat substitutes

*Sunflower seeds may be processed on equipment shared with peanuts.

**Marzipan is a paste made of almond and sugar, used on pastry or molded into candy. Marzipan might be made with egg white as well.

***Satay sauce is made with peanuts or peanut butter and soy sauce. It might also be made with other allergenic ingredients such as shrimp paste or fish sauce.

Individuals with a peanut allergy may or may not be allergic to tree nuts (e.g., almonds, cashews, pecans, walnuts) as well. Individuals with tree-nut allergies should be cautious of the foods listed above as well as the following: mixed nuts, artificial nuts, nut oils, nut pastes, nut butters, nut extracts, salad dressings, and amaretto products.

Fish And Seafood

Seafood refers to fish and shellfish. Fish is a potent allergen among children. Shellfish tends to be a more potent allergen among adults. Although seafood might be incorporated into a variety of foods during processing, the product's label generally states this clearly. Certain species of fish contain high levels of histidine (an amino acid), which can be converted into histamine by bacteria. Reactions to histamine can mimic allergic reactions, but are not indicative of a true allergy.

Types of foods that might contain fish/seafood proteins include:

- Worcestershire/ steak sauce
- Caesar salad dressing
- Hot dogs/ bologna/ham

- Pizza toppings
- Fish sauce
- Fish stock
- Surimi*
- Caponata**
- Marinara sauce

- Vitamin supplements (read label)
- Curry paste

*Surimi is a fish protein (most commonly made from pollack), marketed as imitation seafood. Surimi may contain artificial flavor, sweeteners, egg white, starch, and small amounts of real shellfish.

**Caponata is an eggplant relish that can contain anchovies.

Food Additives

Food additives are frequently incorporated into food products during processing. They may be used as a product preservative, a flavor enhancer or sweetener, a coloring agent, a conditioner, or a stabilizer. Over the years, adverse reactions to certain food additives, casually referred to as allergies, have been reported. Most notably:

- Sulfite induced asthma

- Monosodium glutamate induced asthma or MSG symptom complex

- Aspartame induced hives and/or migraines

- FD&C Yellow No. 5 (tartrazine) induced hives and/or asthma

Reactions to these additives are not immunologically mediated. Rather, reactions to these food additives are considered idiosyncratic (affecting different people in different ways) in that the mechanism of these reactions remains unknown.

Sulfites: Sulfites are used as preservatives, to prevent browning reactions. Although sulfite-induced asthma is well documented, its mechanisms are not well understood by experts. So sulfite sensitive individuals should avoid foods with the following terms listed on their label: sulfur dioxide, potassium metabisulfite, sodium metabisulfite, potassium bisulfite, sodium bisulfite, and sodium sulfite.

Monosodium glutamate (MSG): Glutamate, an amino acid, occurs naturally in many foods, with particularly high levels in dairy products, meat, fish and some vegetables. Glutamate has a distinct flavor. Monosodium glutamate (MSG) is added to food as a flavor enhancer. MSG symptom complex includes headaches, nausea, rapid heartbeat, vomiting, a tingling/numbness/burning sensation along the back, neck, arms, face, and chest pains. These MSG induced symptoms tend to occur in sensitive individuals within 1 hour of consuming large amounts (> 3 grams) of MSG or consuming MSG in a liquid (e.g. soup). Individuals with asthma may be predisposed to this syndrome as well as MSG induced asthma attacks. Food products containing MSG will list it on the label. However, MSG may be used in restaurants, especially in oriental cooking.

Aspartame: Aspartame is an artificial sweetener made from two amino acids phenylalanine and aspartic acid. Aspartame is marketed as a low-calorie sweetener (NutraSweet and Equal are among its popular names). Associations have been reported between Aspartame and a list of adverse symptoms including: headaches or migraines; dizziness; rashes; swelling of the lips and/or

> ## ♣ It's A Fact!!
> Anaphylactic allergic reactions can be fatal even when they begin with mild symptoms such as a tingling in the mouth and throat or gastrointestinal discomfort. Antihistamines and bronchodilators can be used to treat less severe symptoms.
>
> Source: From "Food Allergies: When Food Becomes the Enemy," by Ray Formanek, Jr. U.S. Food and Drug Administration (FDA), FDA Consumer, July-August 2001, revised April 2004.

eyelids; difficulty breathing; rapid heartbeat; and depression. Individuals with mood disorders may be particularly vulnerable to these reactions. Aspartame is listed on the label of food products, beverages, and in medications, where it may also be used as a sweetening agent.

FD&C Yellow No. 5 (Tartrazine): FD&C Yellow No. 5 or tartrazine is a dye used as a coloring agent in food processing. Among sensitive individuals, tartrazine appears to be a trigger for asthma, runny nose, and hives. The presence of this dye in a food or drug should be clearly indicated by the terms FD&C Yellow No. 5, tartrazine, or possibly E102 on the food product label or drug package insert. Individuals who are sensitive to aspirin may be sensitive to tartrazine as well.

Cross-Contamination Of Foods In And Away From Home

If you are or live with an allergic individual, then cross-contamination becomes a daily issue. Cross-contamination refers to the situation through which a "safe" food comes in contact with an allergen—even a small amount.

♣ It's A Fact!!

The Federal Food, Drug, and Cosmetic Act requires, in virtually all cases, that all the ingredients of a food be listed on the food label. Two exemptions to the labeling requirements recently have been involved in a number of reported food allergen reactions: the collective naming of spices, flavorings, and colorings; and insignificant levels of additives in a food that do not have a technical or functional effect on the final product. The FDA, however, does not consider food allergens eligible for the latter labeling exemption. The agency also strongly encourages the declaration of an allergenic ingredient in a spice, flavor, or color.

Source: From "Food Allergies: When Food Becomes the Enemy," by Ray Formanek, Jr. U.S. Food and Drug Administration (FDA), FDA Consumer, July-August 2001, revised April 2004.

At home, this could occur by cutting a peanut butter sandwich on a cutting board. The board is effectively contaminated with enough peanut allergen to elicit a reaction from the next allergic user. In a bakery, this could occur when an employee removes a sugar cookie for an allergic customer, with the same tongs that were used to remove a peanut-butter cookie. In a restaurant, this could occur if the steak you ordered is grilled alongside the fish you are allergic to.

To Avoid Cross-Contamination At Home

- Separate allergenic foods from other foods by storing them in a plastic box or container in the refrigerator or on the pantry shelf.

- Clean all pots, pans, and utensils thoroughly with soap and hot water, immediately after use with an allergen.

- Wash plates and utensils used with allergenic foods, separately and with a separate set of washing and drying cloths.

♣ It's A Fact!!

Many large food companies have long been aware of how serious food allergies can be, and have made appropriate changes in their manufacturing and labeling practices. There are still many more companies that have yet to take the issue seriously.

For example, today there are more than a dozen ways to indicate the presence of milk protein without using the word "milk." Another common problem is the term "nondairy." Many consumers mistakenly believe that nondairy means there is no milk in a product. Current labeling guidelines allow the use of "nondairy" when the foods contain milk byproducts.

In addition, manufacturers may use the term "natural flavors" even when the product contains major allergens. To avoid a major allergen, a food-allergic consumer would need to call the manufacturer before purchasing the product to confirm that an allergen was present.

A review of food labels indicates an overuse of "may contain" statements, leaving food-allergic people to wonder whether food companies are really looking after their best interest.

Source: From "Food Allergies: When Food Becomes the Enemy," by Ray Formanek, Jr. U.S. Food and Drug Administration (FDA), FDA Consumer, July-August 2001, revised April 2004.

- Do not use wooden bowls or utensils because they absorb contaminants.

- Wash hands after contact with an allergen or wear non-latex food gloves during food preparation.

To Avoid Cross-Contamination In Restaurants

- Avoid buffet-style dining.

- Avoid stores or cafes where food products are stored in bulk bins.

- Avoid sliced deli meats because slicers are used with a variety of products.

- Avoid seafood restaurants if you are allergic to any type of seafood.

- Avoid Asian restaurants (Thai, Indonesian) if you have a peanut or soy allergy.

- Tell your server about your allergy.

- Ask about possible hidden ingredients, especially in salad dressings and sauces.

- Ask about other foods being prepared in the kitchen simultaneously.

- Order simple dishes with sauces on the side.

- Carry a *Chef Card*—a personalized card with simple instructions to the chef and others, describing your allergy, related ingredients, and cross-contamination issues.

- Don't be afraid to leave a restaurant if you don't feel "safe".

Disclaimer: Not all foods and potential allergens have been included in this chapter. Check with your physician or specialist to make sure you have a complete, individualized list. If you are in doubt regarding food label information or product ingredients, contact the food manufacturer.

References

1. Food Allergen Labeling and Consumer Protection Act of 2003 (HR 3684 IH).

2. IFT—Scientific Status Summary: Seafood Allergy and Allergens—A review. October 1995.

3. Sicherer SH, Sampson HA. Prevalence of peanut and tree nut allergy in the United States determined by means of a random digit dial telephone survey: a five-year follow-up study. *Journal of Allergy and Clinical Immunology*. 2003;112(6):1203–7.

4. Steinman HA. Hidden allergens in foods. *Journal of Allergy and Clinical Immunology*. 1996;98(2):241–250.

5. Taylor SL, Hefle SL. Food allergies and other food sensitivities. *Food Technology*. 2001;55(9):68–83.

6. Taylor SL, Stratton JE, Nordlee JA. Histamine poisoning (scombroid fish poisoning): an allergylike intoxication. *J Toxicol Clin Toxicol*. 1989;27(4-5):225–240.

7. U.S. Food and Drug Administration. FDA Medical Bulletin. Monosodium Glutamate. 1996; vol 26(1). http://www.fda.gov/medbull/january96/msg.html.

8. U.S. Food and Drug Administration. Food allergies rare but risky. *FDA Consumer* May 1994. http://vm.cfsan.fda.gov/~dms/wh-alrg1.html.

9. U.S. Food and Drug Administration. When food becomes the enemy. *FDA Consumer* July-August 2001 revised April 2004. www.fda.gov/fdac/features/2001/401_food.html.

10. Walton RG, Hudak R, Green-Waite RJ. Adverse reactions to aspartame: double-blind challenge in patients from a vulnerable population. *Biol Psychiatry*. 1993 Jul 1–15; (34(1-2): 13–7.

11. William, J., Jr. Food Allergens: Effectively managing processing risks. *Food Protection Trends*. 2004. Vol. 24(1):20–22.

Chapter 31

Food Allergies And Your Social Life

Dining Out With A Food Allergy

If you have a food allergy, you know that dining out can be risky business. After all, you don't have the ingredient labels available to scrutinize. Often, dishes can contain surprise ingredients...and the surprise may be that it's a food you are allergic to!

In addition to asking a lot of questions about ingredients and preparation methods, many food-allergic teens and adults carry a "chef card" with them that outlines the foods that they must to avoid. The card is presented to the chef or manager for review, and serves as a reminder of the food allergy.

Some people have made their information a little smaller and have had it printed on business cards.

To create your own customized card with your doctor's help. Once you have done so, consider these options:

• Print the information on brightly colored paper.

About This Chapter: This chapter includes "Dining Out with a Food Allergy," "Managing Food Allergies and Outdoor Activities," "Dating and Food Allergies: Do They Go Hand-in-Hand?" "Camping with a Food "Allergy," and "Participating in Specialty Camps," © 2005 The Food Allergy & Anaphylaxis Network. All Rights Reserved. Reprinted with permission. For additional information, visit http://www.foodallergy.org or http://www.fankids.org.

- Print several copies of the chef card so that if you forget to get your card back, you have extra copies available.

- Laminate your chef card so that it doesn't get damaged or stained.

Always remember to ask questions about ingredients and preparation methods. Don't rely on your chef card to take the place of talking to the waitstaff and/or management of a restaurant.

Finally, the chef card is designed to help you convey food allergy information to the chef. It will not prevent a reaction...you must make careful food choices.

To the Chef:
WARNING! I am allergic to _____. In order to avoid a life-threatening reaction, I must avoid all foods that might contain _____, including these ingredients:

_____	_____
_____	_____
_____	_____
_____	_____
_____	_____
_____	_____

Please please ensure that my food does not contain any of these ingredients, and that any utensils and equipment used to prepare my meal, as well as prep surfaces are thoroughly cleaned prior to use. Thanks for your cooperation.
                      Blank form courtesy of the Food Allergy & Anaphylaxis Network

---

Figure 31.1. Sample Chef Card (Source: © 2005 The Food Allergy & Anaphylaxis Network. All Rights Reserved. Reprinted with permission. For additional information, visit http://www.foodallergy.org or http://www.fankids.org.)

Managing Food Allergies And Outdoor Activities

As the weather warms up, activities and meals tend to move outdoors, so you may find yourself invited to picnics, backyard barbecues, graduation and end-of-school parties, pool parties, and amusement parks.

How do teens handle their food allergies at these social events? They do so by planning, by using common sense, and by being determined not to take chances with risky foods.

Picnics And Barbecues

If you'll be attending a picnic or barbecue, talk to those in charge of the food to be sure they know about your food allergy. Keep in mind that those who do not have food allergies may not be as well-versed in shopping or cooking for an allergy as you are. Offer suggestions, or help with the actual shopping.

Don't assume barbecue sauce will be okay for you to eat, at least one brand of barbecue sauce lists pecans on the label. Also, be on the lookout for cooks who make their own barbecue sauce or add "secret" ingredients to store-bought brands. If you don't know all of the ingredients or if you are unsure, do not eat the sauce—avoid it.

You always have the option of bringing your own food. This way you'll know that there will be something you can safely eat. To avoid the chance of cross contact from foods prepared on the grill, consider bringing precooked foods, such as steak, chicken, or burgers. To reheat food, wrap it in aluminum foil to protect it before placing it on the grill or in an oven.

Parties

Depending on the type of party you will be attending, you may find that your food allergy may not be much of an issue. Oftentimes, parties offer a casual eating atmosphere and snack-type foods are offered. Try to fill up on safe foods before the party—you'll be less tempted to snack later. Another option would be to arrive at the party early and offer to help set up. This will give you the opportunity to check out the labels and to serve yourself first to avoid any potential cross contact issues. If something doesn't have a label, don't eat it.

Amusement Parks

Amusement parks may present challenges to those who have food allergies. How do you plan a full day of meals and snacks? Many teens plan to take a picnic lunch packed in a cooler that they keep in the car until they are

Tell And Kiss?

As you know, being a teenager is hard enough. You have school to deal with, peer pressure, and lots of decisions to face every day. One of the more fun and exciting things that teens experience is dating. Most teens, including those who don't have food allergies, are worried about their first kiss. But those who do have food allergies also have their safety to take into consideration before getting romantically involved with someone.

According to a study published in 2003, individuals with food allergies may have a reaction after kissing someone who has eaten the food to which he or she is allergic. Of the cases studied, most of the allergic reactions occurred immediately after the person kissed someone who had eaten the allergy-causing food. In one case, however, a reaction occurred two hours after eating. Symptoms included itchy eyes; itching where close contact had occurred; itchy lips, mouth, and throat; hives; abdominal pain; and redness of skin. Some of the commonly reported offending allergens were milk, eggs, carrots, fruits, tree nuts, and peanuts.

Your food allergy may seem like an "uncool" topic to bring up, but it's much cooler to talk about it than to have a reaction. Be upfront with people you are interested in. If they care about you, they will understand and want to learn about how they can help keep you safe.

If you are in the early stages of a relationship and don't feel quite ready to tell the other person about your food allergy, try to avoid food-related activities. For example, plan dates before or after mealtimes or offer to supply the snack if you are planning a long date. Whichever you decide, avoid close contact with your date until you can be honest with him or her and feel he or she will respect your food restrictions.

Dating is all about spending time with a person you like and finding out if you are compatible and comfortable with each other. If your date isn't understanding about your food allergy or is pressuring you to take chances that would harm you, then it might be time to move on! On the other hand, if your new boyfriend or girlfriend is making an effort to learn about food allergy and is genuinely concerned, let him or her know how much it means to you.

ready to eat. Most parks will allow you to leave and return, making a "car picnic" the easiest option. Call the park in advance to find out its policy. If that plan doesn't appeal to you, you'll have to do some research before you go. Visit the website of the amusement park and look up your meal options. Most amusement parks offer restaurant names and a list of menu items. Some will list the ingredients of their menu items online; others have an ingredients list available at each restaurant. Be sure to enlist the help of the restaurant's manager and chef in selecting safe foods.

Enjoy spring and continue to make smart meal choices. No matter what time of year, remember to carry your emergency treatment plan, contact numbers, and medicines (for example, antihistamines and epinephrine) at all times so that you are prepared to treat a reaction. Read the label for all foods every time, and plan ahead when possible.

Dating And Food Allergies: Do They Go Hand-In-Hand?

While dating can be exciting and fun, it can also prove to be a nerve-wracking experience—even without food allergies. Teens with food allergies just need to take a few extra precautions to ensure their safety.

Let 'em know. First and foremost, clue your date in about your food allergies. Don't feel embarrassed, or shy about it. It is important that he or she knows. John Z., a teen with peanut allergies, offers this outlook. "You gotta tell people about it, and you can't worry about what they think about it. It's either you die or you care what they think about it. And I'd rather just not care what they think about it than die, you know?"

Plan your date in advance. Chances are you will be talking with your date-to-be about the details as the day of your date gets closer. Will you be doing something that involves food? Going out to a restaurant, for example? This would be an ideal time to mention that you have a food allergy. Let your date know that you will need time to talk to the waitstaff in detail about menu choices.

Show him or her how they can help. Don't feel as if you have to go into great detail regarding symptoms you may have, but do let your date know how they will be able to tell if you are having a reaction, and what they can do to help you. Give your date an opportunity to ask you any questions he or she might have.

Here is a list of a few additional things to keep in mind:

- Even if you don't eat anything that contains a food to which you are allergic, you can still have a mild reaction from close contact with someone who does. The best situation would be for your date to avoid eating anything with that ingredient as well. If you're uncomfortable making this request, just make sure your date washes their hands thoroughly before any close contact.

- Kissing can be risky business. Mild reactions can occur with contact. If your date eats a food that you're allergic to, make sure all traces of that food have been thoroughly cleaned up before you kiss.

- No matter what your plans include, don't forget to bring your medicine along.

Camping With A Food Allergy

Whether you are planning on attending camp to participate in activities, working as a camp counselor, or just going on a weekend hiking trip with friends, here are some things to think about when you're planning your trip:

- Will you be able to bring food from home? How and where will that food be stored?

- How will you carry and store your medications?

- Will you have access to a phone at all times? How can you reach emergency help? Can you call 911, or is there another number you must call?

- If you phone for emergency help, how will people know where to locate you? Will you have a map of the area in which you'll be camping?

- Where is the nearest emergency facility? Does the ambulance carry epinephrine at all times, or must it be requested? Can the ambulance crew administer epinephrine?

- Do you have a written Emergency Health Care Plan that you will carry with you? Is the information current?

- Do those with whom you'll be camping know about your food allergy? Do they know how to help you in the event that you have a reaction?

Don't forget to check the expiration date of your medicine before your trip. Finally, consider talking with your doctor, as he or she may want to prescribe additional medicine so that you will have a back-up in case you need it.

Participating In Specialty Camps

Your middle school and high school years bring many opportunities in regards to extracurricular activities. During the summer, school clubs such as athletics, band, or drama to name just a few, may participate in special over-night camps.

✔ Quick Tip

If an allergic reaction occurs:

- don't go off to the bathroom alone;

- don't rely on asthma inhalers for a severe reaction;

- do tell a friend; and

- do get an Emergency Action Plan ready.

Source: © 2005 The Food Allergy & Anaphylaxis Network.

For someone with food allergies, these opportunities can present new challenges. If you belong to a club that offers these camps, here are some things you should consider before participating.

Talk to your parents and the camp director, as well as coaches and chaperones who will be attending the camp. Inform them of any special dietary needs you may require, and be sure they will be able to accommodate your needs.

Create an allergy emergency plan and make sure everyone knows what to do if a reaction occurs. Keep in mind that you may be working with coaches, trainers, and teachers from other schools as well. Make sure they are informed of your allergy, how to spot symptoms of an allergic reaction, and what to do should one occur.

Many sports and music camps are held on college campuses, therefore call the campus' dining services and explain your situation. Ask about ingredients and discuss safe menu options. Find out how meals are served (buffet style, individually, etc.), and if you can be served your meal before the rest of the diners as an extra precaution.

If you don't feel comfortable about eating the food prepared on campus, ask if you can store your own food somewhere in the kitchen.

Whichever you decide, carry some of your own snacks with you in case you get hungry or if a situation arises where you don't feel comfortable eating the food prepared for you.

If you are at an athletic camp where it's popular to carry water bottles, make sure yours is clearly labeled so that it is easily recognizable. This will reduce the risk of someone accidentally drinking out of yours. Try to keep your water bottle separate from those belonging to the other campers.

Carry your meds with you at all times. If you don't want to wear a hip-pack or carry a purse, create a "medicine kit" and carry it in your gym bag. Also, keep copies of insurance and pharmacy cards, as well as a list of who should be called in the event of an emergency.

Make sure that your coach, chaperone, and teammates know where to find your medicine. If you've been prescribed an EpiPen®, make sure several key people know how to use it, too.

If you carry an EpiPen® and plan to participate in outdoor activities, protect this medication from the heat by wrapping it in a towel and storing it in a small cooler. Again, make sure a coach or chaperone knows where it is at all times.

Finally, keep in mind that accidents can and do occur. If you have a reaction, don't be shy about speaking up; the sooner you get help, the better you'll feel. Afterwards, review what went wrong and how you can avoid a similar situation in the future.

Chapter 32

Will Food Proteins In Cosmetics And Bath Products Cause Allergic Reactions?

In recent years, the popularity and use of scented and "natural" bath products, aromatherapy products, and cosmetics have soared. We often do not contemplate what they are made of, and just enjoy their pleasant scents and soothing properties. However, many of these products contain extracts or oils of herbs, plants, or nuts.

Do they contain protein?

For the most part, extracts and oils contain only fat, color, and aroma components, and little or no protein. This could explain why, to date, we have not received reports of allergic reactions to these types of products. Yet you cannot always be confident that a product does not contain protein. Each product should be evaluated on an individual basis.

Ingredients such as hydrolyzed soy and wheat proteins, hops, and other plant proteins can be found in some bath and skincare products. Some products contain large quantities of food proteins. Many "volumizing" shampoos contain milk protein, to help add body to the hair. Egg proteins are sometimes used in shampoos to give more shine to the hair. These products could possibly cause a severe reaction if accidentally ingested by a milk- or egg-allergic child.

About This Chapter: "Will Food Proteins in Cosmetics and Bath Products Cause Reactions?" by Susan L. Hefle, Ph.D. © 2005 The Food Allergy & Anaphylaxis Network. All Rights Reserved. Reprinted with permission. For additional information, visit http://www.foodallergy.org or http://www.fankids.org.

Will contact cause a reaction?

We readily absorb proteins through the skin, particularly when it is wet, as skin is more soft and porous in this state. Children who suffer from atopic dermatitis often have broken and inflamed skin, through which protein can more easily be absorbed. While skin contact with food proteins in hair-care, bath, and cosmetic products will most likely cause only a mild reaction or irritation (such as hives or itching), there is the possibility that a more severe allergic reaction could occur.

What can you do?

Be sure to read all cosmetic, bath product, massage oil, and body lotion ingredient statements just as you would for a food product. If personal-sized packages of these products do not have an ingredient label, ask the store manager or cosmetic department staff to provide you with ingredient information. If you have already purchased the product, call the manufacturer's toll-free number, if one is listed on the package, and inquire about the ingredients. Cosmetic products labeled and marketed with the term "hypoallergenic" can be misleading; some may contain food proteins. Check the ingredient labels of these products very carefully.

Be cautious about trying "testers" of products in cosmetic, bath, and fragrance shops. Remember to ask specific questions about the ingredients in cosmetics when you get a makeover at a department store, another cosmetic supplier, or an at-home demonstration party. Ask your hair stylist or barber about ingredients in any new shampoo, conditioner, styling gel, or mousse he or she wishes to use. Review the labels of bath and hair products you currently have at home before using them. Remember not to share lip balms and other cosmetic products with others.

👉 Remember!

The general rule for managing food allergies is to read ingredient labels carefully. The new varieties of bath and beauty products currently on the market make it necessary for all of us to read those labels carefully, too. Consult your allergist about any allergic reaction caused by a new cosmetic, shampoo, lotion, or other body-care product.

Part 4

Allergens In The Air

Chapter 33

Are You Allergic To Something In The Air?

Introduction

Sneezing is not always the symptom of a cold. Sometimes, it is an allergic reaction to something in the air. Health experts estimate that 35 million Americans suffer from upper respiratory tract symptoms that are allergic reactions to airborne allergens. Pollen allergy, commonly called hay fever, is one of the most common chronic diseases in the United States. Worldwide, airborne allergens cause the most problems for people with allergies. The respiratory symptoms of asthma, which affect approximately 11 million Americans, are often provoked by airborne allergens.

Overall, allergic diseases are among the major causes of illness and disability in the United States, affecting as many as 40 to 50 million Americans.

The National Institute of Allergy and Infectious Diseases (NIAID) of the National Institutes of Health (an agency of the U.S. Department of Health and Human Services) supports and conducts research on allergic diseases. The goals of this research are to provide a better understanding of the causes of allergy, to improve methods for diagnosing and treating allergic reactions, and eventually to prevent allergies.

About This Chapter: From "Airborne Allergens: Something in the Air," National Institute of Allergy and Infectious Diseases (NIAID), NIH Pub. No. 03-7045, April 2003.

✎ What's It Mean?

Allergen: Substance that causes an allergic reaction.

Allergenic: Describes a substance which produces an allergic reaction.

Antibody: Molecule tailor-made by the immune system to lock onto and destroy specific germs.

Basophils: White blood cells that contribute to inflammatory reactions.

Conjunctivitis: Inflammation of the lining of the eyelid, causing red-rimmed, swollen eyes, and crusting of the eyelids.

Genes: Units of genetic material that carry the directions a cell uses to perform a specific function.

Granules: Small particles; in cells the particles typically include enzymes and other chemicals.

Immune System: A complex network of specialized cells, tissues, and organs that defends the body against attacks by disease-causing organisms.

Inflammation: An immune system process that stops the progression of disease-causing organisms.

Lymphocytes: Small white blood cells which are important parts of the immune system.

Mast Cells: Granule-containing cells found in tissue.

Molecules: The building blocks of a cell. Some examples are proteins, fats, and carbohydrates.

Organism: An individual living thing.

Perennial: Describes something that occurs throughout the year.

Rhinitis: Inflammation of the nasal passages, which can cause a runny nose.

Sinuses: Hollow air spaces located within the bones of the skull surrounding the nose.

Sputum: Matter ejected from the lungs and windpipe through the mouth.

Tissues: Groups of similar cells joined to perform the same function.

Upper Respiratory Tract: Area of the body which includes the nasal passages, mouth, and throat.

This chapter summarizes what health experts know about the causes and symptoms of allergic reactions to airborne allergens, how health care providers diagnose and treat these reactions, and what medical researchers are doing to help people who suffer from these allergies.

Why are some people allergic?

Scientists think that some people inherit a tendency to be allergic from one or both parents. This means they are more likely to have allergies. They probably, however, do not inherit a tendency to be allergic to any specific allergen. Children are more likely to develop allergies if one or both parents have allergies. In addition, exposure to allergens at times when the body's defenses are lowered or weakened, such as after a viral infection or during pregnancy, seems to contribute to developing allergies.

What is an allergic reaction?

Normally, the immune system functions as the body's defense against invading germs such as bacteria and viruses. In most allergic reactions, however, the immune system is responding to a false alarm. When an allergic person first comes into contact with an allergen, the immune system treats the allergen as an invader and gets ready to attack.

The immune system does this by generating large amounts of a type of antibody called immunoglobulin E, or IgE. Each IgE antibody is specific for one particular substance. In the case of pollen allergy, each antibody is specific for one type of pollen. For example, the immune system may produce one type of antibody to react against oak pollen and another against ragweed pollen.

The IgE molecules are special because IgE is the only type of antibody that attaches tightly to the body's mast cells, which are tissue cells, and to basophils, which are blood cells. When the allergen next encounters its specific IgE, it attaches to the antibody like a key fitting into a lock. This action signals the cell to which the IgE is attached to release (and, in some cases, to produce) powerful chemicals like histamine, which cause inflammation. These chemicals act on tissues in various parts of the body, such as the respiratory system, and cause the symptoms of allergy.

Symptoms

The signs and symptoms of airborne allergies are familiar to many.

- Sneezing, often with a runny or clogged nose

- Coughing and postnasal drip

- Itching eyes, nose, and throat

- Watering eyes

- Conjunctivitis

- "Allergic shiners" (dark circles under the eyes caused by increased blood flow near the sinuses)

- "Allergic salute" (in a child, persistent upward rubbing of the nose that causes a crease mark on the nose)

> ### ♣ It's A Fact!!
> #### What is an allergy?
>
> An allergy is a specific reaction of the body's immune system to a normally harmless substance, one that does not bother most people. People who have allergies often are sensitive to more than one substance. Types of allergens that cause allergic reactions include the following:
>
> - Pollens
> - House dust mites
> - Mold spores
> - Food
> - Latex rubber
> - Insect venom
> - Medicines

In people who are not allergic, the mucus in the nasal passages simply moves foreign particles to the throat, where they are swallowed or coughed out. But something different happens in a person who is sensitive to airborne allergens.

In sensitive people, as soon as the allergen lands on the lining inside the nose, a chain reaction occurs that leads the mast cells in these tissues to release histamine and other chemicals. The powerful chemicals contract certain cells that line some small blood vessels in the nose. This allows fluids to escape, which causes the nasal passages to swell—resulting in nasal congestion. Histamine also can cause sneezing, itching, irritation, and excess mucus production, which can result in allergic rhinitis.

Other chemicals released by mast cells, including cytokines and leukotrienes, also contribute to allergic symptoms.

Some people with allergy develop asthma, which can be a very serious condition. The symptoms of asthma include coughing, wheezing, and shortness of breath. The shortness of breath is due to a narrowing of the airways in the lungs and to excess mucus production and inflammation. Asthma can be disabling and sometimes fatal. If wheezing and shortness of breath accompany allergy symptoms, it is a signal that the airways also have become involved.

Pollen Allergy

Each spring, summer, and fall, tiny pollen grains are released from trees, weeds, and grasses. These grains hitch rides on currents of air. Although the mission of pollen is to fertilize parts of other plants, many never reach their targets. Instead, pollen enters human noses and throats, triggering a type of seasonal allergic rhinitis called pollen allergy. Many people know this as hay fever.

Of all the things that can cause an allergy, pollen is one of the most common. Many of the foods, medicines, or animals that cause allergies can be avoided to a great extent. Even insects and household dust are escapable. But short of staying indoors, with the windows closed, when the pollen count is high—and even that may not help—there is no easy way to avoid airborne pollen.

♣ It's A Fact!!
Is it an allergy or a cold?

There is no good way to tell the difference between allergy symptoms of runny nose, coughing, and sneezing and cold symptoms. Allergy symptoms, however, may last longer than cold symptoms. Anyone who has any respiratory illness that lasts longer than a week or two should consult a health care provider.

What is pollen?

Plants produce tiny—too tiny to see with the naked eye—round or oval pollen grains to reproduce. In some species, the plant uses the pollen from its own flowers to fertilize itself. Other types must be cross-pollinated. Cross-pollination means that for fertilization to take place and seeds to form, pollen must be transferred from the flower of one plant to that of another of the same species. Insects do this job for certain flowering plants, while other plants rely on wind for transport.

The types of pollen that most commonly cause allergic reactions are produced by the plain-looking plants (trees, grasses, and weeds) that do not have showy flowers. These plants make small, light, dry pollen grains that are custom-made for wind transport.

Amazingly, scientists have collected samples of ragweed pollen 400 miles out at sea and two miles high in the air. Because airborne pollen can drift for many miles, it does little good to rid an area of an offending plant. In addition, most allergenic pollen comes from plants that produce it in huge quantities. For example, a single ragweed plant can generate a million grains of pollen a day.

The type of allergens in the pollen is the main factor that determines whether the pollen is likely to cause hay fever. For example, pine tree pollen is produced in large amounts by a common tree, which would make it a good candidate for causing allergy. It is, however, a relatively rare cause of allergy because the type of allergens in pine pollen appear to make it less allergenic. In addition, because pine pollen is heavy, it tends to fall straight down from the tree and does not scatter in the wind, rarely reaching human noses.

Among North American plants, weeds are the most prolific producers of allergenic pollen. Ragweed is the major culprit, but other important sources are sagebrush, redroot pigweed, lamb's quarters, Russian thistle (tumbleweed), and English plantain.

Grasses and trees, too, are important sources of allergenic pollens. Although more than 1,000 species of grass grow in North America, only a few produce highly allergenic pollen.

It is common to hear people say they are allergic to colorful or scented flowers like roses. In fact, only florists, gardeners, and others who have prolonged, close contact with flowers are likely to be sensitive to pollen from these plants. Most people have little contact with the large, heavy, waxy pollen grains of such flowering plants because this type of pollen is not carried by wind but by insects such as butterflies and bees.

When do plants make pollen?

One of the most obvious features of pollen allergy is its seasonal nature—people have symptoms only when the pollen grains to which they are allergic are in the air. Each plant has a pollinating period that is more or less the same from year to year. Exactly when a plant starts to pollinate seems to depend on the relative length of night and day—and therefore on geographical location—rather than on the weather. On the other hand, weather conditions during pollination can affect the amount of pollen produced and distributed in a specific year. Thus, in the Northern Hemisphere, the farther north you go, the later the start of the pollinating period and the later the start of the allergy season.

A pollen count, familiar to many people from local weather reports, is a measure of how much pollen is in the air. This count represents the concentration of all the pollen (or of one particular type, like ragweed) in the air in a certain area at a specific time. It is shown in grains of pollen per square meter of air collected over 24 hours. Pollen counts tend to be the highest early in the morning on warm, dry, breezy days and lowest during chilly, wet periods. Although the pollen count is an approximate measure that changes, it is useful as a general guide for when it may be wise to stay indoors and avoid contact with the pollen.

Mold Allergy

What is mold?

There are thousands of types of molds and yeasts in the fungus family. Yeasts are single cells that divide to form clusters. Molds are made of many cells that grow as branching threads called hyphae. Although both can probably cause allergic reactions, only a small number of molds are widely recognized offenders.

The seeds or reproductive pieces of fungi are called spores. Spores differ in size, shape, and color among types of mold. Each spore that germinates can give rise to new mold growth, which in turn can produce millions of spores.

What is mold allergy?

When inhaled, tiny fungal spores, or sometimes pieces of fungi, may cause allergic rhinitis. Because they are so small, mold spores also can reach the lungs.

> ♣ **It's A Fact!!**
> There is no relationship between a respiratory allergy to the mold *Penicillium* and an allergy to the drug penicillin, which is made from mold.

In a small number of people, symptoms of mold allergy may be brought on or worsened by eating certain foods such as cheeses processed with fungi. Occasionally, mushrooms, dried fruits, and foods containing yeast, soy sauce, or vinegar will produce allergy symptoms.

Where do molds grow?

Molds can be found wherever there is moisture, oxygen, and a source of the few other chemicals they need. In the fall, they grow on rotting logs and fallen leaves, especially in moist, shady areas. In gardens they can be found in compost piles and on certain grasses and weeds. Some molds attach to grains such as wheat, oats, barley, and corn, which makes farms, grain bins, and silos likely places to find mold.

Hot spots of mold growth in the home include damp basements and closets, bathrooms (especially shower stalls), places where fresh food is stored, refrigerator drip trays, house plants, air conditioners, humidifiers, garbage pails, mattresses, upholstered furniture, and old foam rubber pillows.

Molds also like bakeries, breweries, barns, dairies, and greenhouses. Loggers, mill workers, carpenters, furniture repairers, and upholsterers often work in moldy environments.

What molds are allergenic?

Like pollens, mold spores are important airborne allergens only if they are abundant, easily carried by air currents, and allergenic in their chemical makeup. Found almost everywhere, mold spores in some areas are so numerous they often outnumber the pollens in the air. Fortunately, however, only a few dozen different types are significant allergens.

In general, *Alternaria* and *Cladosporium* (*Hormodendrum*) are the molds most commonly found both indoors and outdoors in the United States. *Aspergillus, Penicillium, Helminthosporium, Epicoccum, Fusarium, Mucor, Rhizopus,* and *Aureobasidium* (*Pullularia*) are common as well.

Are mold counts helpful?

Similar to pollen counts, mold counts may suggest the types and number of fungi present at a certain time and place. For several reasons, however, these counts probably cannot be used as a constant guide for daily activities.

One reason is that the number and types of spores actually present in the mold count may have changed considerably in 24 hours because weather and spore distribution are directly related. Many common allergenic molds are of the dry spore type. They release their spores during dry, windy weather. Other fungi need high humidity, fog, or dew to release their spores. Although rain washes many larger spores out of the air, it also causes some smaller spores to be propelled into the air.

In addition to the effect of weather changes during 24-hour periods on mold counts, spore populations may also differ between day and night. Dry spore types are usually released during daytime, and wet spore types are usually released at night.

Are there other mold-related disorders?

Fungi or organisms related to them may cause other health problems similar to allergic diseases. Some kinds of *Aspergillus* may cause several different illnesses, including both infections and allergies. These fungi may lodge in the airways or a distant part of the lung and grow until they form a compact sphere known as a "fungus ball." In people with lung damage or serious underlying illnesses, *Aspergillus* may grasp the opportunity to invade the lungs or the whole body.

In some people, exposure to these fungi also can lead to asthma or to a lung disease resembling severe inflammatory asthma called allergic bronchopulmonary aspergillosis. This latter condition, which occurs only in a small number of people with asthma, causes wheezing, low-grade fever, and coughing up of brown-flecked masses or mucus plugs. Skin testing, blood tests, x-rays, and examination of the sputum for fungi can help establish the diagnosis. Corticosteroid drugs usually treat this reaction effectively. Immunotherapy (allergy shots) is not helpful.

Dust Mite Allergy

Dust mite allergy is an allergy to a microscopic organism that lives in the dust found in all dwellings and workplaces. House dust, as well as some house furnishings, contains microscopic mites. Dust mites are perhaps the most common cause of perennial allergic rhinitis. House dust mite allergy usually produces symptoms similar to pollen allergy and also can produce symptoms of asthma.

House dust mites, which live in bedding, upholstered furniture, and carpets, thrive in summer and die in winter. In a warm, humid house, however, they continue to thrive even in the coldest months. The particles seen floating in a shaft of sunlight include dead dust mites and their waste products. These waste products, which are proteins, actually provoke the allergic reaction.

What is house dust?

Rather than a single substance, so-called house dust is a varied mixture of potentially allergenic materials. It may contain fibers from different types of fabrics and materials. The following list provides some examples:

- Cotton lint, feathers, and other stuffing materials
- Dander from cats, dogs, and other animals
- Bacteria

- Mold and fungus spores (especially in damp areas)

- Food particles

- Bits of plants and insects

- Other allergens peculiar to an individual house or building

Cockroaches are commonly found in crowded cities and in the southern United States. Certain proteins in cockroach feces and saliva also can be found in house dust. These proteins can cause allergic reactions or trigger asthma symptoms in some people, especially children. Cockroach allergens likely play a significant role in causing asthma in many inner-city populations.

Animal Allergy

Household pets are the most common source of allergic reactions to animals.

Many people think that pet allergy is provoked by the fur of cats and dogs. Researchers have found, however, that the major allergens are proteins in the saliva. These proteins stick to the fur when the animal licks itself.

Urine is also a source of allergy-causing proteins, as is the skin. When the substance carrying the proteins dries, the proteins can then float into the air. Cats may be more likely than dogs to cause allergic reactions because hey lick themselves more, may be held more, and spend more time in the house, close to humans.

Some rodents, such as guinea pigs and gerbils, have become increasingly popular as household pets. They, too, can cause allergic reactions in some people, as can mice and rats. Urine is the major source of allergens from these animals.

Allergies to animals can take two years or more to develop and may not decrease until six months or more after ending contact with the animal. Carpet and furniture are a reservoir for pet allergens, and the allergens can remain in them for four to six weeks. In addition, these allergens can stay in household air for months after the animal has been removed. Therefore, it is wise for people with an animal allergy to check with the landlord or previous owner to find out if furry pets lived on the premises.

Diagnosis

People with allergy symptoms—such as the runny nose of allergic rhinitis—say at first suspect they have a cold, but the "cold" lingers on. Testing for allergies is the best way to find out if a person is allergic.

Skin Tests

Allergists (doctors who specialize in allergic diseases) use skin tests to determine whether a person has IgE antibodies in the skin that react to a specific allergen. The allergist will use weakened extracts from allergens such as dust mites, pollens, or molds commonly found in the local area. The extract of each kind of allergen is injected under a person's skin or is applied to a tiny scratch or puncture made on the arm or back.

Skin tests are one way of measuring the level of IgE antibody in a person. With a positive reaction, a small, raised, reddened area, called a wheal (hive), with a surrounding flush, called a flare, will appear at the test site. The size of the wheal can give the doctor an important diagnostic clue, but a positive reaction does not prove that a particular allergen is the cause of symptoms. Although such a reaction indicates that IgE antibody to a specific allergen is present, respiratory symptoms do not necessarily result.

♣ It's A Fact!!
Chemical Sensitivity

Some people report that they react to chemicals in their environments and that these allergy-like reactions seem to result from exposure to a wide variety of synthetic and natural substances. Such substances can include those found in many products, including the following:

- Paints
- Carpeting
- Plastics
- Perfumes
- Cigarette smoke
- Plants

Although the symptoms may resemble those of allergies, sensitivity to chemicals does not represent a true allergic reaction involving IgE and the release of histamine or other chemicals. Rather than a reaction to an allergen, it is a reaction to a chemical irritant, which may affect people with allergies more than others.

Blood Tests

Skin testing is the most sensitive and least costly way to identify allergies. People with widespread skin conditions like eczema, however, should not be tested using this method.

There are other diagnostic tests that use a blood sample to detect levels of IgE antibody to a particular allergen. One such blood test is called the radioallergosorbent test (RAST), which can be performed when eczema is present or if a person has taken medicines that interfere with skin testing.

Prevention

Avoid Pollen And Molds

Complete avoidance of allergenic pollen or mold means moving to a place where the offending substance does not grow and where it is not present in the air. Even this extreme solution may offer only temporary relief because a person sensitive to a specific pollen or mold may develop allergies to new allergens after repeated exposure to them. For example, people allergic to ragweed may leave their ragweed-ridden communities and relocate to areas where ragweed does not grow, only to develop allergies to other weeds or even to grasses or trees in their new surroundings. Because relocating is not a reliable solution, allergy specialists do not encourage this approach.

There are other ways to reduce exposure to offending pollens.

- Remain indoors with the windows closed in the morning, for example, when the outdoor pollen levels are highest. Sunny, windy days can be especially troublesome.

- Wear a face mask designed to filter pollen out of the air and keep it from reaching nasal passages, if you must work outdoors.

- Take your vacation at the height of the expected pollinating period and choose a location where such exposure would be minimal.

Vacationing at the seashore or on a cruise, for example, may be effective retreats for avoiding pollen allergies.

Avoid House Dust

If you have dust mite allergy, pay careful attention to dust-proofing your bedroom. The worst things to have in the bedroom include these items:

- Wall-to-wall carpet

- Blinds

- Down-filled blankets

- Feather pillows

- Stuffed animals

- Heating vents with forced hot air

- Dogs and cats

- Closets full of clothing

> ✔ **Quick Tip**
>
> **Pets**
>
> If you are allergic to furry pets, especially cats, the best way to avoid allergic reactions is to find them another home. If you are like most people who are attached to their pets, that is usually not a desirable option. There are ways, however, to help lower the levels of animal allergens in the air, which may reduce allergic reactions.
>
> - Bathe your cat weekly and brush it more frequently (ideally, a non-allergic person should do this).
> - Keep cats out of your bedroom.
> - Remove carpets and soft furnishings, which collect animal allergens.
> - Use a vacuum cleaner and room air cleaners with HEPA filters.
> - Wear a face mask while house and cat cleaning.

Carpets trap dust and make dust control impossible.

- Shag carpets are the worst type of carpet for people who are sensitive to dust mites.

- Vacuuming doesn't get rid of dust mite proteins in furniture and carpeting, but redistributes them back into the room, unless the vacuum has a special HEPA (high-efficiency particulate air) filter.

- Rugs on concrete floors encourage dust mite growth.

If possible, replace wall-to-wall carpets with washable throw rugs over hardwood, tile, or linoleum floors, and wash the rugs frequently.

Reducing the amount of dust mites in your home may mean new cleaning techniques as well as some changes in furnishings to eliminate dust collectors. Water is often the secret to effective dust removal.

- Clean washable items, including throw rugs, often, using water hotter than 130 degrees Fahrenheit. Lower temperatures will not kill dust mites.

- Clean washable items at a commercial establishment that uses high water temperature, if you cannot or do not want to set water temperature in your home at 130 degrees. (There is a danger of getting scalded if the water is more than 120 degrees.)

- Dust frequently with a damp cloth or oiled mop.

If cockroaches are a problem in your home, the U.S. Environmental Protection Agency suggests some ways to get rid of them:

- Do not leave food or garbage out.

- Store food in airtight containers.

- Clean all food crumbs or spilled liquids right away.

- Try using poison baits, boric acid (for cockroaches), or traps first, before using pesticide sprays.

If you use pesticide sprays, take the following precautions:

- Do not spray in food preparation or storage areas.

- Do not spray in areas where children play or sleep.

- Limit the spray to the infested area.

- Follow instructions on the label carefully.

- Make sure there is plenty of fresh air when you spray.

- Keep the person with allergies or asthma out of the room while spraying.

✔ **Quick Tip**

Some Ways to Handle Airborne Allergies

- Avoid the allergen
- Take medicine
- Get allergy shots

Avoid Chemical Irritants

Irritants such as chemicals can worsen airborne allergy symptoms, and you should avoid them as much as possible. For example, if you have pollen allergy, avoid unnecessary exposure to irritants such as insect sprays, tobacco smoke, air pollution, and fresh tar or paint during periods of high pollen levels.

Use Air Conditioners And Appropriate Air Filters

When possible, use air conditioners inside your home or car to help prevent pollen and mold allergens from entering. Various types of air-filtering devices made with fiberglass or electrically charged plates may help reduce allergens produced in the home. You can add these to your present heating and cooling system. In addition, portable devices that can be used in individual rooms are especially helpful in reducing animal allergens.

An allergist can suggest which kind of filter is best for your home. Before buying a filtering device, rent one and use it in a closed room (the bedroom, for instance) for a month or two to see whether your allergy symptoms diminish. The airflow should be sufficient to exchange the air in the room five or six times per hour. Therefore, the size and efficiency of the filtering device should be determined in part by the size of the room.

You should be wary of exaggerated claims for appliances that cannot really clean the air. Very small air cleaners cannot remove dust and pollen. No air purifier can prevent viral or bacterial diseases such as the flu, pneumonia, or tuberculosis.

Before buying an electrostatic precipitator, you should compare the machine's ozone output with Federal standards. Ozone can irritate the noses and airways of people with allergies, especially those with asthma, and can increase their allergy symptoms. Other kinds of air filters, such as HEPA filters, do not release ozone into the air. HEPA filters, however, require adequate air flow to force air through them.

Treatment

Medicines

If you cannot adequately avoid airborne allergens, your symptoms often can be controlled by medicines. You can buy medicines without a prescription that can relieve allergy symptoms. If, however, they don't give you relief or they cause unwanted side effects such as sleepiness, your health care provider can prescribe antihistamines and topical nasal steroids. You can use either medicine alone or together.

Antihistamines: As the name indicates, an antihistamine counters the effects of histamine, which is released by the mast cells in your body's tissues and contributes to your allergy symptoms. For many years, antihistamines have proven useful in relieving itching in the nose and eyes; sneezing; and in reducing nasal swelling and drainage.

Many people who take antihistamines have some distressing side effects such as drowsiness and loss of alertness and coordination. Adults may interpret such reactions in children as behavior problems.

Antihistamines that cause fewer of these side effects are available over-the-counter or by prescription. These non-sedating antihistamines are as effective as other antihistamines in preventing histamine-induced symptoms, but most do so without causing sleepiness.

Topical Nasal Steroids: You should not confuse topical nasal steroids with anabolic steroids, which athletes sometimes use to enlarge muscle mass and which can have serious side effects. The chemicals in nasal steroids are different from those in anabolic steroids.

Topical nasal steroids are anti-inflammatory medicines that stop the allergic reaction. In addition to other helpful actions, they decrease the number of mast cells in the nose and reduce mucus secretion and nasal swelling. The combination of antihistamines and nasal steroids is a very effective way to treat allergic rhinitis, especially if you have moderate or severe allergic rhinitis.

Although topical nasal steroids can have side effects, they are safe when used at recommended doses.

Cromolyn Sodium: Cromolyn sodium is a nasal spray that in some people helps prevent allergic rhinitis from starting. When used as a nasal spray, it can safely stop the release of chemicals like histamine from mast cells. It has few side effects when used as directed and significantly helps some people manage their allergies.

Decongestants: Sometimes helping the nasal passages to drain away mucus will help relieve symptoms such as congestion, swelling, excess secretions, and discomfort in the sinus areas that can be caused by nasal allergies. Your doctor may recommend using oral or nasal decongestants to reduce congestion along with an antihistamine to control allergic symptoms.

You should not, however, use over-the-counter or prescription decongestant nose drops and sprays for more than a few days. When used for longer periods, these medicines can lead to even more congestion and swelling of the nasal passages. Because of recent concern about the bad effects of decongestant sprays and drops, some have been removed from store shelves.

Immunotherapy

Immunotherapy, or a series of allergy shots, is the only available treatment that has a chance of reducing your allergy symptoms over a longer period of time. You would receive subcutaneous (under the skin) injections of increasing concentrations of the allergen(s) to which you are sensitive. These injections reduce the level of IgE antibodies in the blood and cause the body to make a protective antibody called IgG.

About 85 percent of people with allergic rhinitis will see their hay fever symptoms and need for medicines drop significantly within 12 months of starting immunotherapy. Those who benefit from allergy shots may continue it for three years and then consider stopping. While many are able to stop the injections with good results lasting for several years, others do get worse after the shots are stopped.

One research study shows that children treated for allergic rhinitis with immunotherapy were less likely to develop asthma. Researchers need to study this further, however.

As researchers produce better allergens for immunotherapy, this technique will be become an even more effective treatment.

Allergy Research

Research on allergies is focused on understanding what happens to the human body during the allergic process—the sequence of events leading to the allergic response and the factors responsible for allergic diseases.

Scientists supported by the National Institute of Allergy and Infectious Diseases (NIAID) found that, during the first years of their lives, children raised in a house with two or more dogs or cats may be less likely to develop allergic diseases as compared with children raised without pets. The striking finding here is that high pet exposure early in life appears to protect some children from not only pet allergy but also other types of common allergies, such as allergy to house dust mites, ragweed, and grass. This new finding is changing the way scientists think about pet exposure. Scientists must now figure out how pet exposure causes a general shift of the immune system away from an allergic response.

The results of this and a number of other studies suggest that bacteria carried by pets may be responsible for holding back the immune system's allergic response. These bacteria release molecules called endotoxin. Some researchers think endotoxin is the molecule responsible for shifting the developing immune system away from responding to allergens through a class of lymphocytes called Th-2 cells. (These cells are associated with allergic reactions.) Instead, endotoxin may stimulate the immune system to block allergic reactions.

If scientists can find out exactly what it is about pets or the bacteria they carry that prevents the allergic response, they might be able to develop a new allergy treatment.

Some studies are seeking better ways to diagnose as well as treat people with allergic diseases and to better understand the factors that regulate IgE production to reduce the allergic response. Several research institutions are focusing on ways to influence the cells that participate in the allergic response.

NIAID supports a network of Asthma, Allergic and Immunologic Diseases Cooperative Research Centers throughout the United States. The centers encourage close coordination among scientists studying basic and clinical immunology, genetics, biochemistry, pharmacology, and environmental science. This interdisciplinary approach helps move research knowledge as quickly as possible from the lab into the hands of doctors and their allergy patients.

Educating patients and health care providers is an important tool in controlling allergic diseases. All of these research centers conduct and evaluate education programs focused on methods to control allergic diseases.

Since 1991, researchers participating in NIAID's Inner-City Asthma Study have been examining ways to treat asthma in minority children living in inner-city environments. Asthma, a major cause of illness and hospitalizations among these children, is provoked by a number of possible factors, including allergies to airborne substances.

The success of NIAID's model asthma program led the U.S. Centers for Disease Control and Prevention to award grants to help community-based health organizations throughout the United States implement the program.

Based on the success of the first National Cooperative Inner-City Asthma Study, NIAID and the National Institute of Environmental Health Sciences, also part of NIH, started a second cooperative multicenter study in 1996. This study recruited children with asthma, aged 4 to 11, to test the effectiveness of two interventions. One intervention uses a novel communication and doctor education system. Information about the children's asthma severity is provided to their primary care physicians, with the intent that this information will help the doctors give the children the best care possible.

The other intervention involves educating families about reducing exposure to passive cigarette smoke and to indoor allergens, including cockroach, house dust mite, and mold. Researchers are assessing the effectiveness of both interventions by evaluating their capacity to reduce the severity of asthma in these children.

Early data show that by reducing allergen levels in children's beds by one-third, investigators reduced by nearly one-quarter (22 percent) both the number of days the children wheezed and the number of days the children missed school.

Although several factors provoke allergic responses, scientists know that heredity plays a major role in determining who will develop an allergy. Therefore, scientists are trying to identify and describe the genes that make a person susceptible to allergic diseases.

Because researchers are becoming increasingly aware of the role of environmental factors in allergies, they are evaluating ways to control environmental exposures to allergens and pollutants to prevent allergic disease.

These studies offer the promise of improving the treatment and control of allergic diseases and the hope that one day allergic diseases will be preventable.

Chapter 34

Pollen Allergies

What Is Hay Fever?

Hay fever is the name given to pollen allergy. Other terms for hay fever include "seasonal allergic rhinitis" or "pollinosis." If you have hay fever, you are not alone. An estimated 26.1 million Americans have hay fever symptoms each year. 14.6 million Americans have asthma, which can often accompany hay fever.

How Hay Fever Occurs

Anyone can develop an allergy to a common substance, but those who do usually have inherited the tendency as a family trait. The sensitivity is developed after exposure to the substance. Hay fever is a good example of this process.

During the seasons when plants are pollinating, everyone in the surrounding area is exposed. People with allergic tendency may develop sensitivity to any one or more of the pollens, although certain pollens are more likely to cause an allergic reaction than others.

About This Chapter: This chapter begins with text from "Facts about Hay Fever," reprinted with permission; © 2005 American Lung Association. For more information about the American Lung Association or to support the work it does, call 1-800-LUNG-USA (1-800-586-4872) or log on to www.lungusa.org. "Questions And Answers About Pollen Allergy" is from a fact sheet produced by the National Institute of Allergy and Infectious Diseases, updated March 2005.

Pollens that are light enough to be wind-borne are what cause the problem for most hay-fever sufferers. Heavier pollens that are carried from plant to plant by bees and by other insects can also be allergens, but they cause trouble only when a person comes into direct contact with the plant. Airborne pollens can penetrate anywhere, indoors and out, and are most numerous at the height of the pollinating season for the particular plant.

What Are The Symptoms For Hay Fever?

Sneezing that is repeated and prolonged is the most common mark of the hay fever sufferer. A stuffy and watery nose is also a main sign of hay fever. Other symptoms include redness, swelling and itching of the eyes; itching of the nose, throat and mouth and itching of the ears, or other ear problems. Breathing difficulties at night due to obstruction of the nose may interfere with sleep.

These symptoms differ in degree according to the individual, ranging from mild to severe. When severe, they are very uncomfortable, make it difficult to carry out daily tasks, and may cause loss of time from work and school.

Health complications from repeated hay fever attacks, year after year, may be an even more serious problem. Chronic sinusitis—inflammation of the sinus cavities—is one of these problems. Another is nasal polyps, or growths. In addition, a significant percentage of people with hay fever have or develop asthma.

The Seasons For Hay Fever

The "hay fever season" can be a different time of year for different people. In part, this is because trees, grasses, and weeds produce pollens during different seasons. For example, people in the eastern and Midwestern United States who are sensitive to tree pollen may suffer in the early spring when trees such as elm, maple, birch and poplar are producing pollen. People who are sensitive to pollens produced by grasses may suffer in the late spring, and early summer, the time when most grasses are pollinating. About half of all hay fever sufferers are sensitive to grass pollens.

Weeds flourish in most parts of the country from midsummer to late fall. In the late fall, ragweed is the most common problem. In fact, ragweed is the plant that causes the most hay fever. But an individual may react to one or more pollens in more than one of these groups, so the person's "season" may be from early spring to the first frost.

For that matter, people who are sensitive to dust, to dog or cat dander (tiny scales or particles that fall off hair, feathers, or skin) or to other some other airborne material that they cannot protect themselves from may suffer all year round.

Mold and fungus spores ("seeds"), also airborne during the summer and fall months, cause reactions in many people. Frequently found around hay, straw, and dead leaves, their growth is encouraged by humid weather and by places with poor air circulation—damp basements for instance.

Sensitivity And How It Works

"Sensitivity" is the term used to describe the process by which you develop an allergy. Sensitivity is established when the tissues that form antibodies (lymphoid tissues) are stimulated to make specialized antibodies to otherwise harmless pollens, spores, etc. These antibodies fix to other specialized cells throughout the body that contain powerful defensive substances such as histamine. When the individual next is exposed to the pollen (as in the nose, for instance), the antibodies trigger the cells to secrete their defensive substances. This in turn causes the dilation of blood vessels, increased secretions of fluids, swelling of tissues, itching, sneezing, and other reactions that add up to hay fever.

The inflammation and other symptoms—while real enough—actually are not of the same destructive nature as those carried by more serious diseases. Removing the cause of the reaction results in immediate relief.

How To Control Hay Fever

Avoiding the substance that causes a reaction is the best way to control hay fever. Moving to a different part of the country is sometimes suggested, but taking this drastic and expensive step may prove useless if the person has or develops sensitivity to a substance common in the new location.

Using air conditioning and air purifying devices may help cut down on suffering during the hay fever season, so that normal sleep and work are

possible. Dust masks should be used during outdoor work if the work cannot be avoided.

Antihistamines—drugs that counteract the histamine released by the
allergen-antibody reaction (see "Sensitivity And How It Works," previous
section)—usually serve to give relief from some symptoms. Decongestants
may help, as well. However, they don't affect the underlying sensitivity.
Each individual has to depend on his or her doctor to find out what drug or
combination of drugs works best.

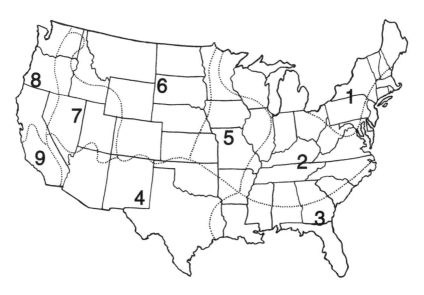

Figure 34.1. When do allergy causing pollens bloom in your backyard?

Area	Ragweed	Trees	Grasses
1	July–September	February–June	May–November
2	August–September	March–June	June–November
3	August–October	April–June	May–September
4	July–October	March–July	May–November
5	August–October	March–June	May–October
6	June–November	January–July	April–November
7	June–September	January–April	April–October
8	June–November	March–June	May–October
9	August–September	March–June	May–August

Over-the-counter nose sprays are usually of limited value and their prolonged use may actually cause symptoms or make them worse. Inhaled steroids are often effective and may be prescribed by a doctor. Specific desensitizing injections are a commonly used treatment.

Questions And Answers About Pollen Allergy

Do pollen allergies occur only in the spring?

No. Pollen grains can be dispersed into the air in the spring, summer and fall, depending on the type of tree, grass or weed. For example, ragweed is a common cause of pollen allergy reactions in the fall. In mild climates, some plants pollinate in the winter as well.

Why are some people allergic to pollen while others are not?

People inherit a tendency to be allergic, meaning an increased likelihood of being allergic to one or more allergens (such as pollen), although they probably do not inherit a tendency to be allergic to any specific allergens. Children are much more likely to develop allergies if their parents have allergies, even if only one parent is allergic. Exposure to allergens at certain times when the body's defenses are lowered or weakened, such as after a viral infection or during pregnancy, also seems to contribute to the development of allergies.

Which trees and grasses produce the most allergens?

Plain-looking trees, grasses and weeds, which do not have showy flowers, produce the types of pollen that most commonly cause allergic reactions. These plants manufacture small, light, dry pollen granules that are custom-made for wind transport. Although most allergenic pollen comes from plants that produce it in huge quantities, it's the chemical makeup of the pollen that determines whether it is likely to cause hay fever.

Where can I get information on the pollen count where I live?

The National Allergy Bureau monitors pollen counts in many locations throughout the United States. Their phone number for pollen counts is 1-800-9-POLLEN.

Table 34.1. Pollens in the United States

In the United States, the following trees, grasses and weeds can cause significant allergic reactions. The intensity of pollens varies within broad geographic areas and by season.

Grasses	Trees	Weeds
Bermuda	Alder	Burroweed
Blue	Ash	Greasewood
Brome	Australian Pine	Hemps
Canary	Beech	Marsh Elder
Johnson	Birch	Burweed and Rough
Orchard	Box Elder	Mugworts
Red Top	Cedar, Mountain	Nettle
Rye	and Red Cypress	Pigweeds (Amaranths)
Salt	Arizona and Bald Elm	Plantain
Sudan	Hackberry	Poverty Weed
Sweet Vernal	Hazelnut	Rabbit Bush
Wild Oats	Hickories	Ragweeds
	Juniper	Russian Thistle
	Maples	Sages
	Mulberry	Sagebrush
	Oak	Shadscale
	Olive	Sheep (Red) Sorrel
	Osage Orange	Smotherwood
	Palm	Sugarbeet
	Paper Mulberry	
	Poplar	
	Sweet Gum	
	Sycamore	
	Walnut	
	Willow	

Reference: Solomon WR and Matthews KP, Aerobiology and Inhalant Allergies. In: Middleton E, Reed CE, Ellis EF, eds. *Allergy: Principles and Practice*, vol. 2; 2nd edition. St. Louis, MO: Mosby, 1983; 1143–1202.

Source: "Pollens in the United States," National Institute of Allergy and Infectious Diseases, April 2003.

What time of day and weather conditions are worst for people with pollen allergy?

Generally, pollen is most abundant in the early morning, especially between 5:00 a.m. and 10:00 a.m. Other considerations, however, also determine exposure, such as wind velocity. Also, rain can wash pollen out of the air for a time, and some plants may not pollinate in damp weather.

How can I get tested to find out if I have pollen allergy?

A doctor can use a skin test to see if you will react to specific pollen allergens. A diluted extract is injected under the patient's skin or is applied to a tiny scratch or puncture made on the arm or back. Skin testing is the most common method used to test for allergic reactions. Blood tests are also available to determine if you have a pollen allergy.

What are the best treatments for pollen allergy?

The best treatment for pollen allergy is to avoid coming into contact with pollen. Because that is usually not possible, certain medications can control allergic reactions in most people. Several oral antihistamine medications are available over-the-counter or by a doctor's prescription. Topical nasal steroid sprays are anti-inflammatory drugs that stop the allergic rhinitis. Using a combination of antihistamines and nasal steroids can effectively treat allergic symptoms, especially in people with moderate or severe allergic symptoms.

Cromolyn sodium, a nasal spray, helps prevent allergic reactions from starting. It significantly helps some people with allergies.

Oral and nasal decongestants reduce congestion sometimes caused by the allergic reaction. Doctors sometimes recommend their use along with an antihistamine which controls the allergic symptoms. Nose drops and sprays, however, should not be used for more than a few days at a time because they can lead to even more congestion and swelling of the nasal passages.

Allergy drugs make me sleepy. Is there anything I can take that won't do that?

There are several non-sedating antihistamines on the market that are available with a doctor's prescription.

♣ It's A Fact!!

What is the pollen count?

The pollen count tells us how many grains of plant pollen were in a certain amount of air (often one cubic meter) during a set period of time (usually 24 hours). Pollen is a very fine powder released by trees, weeds and grasses. It is carried to another plant of the same kind, to fertilize the forerunner of new seeds. This is called pollination.

The pollen of some plants is carried from plant to plant by bees and other insects. These plants usually have brightly colored flowers and sweet scents to attract insects. They seldom cause allergic reactions. Other plants rely on the wind to carry pollen from plant to plant. These plants have small, drab flowers and little scent. These are the plants that cause most allergic reactions, or hay fever.

When conditions are right, a plant starts to pollinate. Weather affects how much pollen is carried in the air each year, but it has less effect on when pollination occurs. As a rule, weeds pollinate in late summer and fall. The weed that causes 75 percent of all hay fever is ragweed which has numerous species. One ragweed plant is estimated to produce up to 1 billion pollen grains. Other weeds that cause allergic reactions are cocklebur, lamb's quarters, plantain, pigweed, tumbleweed or Russian thistle and sagebrush.

Trees pollinate in late winter and spring. Ash, beech, birch, cedar, cottonwood, box, elder, elm, hickory, maple and oak pollen can trigger allergies.

Grasses pollinate in late spring and summer. Those that cause allergic reactions include Kentucky bluegrass, timothy, Johnson, Bermuda, redtop, orchard, rye and sweet vernal grasses.

Much pollen is released early in the morning, shortly after dawn. This results in high counts near the source plants. Pollen travels best on warm, dry, breezy days and peaks in urban areas midday. Pollen counts are lowest during chilly, wet periods.

Source: Excerpted from "Pollen and Mold Counts," reprinted with permission from the Asthma and Allergy Foundation of America, © 2005. All rights reserved.

Can I take shots to get rid of my pollen allergy?

Immunotherapy, or a series of allergy shots, is the only available treatment that has a chance of reducing allergy symptoms over the long term. About 80 percent of people with hay fever will have a significant reduction in their symptoms and in their need for medication within 12 months of starting allergy shots.

Do air filters help?

Various types of air-filtering devices made with fiberglass or electrically charged plates may help reduce pollen allergens. An allergy specialist can suggest which kind of filter is best for your home.

Should I consider moving to another geographic area where I would have less exposure to the trees, grasses, etc., that I am allergic to?

Most people who relocate to get away from the pollens that cause their allergic symptoms find that they eventually develop allergies to the plant pollens in the new area. In addition, other airborne allergens, such as dust or mold, in the new area also might cause allergic rhinitis in a person. Therefore, doctors usually do not recommend that their patients move.

What new treatments and vaccines are being studied?

New treatments under investigation include anti-IgE, a compound designed to block IgE antibodies, which are produced in massive quantities by allergic individuals. Researchers also are exploring the use of agents designed to antagonize other molecules that participate in allergic reactions. An exciting area of vaccine research involves the use of DNA encoding allergy-inducing substances. Other researchers are developing allergy vaccines composed of molecularly modified allergens.

Has the number of individuals with allergies been increasing in recent years?

There are very little data available on this issue. Some researchers hypothesize that environmental pollutants can stimulate the immune system in such a way as to make people more vulnerable to allergies. Still, there is insufficient evidence at this time to say that allergies have truly increased within the population. This question requires additional study. Any increase in new commercial products, anecdotal stories, etc., does not necessarily mean that there is a scientifically proven increase in the rate of allergies.

👉 Remember!!

Avoiding exposure to pollen is the best way to decrease allergic symptoms.

- Remain indoors in the morning when outdoor pollen levels are highest.

- Wear face masks designed to filter out pollen if you must be outdoors.

- Keep windows closed and use the air conditioner if possible in the house and car.

- Do not dry clothes outdoors.

- Avoid unnecessary exposure to other environmental irritants such as insect sprays, tobacco smoke, air pollution, and fresh tar or paint.

- Avoid mowing the grass or doing other yard work, if possible.

Source: National Institute of Allergy and Infectious Diseases, 2005.

Chapter 35

Allergies To Mold

If you have an allergy that never ends when seasons change, you may be allergic to the spores of molds or other fungi. Molds live everywhere, and disturbing a mold source can disperse the spores into the air.

What is mold allergy?

Mold and mildew are fungi. They differ from plants or animals in how they reproduce and grow. The "seeds," called spores, are spread by the wind outdoors and by air indoors. Some spores are released in dry, windy weather. Others are released with the fog or dew when humidity is high.

Inhaling the spores causes allergic reactions in some people. Allergic symptoms from fungus spores are most common from July to late summer. But with fungi growing in so many places, allergic reactions can occur year round.

Although there are many types of molds, only a few dozen cause allergic reactions. *Alternaria*, *Cladosporium* (*Hormodendrum*), *Aspergillus*, *Penicillium*, *Helminthosporium*, *Epicoccum*, *Fusarium*, *Mucor*, *Rhizopus* and *Aureobasidium* (*Pullularia*) are the major culprits. Some common spores can be identified when viewed under a microscope. Some form recognizable growth or colonies.

About This Chapter: "Mold Allergy," Reprinted with permission from the Asthma and Allergy Foundation of America, © 2005. All rights reserved.

Many molds grow on rotting logs and fallen leaves, in compost piles and on grasses and grains. Unlike pollens, molds do not die with the first killing frost. Most outdoor molds become dormant during the winter. In the spring they grow on plants killed by the cold.

Indoors, fungi grow in damp areas, particularly in the bathroom, kitchen or basement.

♣ It's A Fact!!

Molds are simple, microscopic organisms called fungi that are found virtually everywhere, indoors and out. Most live on plant or animal matter. According to the Centers for Disease Control and Prevention (CDC), the number of mold species isn't known. Estimates range from tens of thousands to perhaps 300,000 or more.

Source: Excerpted from "Battling Mold," Reprinted courtesy of Allergy & Asthma Network Mothers of Asthmatics (AANMA), 800-878-4403, www.breatherville .org, © 2000.

Who gets the allergy?

It is common for people to get mold allergy if they or other family members are allergic to substances such as pollen or animal dander. People may become allergic to only mold or fungi, or they may also have problems with dust mites, pollens and other spores. If you are allergic to only fungi, it is unlikely that you would be bothered by all fungi. The different types of fungi spores have only limited similarities.

People in some occupations have more exposure to mold and are at greater risk of developing allergies. Farmers, dairymen, loggers, bakers, mill workers, carpenters, greenhouse employees, wine makers and furniture repairers are at increased risk.

There is only weak evidence that allergic symptoms are caused by food fungi (for example, mushrooms, dried fruit, foods containing yeast, vinegar or soy sauce). It is more likely that reactions to food fungi are caused by the food's direct effect on blood vessels. For example, histamine may be present because of the fermentation of red wines.

Fungi on house plants can cause an allergic reaction, but this is only likely to happen if the soil is disturbed.

Fungi can even grow in the human body. If not properly treated, intense inflammation can recur often. It can permanently damage airway walls. This is not common, though.

What are the symptoms?

The symptoms of mold allergy are very similar to the symptoms of other allergies, such as sneezing, itching, nasal discharge, congestion and dry, scaling skin. Some people with mold allergies may have allergy symptoms the entire summer because of outdoor molds or year-round if symptoms are due to indoor molds.

Mold spores can deposit on the lining of the nose and cause hay fever symptoms. They also can reach the lungs, to cause asthma or another serious illness called allergic bronchopulmonary aspergillosis.

Sometimes the reaction is immediate, and sometimes the reaction is delayed. Symptoms often worsen in a damp or moldy room such as a basement; this may suggest mold allergy.

How is mold allergy diagnosed?

To diagnose an allergy to mold or fungi, the doctor will take a complete medical history. If mold allergy is suspected, the doctor often will do skin tests. Extracts of different types of fungi will be used to scratch or prick the skin. If there is no reaction, allergy is not suggested. In some people with allergy, irritation alone can cause a reaction. Therefore the doctor uses the patient's medical history, the skin testing results, and the physical examination combined to diagnose mold allergy.

How is mold allergy treated?

As with most allergies, patients should:

- **Avoid contact with the spores:** Wear a dust mask when cutting grass, digging around plants, picking up leaves and disturbing other plant materials. Reduce the humidity indoors to prevent fungi from growing. These measures will reduce symptoms.

- **Take medications for nasal or other allergic symptoms:** Antihistamines and decongestants are available over the counter—without a prescription. Because these antihistamines can cause drowsiness, they are best taken at bedtime. If drowsiness continues to be a problem, talk to your doctor about taking non-sedating antihistamines, which require a prescription. For moderate and severe allergy symptoms, your doctor may prescribe corticosteroid nasal sprays.

♣ **It's A Fact!!**

What is the mold count?

Mold and mildew are fungi. They differ from plants or animals in how they reproduce and grow. The "seeds," called spores, are spread by the wind. Allergic reactions to mold are most common from July to late summer.

Mold counts are likely to change quickly, depending on the weather. Certain spore types reach peak levels in dry, breezy weather. Some need high humidity, fog, or dew to release spores. This group is abundant at night and during rainy periods.

To collect a sample of particulates in the air, a plastic rod or similar device is covered with a greasy substance. The device spins in the air at a controlled speed for a set amount of time—usually over a 24-hour period. At the end of that time a trained analyst studies the surface under a microscope. A formula is then used to calculate that day's particle count.

The counts reported are always for a past time period and may not describe what is currently in the air.

Source: Excerpted from "Pollen and Mold Counts," reprinted with permission from the Asthma and Allergy Foundation of America, © 2005. All rights reserved.

- **If these medications are inadequate:** talk to your doctor or allergist about taking allergy shots (immunotherapy). This works for some carefully selected patients.

How can I prevent a reaction to mold?

Allergies cannot be cured. But the symptoms of the allergy can be reduced by avoiding contact with the spores. Several measures will help:

Staying indoors: Stay indoors during periods when the published mold count is high. This will lessen the amount you inhale. Mold spores are "counted" by collecting a sample of particulates in the air then identifying and counting the mold spores in the sample.

The amount of airborne spores are likely to change quickly, depending on the weather. The counts reported are always for a past time period and may not reflect what is currently in the air. The mold that causes your allergic reaction may not be counted separately. This means that allergy symptoms may not relate closely to the published count. But knowing the count can help you decide when to stay indoors.

Using air conditioning and air filters: Use central air conditioning with a HEPA (high efficiency particulate air) filter attachment. It will help trap spores before they reach you. Air conditioning with a HEPA filter attached works better than electrostatic air-cleaning devices and much better than freestanding air cleaners. Devices that treat air with heat, ions or ozone are not recommended.

Controlling moisture: No air cleaners will help if excess moisture remains. If indoor humidity is above 50 percent, risks of fungus growth rise steeply. Hygrometers can be used to measure humidity accurately. The goal is to keep humidity below 45 percent, and preferably about 35 percent.

If humidifiers are necessary, scrub the fluid reservoirs at least twice a week to prevent mold growth. Air conditioners and dehumidifiers can also be a source of mold and should be cleaned.

To prevent mold and mildew build up inside the home, especially in bathrooms, basements and laundry areas, be aggressive about reducing dampness:

- Put an exhaust fan or open a window in the bathroom.

- Quickly repair any plumbing leaks.

- Remove bathroom carpeting where moisture is a concern.

- Scour sinks and tubs at least monthly. Fungi thrive on soap and other films that coat tiles and grout. For problem areas, use ordinary laundry bleach (1 ounce diluted in a quart of water). Fungicides (chemicals that kill fungus) are less important than a good scrubbing. Fungicides may be added to paint, primer or wallpaper paste to slow fungus growth on treated areas. But this will have little effect if excess moisture remains.

- Clean garbage pails frequently.

- Clean refrigerator door gaskets and drip pans.

- Repair basement plumbing leaks, blocked drains, poorly vented clothes dryers and water seepage through walls.

- Use an electric dehumidifier to remove moisture from the basement. Be sure to drain the dehumidifier regularly and clean the condensation coils and collection bucket.

- Raise the temperature in the basement to help lower humidity levels. Small space heaters or a low-wattage light bulb may be useful in damp

✤ It's A Fact!!

When inhaled, molds typically cause nasal and lung symptoms similar to those due to plant pollens, says Warren V. Filley, M.D., an Oklahoma City allergy and asthma specialist and clinical professor of internal medicine at the University of Oklahoma Medical School. Typical symptoms can include nasal and sinus congestion, sore throat, sneezing, watery or burning eyes, dry cough, shortness of breath, and irritation of the nose, throat, or even skin.

Source: Excerpted from "Battling Mold," Reprinted courtesy of Allergy & Asthma Network Mothers of Asthmatics (AANMA), 800-878-4403, www.breatherville.org, © 2000.

closets. Be careful where they are placed, though, to avoid creating a fire hazard.

- Polyurethane and rubber foams seem especially prone to fungus invasion. If bedding is made with these foams, it should be covered in plastic.

- Throw away or recycle old books, newspapers, clothing or bedding.

- Promote ground water drainage away from a house. Remove leaves and dead vegetation near the foundation and in the rain gutters. Completely shaded homes dry out slowly, and dense bushes and other plants around the foundation often promote dampness. In the winter, condensation on cold walls encourages mold growth, but even thick insulation can be invaded if vapor barriers in exterior walls are not effective.

Chapter 36

Cockroach Allergy

What is cockroach allergy?

When most people think of allergy "triggers," they often focus on plant pollens, dust, animals, and stinging insects. In fact, cockroaches also can trigger allergies and asthma.

Cockroach allergy was first reported in 1943, when skin rashes appeared immediately after the insects crawled over patients' skin. Skin tests first confirmed patients had cockroach allergy in 1959.

In the 1970s, studies made it clear that patients with cockroach allergies develop acute asthma attacks. The attacks occur after inhaling cockroach allergens and last for hours. Asthma has steadily increased over the past 30 years. It is the most common chronic disease of childhood. Now we know that the frequent hospital admissions of inner-city children with asthma often is directly related to their contact with cockroach allergens—the substances that cause allergies. From 23 percent to 60 percent of urban residents with asthma are sensitive to the cockroach allergen.

The increase in asthma is not fully understood. Experts think one reason for the increase among children is that they play indoors more than in past years and thus have increased contact with the allergen. This is especially true in the inner cities where they stay inside because of safety concerns.

What causes the allergic reaction?

The job of immune system cells is to find foreign substances such as viruses and bacteria and get rid of them. Normally, this response protects us from dangerous diseases. People with allergies have supersensitive immune

---

✤ It's A Fact!!

Can people develop asthma from cockroach allergy?

There is strong evidence in the scientific literature that exposure to cockroach allergens can cause asthma in susceptible children and adults. Cockroach allergens are proteins found in cockroach droppings. One in five children in the U.S. is allergic to cockroach allergens, as indicated by a positive skin prick test. Exposure to cockroach allergens is believed to be a major risk factor for asthma among children in inner-city homes where cockroaches are common.

One study, the National Cooperative Inner-City Asthma Study, found that asthmatic children with both a positive skin prick test to cockroach allergen and a high exposure to cockroach allergen in the bedroom were more likely to have wheezing, missed school days, nights without sleep, and unscheduled medical visits and hospitalizations for asthma. However, the risk of asthma from cockroach allergen exposure and allergy is not limited to children. A study of elderly asthmatics in New York City found that cockroach allergy was associated with more severe asthma.

While scientific data strongly suggest that cockroach allergy can cause asthma, it is important to point out that not everyone who is allergic to cockroach allergens has asthma and not everyone who has asthma is allergic to cockroach allergens. The same is true for allergies to other indoor allergens as well. Researchers believe that asthma is the result of hereditary as well as environmental factors. It is known that children with asthma are more likely to have at least one parent with asthma. Researchers are working to unravel the complex relationship between heredity, exposure to indoor allergens, and the development of asthma.

Source: "Cockroach Allergy and Asthma," National Institute of Environmental Health Sciences, October 2004.

systems that react when they inhale, swallow, or touch certain harmless substances such as pollen or cockroaches. These substances are the allergens.

Cockroach allergen is believed to derive from feces, saliva, and the bodies of these insects. Cockroaches live all over the world, from tropical areas to the coldest spots on earth. Studies show that 78 percent to 98 percent of urban homes have cockroaches. Each home has from 900 to 330,000 of the insects.

Private homes also harbor them, especially if the homes are well insulated. When one roach is seen in the basement or kitchen, it is safe to assume that at least 800 roaches are hidden under the kitchen sink, in closets, and the like. They are carried in with groceries, furniture, and luggage used on trips. Once they are in the home, they are hard to get rid of.

The amount of roach allergen in house dust or air can be measured. In dwellings where the amount is high, exposure is high and the rate of hospitalization for asthma goes up. Allergen particles are large and settle rapidly on surfaces. They become airborne when the air is stirred by people moving around or by children at play.

Who develops cockroach allergy?

People with chronic severe bronchial asthma are most likely to have cockroach allergy. Also likely to have it are people with a chronic stuffy nose, skin rash, constant sinus infection, repeat ear infection, and asthma.

Cockroach allergy is a problem among people who live in inner-cities or in the South and are of low socioeconomic status. In one study of inner-city children, 37 percent were allergic to cockroaches, 35 percent to dust mites, and 23 percent to cats. Those who were allergic to cockroaches and were exposed to the insects were hospitalized for asthma 3.3 times more often than other children. This was true even when compared with those who were allergic to dust mites or cats.

Cockroach allergy is more common among poor African Americans. Experts believe that this is not because of racial differences; rather, it is because of the disproportionate number of African Americans living in the inner cities.

What are its symptoms?

Symptoms vary. They may be a mildly itchy skin, scratchy throat, or itchy eyes and nose. Or the allergy symptoms can become stronger, including severe, persistent asthma in some people. Asthma symptoms often are a problem all year, not just in some seasons. This can make it hard to determine that a cockroach allergy is the cause of the asthma.

How is cockroach allergy diagnosed?

The National Heart, Lung, and Blood Institute recommends that all patients with persistent asthma be tested for allergic response to cockroach as well as to the other chief allergens, dust mites, cats, dogs, and mold.

Diagnosis can be made only by skin tests. The doctor scratches or pricks the skin with cockroach extract. Redness, an itchy rash, or swelling at the site suggests you are allergic to the insect.

Cockroaches should be suspected, though, when allergy symptoms—stuffy nose, inflamed eyes or ears, skin rash, or bronchial asthma—persist year round.

How can I manage cockroach allergy?

If you have cockroach allergy, avoid contact with roaches and their droppings.

- The first step is to rid your home of the roaches. Because they resist many control measures, it is best to call in pest control experts.

- For ongoing control, use poison baits, boric acid, and traps. Don't use chemical agents. They can irritate allergies and asthma.

- Do not leave food and garbage uncovered.

- To manage nasal and sinus symptoms, use antihistamines, decongestants, and anti-inflammatory medications. Your doctor will also prescribe anti-inflammatory medications and bronchodilators if you have asthma.

- If you keep having serious allergic symptoms, see an allergist about "allergy injections" with the cockroach extract. They can reduce symptoms over time.

Chapter 37

Dust Mite Allergy

Frequently Asked Questions About Dust Mite Allergy

What is dust mite allergy?

If you have allergies or asthma, a tiny creature living in your home could be making big problems for you. Although you can't see them, if you have allergies or asthma you may be feeling their effects only too well. They are dust mites, and they live in many homes throughout the world.

Dust mites may be the most common cause of year-round allergy and asthma. About 20 million Americans have dust mite allergy. Dust mites are well adapted to most areas of the world—they are found on every continent except Antarctica. It may not be possible to rid your home entirely of these creatures, but there are ways in which you can lessen your allergic reactions to them.

What is a dust mite?

Too small to be seen with the naked eye, a dust mite measures only about one-quarter to one-third of a millimeter. Under a microscope, they can be

About This Chapter: This chapter begins with "Frequently Asked Questions About Dust Mite Allergy," from "Dust Mites," reprinted with permission from the Asthma and Allergy Foundation of America, © 2005. All rights reserved. "How to Create a Dust-Free Bedroom," is from a fact sheet produced by the National Institute of Allergy and Infectious Diseases, August 2004.

seen as whitish bugs. Having eight rather than six legs, mites are technically not insects but arthropods, like spiders.

Mites are primitive creatures that have no developed respiratory system and no eyes. They spend their lives moving about, eating, reproducing, and eliminating waste products. A mite's life cycle consists of several stages, from egg to adult. A female may lay as many as 100 eggs in her lifetime. Depending on the species, it takes anywhere from 2 to 5 weeks for an adult mite to develop from an egg. Adults may live for 2 to 4 months.

Dust mites thrive in temperatures of 68 to 77 degrees Fahrenheit and relative humidity levels of 70 percent to 80 percent. There are at least 13 species of mites, all of which are well adapted to the environment inside your home. They feed chiefly on the tiny flakes of human skin that people normally shed each day. These flakes work their way deep into the inner layers of furniture, carpets, bedding, and even stuffed toys. These are the places where mites thrive. An average adult person may shed up to 1.5 grams of skin in a day, this is enough to feed one million dust mites.

What causes allergic reactions to dust mites?

Household dust is not a single substance but rather a mixture of many materials. Dust may contain tiny fibers shed from different kinds of fabric, as well as tiny particles of feathers, dander from pet dogs or cats, bacteria, food, plant and insect parts, and mold and fungus spores. It also contains many microscopic mites and their waste products.

These waste products, not the mites themselves, are what cause allergic reactions. Dust mite waste contains a protein that is an allergen—a substance that provokes an allergic immune reaction—for many people. Throughout its life a single dust mite may produce as much as 200 times its body weight in waste.

Most dust mites die when exposed to low humidity levels or extreme temperatures. But they leave their waste behind, which continues to cause allergic reactions. In a warm, humid house, dust mites can easily survive year round.

What can I do?

Unless you live in Antarctica or in an extremely dry climate, there is probably no practical way to completely rid your home of dust mites. But you can take action to lessen their effects.

Having dust mites doesn't mean that your house isn't clean. In most areas of the world, these creatures are in every house, no matter how immaculate. But it is true that keeping your home as free of dust as possible can lessen dust mite allergy.

Studies show that more dust mites live in the bedroom than anywhere else in the home. So to attack the problem of dust mite allergy, the bedroom is the best place to start.

Unfortunately, vacuuming is not enough to remove mites and mite waste. Up to 95 percent of mites may remain after vacuuming, because they live deep inside the stuffing of sofas, chairs, mattresses, pillows, and carpeting.

The first and most important step to reduce dust mites is to cover mattresses and pillows in zippered dust-proof covers. These covers are made of a material with pores too small to let dust mites and their waste product through and are called allergen-impermeable. Plastic or vinyl covers are the least expensive but some people find them uncomfortable. Other fabric allergen impermeable covers can be purchased from allergy supply companies as well as many regular bedding stores.

The next most important step is to wash the sheets and blankets weekly in hot water. Temperatures of at least 130 degrees F are needed to kill dust mite.

Other desirable, but not as critical, steps are to rid the bedroom of all types of materials that mites love. Avoid having wall-to-wall carpeting, blinds, wool blankets, upholstered furniture, and down-filled covers and pillows in the bedroom. Keep pets out of this room as well. Windows should have roll-type shades for the windows instead of curtains; if you do have curtains, be sure to wash them often.

It is ideal for someone without dust mite allergy to do the cleaning of the bedroom. If this is not possible, wear a filtering mask when dusting or vacuuming. Many drug stores carry these items. Because dusting and vacuuming stir up dust, try to do these chores at a time of day when you can stay out of the bedroom for a while afterward.

Special filters for vacuum cleaners can help to keep mites and mite waste from circulating back into the air. These filters can be bought from an allergy supply company or in some specialty vacuum stores.

Other rooms in your house can be treated similarly to the bedroom. Avoid having wall-to-wall carpeting, if possible. If you do use carpeting, the type with a short, tight pile is less hospitable to mites than the loose-pile or shag type. Better still are washable throw rugs over regularly damp-mopped wood, linoleum, or tiled floors.

Wash rugs in hot water whenever possible. Cold water leaves up to 10 percent of mites behind. Dry cleaning kills all mites and is also good for removing dust from fabrics.

✔ Quick Tip
Tips For Controlling Dust Mites

- Cover mattresses and pillows.

- Wash bedding in hot water (at least 130 degrees F).

- Remove stuffed animals from the bedroom.

- Remove upholstered furniture and fabric-covered items from the bedroom, use washable curtains and area rugs.

- Do not allow furry/feathered pets into the bedroom.

- Wet-mop floors.

- Vacuum regularly, using special allergen-controlling bags or machines.

- Improve ventilation.

- Stop using humidifiers.

- Dehumidify, keep the humidity level below 60%.

- Place filters over heating vents.

- Use high efficiency air filters on heating ducts.

- Use air cleaners.

Source: Excerpted from "Tips for Controlling Dust Mites," and reprinted with permission, © 2005 American Lung Association. For more information about the American Lung Association or to support the work it does, call 1-800-LUNG-USA (1-800-586-4872) or log on to www.lungusa.org.

Reduce the humidity in your home to less than 50 percent by using a dehumidifier and/or air conditioner. If you have taken as many of these actions as practically possible and are still having allergic reactions to house dust mites, allergy shots may help. A dust mite extract can be formulated to boost your immune system's response specifically to dust mite allergen. Shots for this purpose have been shown to be very effective.

Dust mites are probably impossible to avoid completely. Still, they don't have to make your life miserable. There are many ways you can change the environment inside your home to reduce the numbers of these unwanted "guests."

Your doctor is an important resource in helping you to keep dust mite allergies under control. Talk to him or her about measures you can take, sources of more information and of allergy products, and whether immunizing shots may be right for you. Together you can prevail against the effects of house dust mites.

How to Create a Dust-Free Bedroom

Preparation

- Completely empty the room, just as if you were moving.
- Empty and clean all closets and, if possible, store contents elsewhere and seal closets.
- Keep clothing in zippered plastic bags and shoes in boxes off the floor, if you cannot store them elsewhere.
- Remove carpeting, if possible.
- Clean and scrub the woodwork and floors thoroughly to remove all traces of dust.
- Wipe wood, tile, or linoleum floors with water, wax, or oil.
- Cement any linoleum to the floor.
- Close the doors and windows until the dust-sensitive person is ready to use the room.

Maintenance

- Wear a filter mask when cleaning.

- Clean the room thoroughly and completely once a week.

- Clean floors, furniture, tops of doors, window frames and sills, etc., with a damp cloth or oil mop.

- Carefully vacuum carpet and upholstery regularly.

- Use a special filter in the vacuum.

- Wash curtains often at 130 degrees Fahrenheit.

- Air the room thoroughly.

✔ Quick Tip
Carpeting makes dust control impossible. Although shag carpets are the worst type to have if you are dust sensitive, all carpets trap dust. Therefore, health care experts recommend hardwood, tile, or linoleum floors. Treating carpets with tannic acid eliminates some dust mite allergen. Tannic acid, however, is not as effective as removing the carpet, is irritating to some people, and must be applied repeatedly.

Source: NIAID, April 2004.

Beds And Bedding

Keep only one bed in the bedroom. Most importantly, encase box springs and mattress in a zippered dust-proof or allergen-proof cover. Scrub bed springs outside the room. If you must have a second bed in the room, prepare it in the same manner.

Use only washable materials on the bed. Sheets, blankets, and other bedclothes should be washed frequently in water that is at least 130 degrees Fahrenheit. Lower temperatures will not kill dust mites. If your hot water temperature is set lower (commonly done to prevent children from scalding themselves), wash items at a laundromat which uses high wash temperatures.

Use a synthetic (such as Dacron) mattress pad and pillow. Avoid fuzzy wool blankets or feather- or wool-stuffed comforters and mattress pads.

Furniture And Furnishings

- Keep furniture and furnishings to a minimum.
- Avoid upholstered furniture and blinds.
- Use only a wooden or metal chair that you can scrub.
- Use only plain, lightweight curtains on the windows.

Air Control

Air filters—either added to a furnace or a room unit—can reduce the levels of allergens. Electrostatic and HEPA (high-efficiency particulate absorption) filters can effectively remove many allergens from the air. If they don't function right, however, electrostatic filters may give off ozone, which can be harmful to your lungs if you have asthma.

A dehumidifier may help because house mites need high humidity to live and grow. You should take special care to clean the unit frequently with a weak bleach solution (1 cup bleach in 1 gallon water) or a commercial product to prevent mold growth. Although low humidity may reduce dust mite levels, it might irritate your nose and lungs.

Toys

- Keep toys that will accumulate dust out of your bedroom.
- Avoid stuffed toys.
- Use only washable toys of wood, rubber, metal, or plastic.
- Store toys in a closed toy box or chest.

☞ Remember!!

Although these steps may seem difficult at first, experience plus habit will make them easier. The results—better breathing, fewer medicines, and greater freedom from allergy and asthma attacks—will be well worth your effort.

Source: NIAID, April 2004.

Pets

Keep all animals with fur or feathers out of the bedroom. If you are allergic to dust mites, you could also be allergic or develop an allergy to cats, dogs, or other animals.

Chapter 38

Allergies To Pets

Questions And Answers About Pet Allergies

What are the most common symptoms of a dog or cat allergy?

Allergic reactions to cats and dogs are caused by proteins found not only in the animal's dander, but also in their saliva and urine. Because these proteins are small, they become part of house dust that gets airborne and circulates throughout your home. This means it is not necessary to touch the pet to have an allergic reaction to it. Just walking into a room where the cat or dog has been can cause a reaction.

What dog or cat breeds are hypoallergenic or safe for children with asthma?

There are no hypoallergenic (allergen-free) dogs or cats, since all breeds have the offending protein allergens in their saliva and urine and produce dander. Occasionally, patients are more allergic to one breed of dogs than another, but this is an exception.

About This Chapter: This chapter begins with questions and answers from "Allergies: Pet Allergies," and continues with text from "The Real Truth about Cats and Dogs," by Robert A. Wood, M.D. and "Animals in School," by Ellie Goldberg. All three documents are reprinted courtesy of Allergy & Asthma Network Mothers of Asthmatics (AANMA), 800-878-4403, www.breatherville.org, "Allergies: Pet Allergies" and "Animals in School" are © 2005. "The Real Truth about Cats and Dogs" is © 2000.

If you have asthma but are not allergic to cats or dogs, either pet is considered safe, but the question is, for how long? Allergies to pets can develop over time and exposure, and they may not occur until the pet has been in your home for years. If there is any question about you having dog or cat allergies, it is best to see a board-certified allergist prior to the purchase of a pet.

What is the reaction time for an allergic reaction to occur to a pet?

Reactions to pets can be immediate, happening within minutes, or may be delayed for hours after the exposure. To determine whether allergy symptoms are triggered by contact with a pet, see a board-certified allergist for a diagnosis.

I get an itchy rash on my hands whenever my dog licks me. Could I be allergic to the dog's saliva?

Itching and hives are common allergic reactions that can occur when skin comes in contact with an allergen. Dogs have proteins in their dander, saliva, and urine that cause reactions in those allergic to them, so it would be possible for your symptoms to be caused by your dog's saliva. However, to confirm a diagnosis of dog allergy it is best to discuss your situation with your physician.

♣ It's A Fact!!

When airborne, an allergen can cause allergic reactions three different ways:

- When inhaled, the allergen may cause respiratory problems such as wheezing, coughing, sinusitis, and asthma.

- If the allergen comes in contact with the skin from touching the animal or being licked, it may cause hives and itching.

- When the allergen gets in the eyes, itching, burning, swelling, and watering of the eyes may occur.

Source: Reprinted courtesy of Allergy & Asthma Network Mothers of Asthmatics (AANMA), © 2005.

I am allergic to my cat and was wondering if washing her frequently would reduce the amount of cat allergen I am exposed to?

Study results on this subject have been conflicting, showing either no change or only a short-lived improvement in cat allergen with frequent cat washings. The current opinion is that the benefits of cat washing are so transient that it is unlikely to be worth the effort or trauma to the cat.

My family member has allergies to animal dander. Is there a dog breed that is well suited for us?

While some breeds of dogs may produce more allergen than others, there is not a breed that is absolutely hypoallergenic or best for people with pet allergies. All dogs have proteins in their dander, saliva, and urine that can cause difficulties for those allergic to them. If you know your family member is allergic to animal dander, it is best not to purchase a dog.

I recently found out I have cat allergies and have decided to find new homes for my cats. My doctor suggested I have my air ducts cleaned. Is this effective in removing cat allergen?

One of the many environmental controls that helps remove cat allergen once the cat is no longer in your home includes cleaning your home's air ducts and cleaning or replacing furnace filters. In addition, thoroughly washing walls, repeatedly vacuuming upholstery and carpets (reservoirs for cat allergen) with a well-sealed HEPA-equipped (High Efficiency Particulate Air Filter) vacuum cleaner, and using HEPA air cleaners throughout your home will help speed the process as well.

Wash all bedding and draperies even if your cats were not in direct contact with them. Cover your bed with new allergen-proof encasements as cat allergen can linger in mattresses for months or years after the cat has been removed. Cat allergen levels in dust fall slowly, so it may take four to six months to notice a difference.

The Real Truth About Cats And Dogs

Can animal lovers with asthma and allergies learn to co-exist with their pet? Robert A. Wood, M.D., separates fact from fiction.

Fact or Fiction? Find a new home for your pet and your pet-related allergy symptoms will soon disappear.

Dr. Wood: **Fact and Fiction**—There are no convincing studies demonstrating the direct clinical benefits of removing an animal from the home. No research has focused on whether finding a new home for a pet will eliminate the pet-related asthma or allergy symptoms.

However, there is compelling clinical experience to support the best currently available advice: Finding a new home for the pet is likely to reduce levels of pet-allergen exposure in the home. Avoidance of allergens is always the most appropriate advice a physician can give.

Fact or Fiction? Some breeds of cats and dogs are less likely to trigger allergy symptoms in people with pet allergies than others.

Dr. Wood: **Fiction**—While it is true that some breeds of cats or dogs are said to produce much more allergen than others, there is absolutely no breed that is hypoallergenic or can promise to be best for people with asthma or pet allergies. It is not possible to predict with any accuracy which animals are likely to be more or less allergenic based on a particular breed, size, hair length, or propensity to shed. There is no perfect furry pet for people with allergies to cats and dogs.

♣ It's A Fact!!

Once the cat or dog has been removed from the home, symptoms may not improve for weeks or even months, as allergen levels fall quite slowly. In homes with cats, for example, the allergen load typically takes as long as four to six months to reach that of non-cat homes. Levels may fall much more quickly if the homeowner makes extensive environmental changes, such as removing carpets, upholstered furniture, and other allergen reservoirs. It has been shown that cat allergen may persist in mattresses for years after a cat has been removed from a home, so new bedding or impermeable encasements must also be recommended.

Source: Reprinted courtesy of Allergy & Asthma Network Mothers of Asthmatics (AANMA), © 2000.

Fact or Fiction? People who have asthma and exhibit allergy symptoms when exposed to animals tend to have more severe disease.

Dr. Wood: Fact—A diagnosis of cat or dog allergy can be made by a skin test or blood (RAST) test. If the test is negative, it is very unlikely that cat or dog exposure will affect the asthma in any way. However, if the test is positive, then it is very likely that animal exposure will lead to a worsening of asthma or allergic rhinitis.

Fact or Fiction? Washing the cat or dog frequently will reduce the level of allergens in the home.

Dr. Wood: Neither Fact nor Fiction—A number of studies have investigated measures that might help reduce the allergen load in a home. One study demonstrated significant reductions in airborne cat allergen with a combination of air filtration, cat washings, vacuum cleaning, and removal of furnishings. It was a small study and the purpose was to measure the ability to reduce the allergen load, not to establish any clinical improvement in symptoms. When cat washing was evaluated separately in that study, dramatic reductions in airborne cat allergen were seen after cat washes.

Subsequent studies have produced conflicting results demonstrating either no change or only a very transient improvement. The current opinion is that the benefits of cat washing are so transient that it is unlikely to be worth the effort or the trauma to the cat. Preliminary information regarding dogs looks very similar.

Fact or Fiction? Using a HEPA (high-efficiency particulate air) filter in the bedroom while the dog sleeps next to (not on) the bed makes it possible for man and beast to co-exist happily.

Dr. Wood: Fiction—While using a HEPA filter helps to remove allergens flowing through the machine, the best advice is to keep the dog out of the bedroom at all times.

Fact or Fiction? Immunotherapy (allergy shots) makes it possible for pet lovers to keep their pets.

Dr. Wood: Neither Fact nor Fiction—Most studies over the last 20 years demonstrate a positive effect, particularly for cat allergen. However, the outcomes of these studies have been based largely on laboratory studies, so what this means for the average allergic pet owner remains a question. Based on available studies, it is most likely that immunotherapy will not allow allergic pet owners to live with a cat or dog more comfortably. More studies are needed to fully define the strategies, both immunologic and environmental, that will be most effective.

Although most asthma and allergies can be controlled by medication, it makes far more sense to begin treatment with allergy avoidance and then to use the least amount of medication possible to control the disease. This approach can have dramatic short-term effects in asthma control and potentially even more important long-term effects in improving the eventual outcome of the asthma.

In the meanwhile, it is best for patients with significant animal allergy, especially if they have asthma, to find new homes for their pets.

✔ Quick Tip

For pet-allergic families who insist on keeping pets, the following recommendations are the best available until pending studies are concluded:

- Restrict pets to one area of the home when inside.
- Keep pets out of the bedroom.
- Use HEPA or electrostatic air cleaners, especially in the room(s) of the person(s) with pet allergies.
- Remove carpets, upholstered furniture, heavy drapes (that cannot be washed), with a focus on the bedroom—even though the pet is not allowed in the room.
- Encase pillows, mattress, and box spring with allergen-proof encasings.

Although tannic acid (chemical product used to typically reduce dust mite allergens) has been shown to reduce cat allergen levels, the effects are modest and short-lived when a cat is present so this treatment should not be routinely recommended.

Source: Reprinted courtesy of Allergy & Asthma Network Mothers of Asthmatics (AANMA), © 2000.

Animals In School

Know The Facts

All warm-blooded animals can cause allergic reactions. Animal allergen is in the dander, saliva, and urine. Allergen particles become airborne and accumulate in carpets, upholstery, and fabrics and on books, desks, and walls.

Allergen particles land in the eyes and are inhaled into the nose and lungs. On the skin they can cause itchy rashes, eczema, and hives. They can cause a range of allergies and illnesses such as allergic rhinitis, asthma, hypersensitivity pneumonitis, conjunctivitis, and chronic sinus and ear infections.

Damp or wet surfaces are a breeding ground for molds, mildews, bacteria, and insects, especially if cages or other animal areas are not cleaned properly. Sensitive airways are also affected by the odors from urine, cedar chips, room deodorizers, disinfectant sprays, and the flea powders or insecticides used to control fleas and ticks.

"Carpets in the room become a trap for animal dander and are a potential reservoir for biological contaminants," says Martin A. Cohen, S.C.D., C.I.H., senior scientist for Environmental Health and Engineering, a company that specializes in indoor air quality. Animal biology labs with independent room ventilation units that exhaust the air to the outside are less likely to cause problems. Cohen knows one school system that houses its animals in a separate building. Some schools allow only turtles, hermit crabs, fish, lizards, or snakes. Others limit animal visits and pet parades to outdoor areas.

Once furry animals are introduced into a school, removal does not immediately stop allergy problems. A central ventilating system can contaminate the entire school. Even after a thorough cleaning, the allergens persist for months. Vacuuming just stirs up the particles. Steam cleaning and vacuuming with a vacuum enhanced by an HEPA (high efficiency particle accumulator) filter may reduce, but not totally eliminate, the allergens.

Know Your School

Read the school manual. Knowing the district's official position on animals can help you identify your goal. Find out who is responsible for decisions that affect you. Start with a letter to the principal. Explain that furry animals undermine your health and ability to attend school. If your school principal isn't helpful, go higher.

You can ask the pupil services or special education director how to get consideration for your allergies or to influence practices that you feel disadvantage yourself.

Is your school ignoring district policy? Contact the superintendent about implementing policies. Is there no policy or does the policy need updating? (Some school policies only provide for advance notice of animal visits so that allergic students can stay home.) Contact the town's board of education about changing policies or developing new ones.

Be Pro-Health, Not Anti-Animal

The experts agree: "Environmental control to reduce exposure to indoor allergens is a critical component of asthma management... Avoiding allergen exposure reduces symptoms, the need for medication, and the level of airway hyper-responsiveness." (National Heart, Lung, and Blood Institute, National Asthma Education and Prevention Program, Guidelines for the Diagnosis and Management of Asthma.) In other words, exposure to an animal can make allergic people sick. Avoiding animals helps them get better.

Your physician's letter for the school records should be more than a list of allergies and medications. The letter should read something like this: "Eliminating allergens and irritants at school is a necessary part of Mary's asthma and allergy treatment."

Work With Your School Nurse

Her professional license and practice standards make this person your best ally and advocate. Her role is to document student health needs and plan necessary services and adaptations. Your physician's letter is her guide to eliminating your allergic triggers and asthma aggravators at school. Where there is no school nurse, contact the health officer at your local board of health who investigates environmental health problems and enforces standards.

Keep track of peak expiratory flow rates as measured by a peak flow meter both at home and at school. Good records teach school staff about a child's airway changes and demonstrate the effect of allergens and irritants in the classroom. If you have an individualized health plan (IHP), be sure it includes a peak flow meter and a daily symptom diary.

Provide resources that help the school nurse educate the school community about allergies, and advocate for health and environmental standards that benefit everyone.

Many teachers and parents may not be aware that coughing, wheezing, sneezing, shortness of breath, rashes, hives, red and watery eyes, a runny nose, or unusual irritability may be signs of allergy.

☞ **Remember!!**
You Are Not Alone

Allergies to animals are common. Work as a team to share concerns, get input from staff and other parents and students, review standards in other districts, and develop recommendations for your school.

Source: Reprinted courtesy of Allergy & Asthma Network Mothers of Asthmatics (AANMA), © 2005.

To cope with occasional animal visits, your doctor may recommend using cromolyn eye drops and a few puffs of cromolyn sodium (Intal®) to block an allergic reaction. Whether this approach may help you depends on his current health and the intensity of the exposure. Someone should stand by prepared to administer the appropriate medication if you have a severe reaction.

Be an Advocate

By law, schools must be accessible and safe for all students. If you are allergic to animals, you have the right to ask the school to prohibit or remove animals that make you sick.

Some administrators may be unsure what to do when the school environment or staff practices affect someone's health. They may not know that federal law protects students with allergies and asthma. Share the free pamphlet "The Civil Rights of Students with Hidden Disabilities under Section

504 of the Rehabilitation Act of 1973" (U.S. Department of Education, Office for Civil Rights, Washington, DC 20202).

If you get no support from the principal or district authorities, contact your state department of education. Tell your story to the Section 504 specialist in the pupil services or law division. You can also call your regional office of the U.S. Department of Education, Office for Civil Rights (DOE-OCR) for information and advice. If all else fails, make a formal complaint to OCR that the school is violating your right to a free and appropriate public education.

♣ It's A Fact!!

Companion Dogs

Both Section 504 and the Americans with Disabilities Act (ADA) require schools to serve students who have a companion dog or service animal and students with allergies. Before class placements, schedules, and other decisions are made, schools must take into account all students who need individual consideration. A collaborative approach to problem solving can expand the school's options and help avoid potential conflicts.

Source: Reprinted courtesy of Allergy & Asthma Network Mothers of Asthmatics (AANMA), © 2005.

Chapter 39

Pets Can Have Allergies, Too

Is your cat grooming half her hair off or your dog licking his paws raw? It may well be your pet is experiencing allergies, one of the most common health problems for pets. Just like people, animals have allergic reactions because their immune system—the system that protects the body from foreign and potentially infectious substances—overreacts to some material. Almost anything—pollen, dust, an ingredient in pet food, a household chemical, an insect bite—can set off an alarm in the immune system, causing it to pump out large amounts of white blood cells, hormones, and other material called histamines into the bloodstream. The result for animals can be a range of different effects, including itchy, swollen skin—known as pruritus—difficulty breathing, or a disruption of the digestive tract such as vomiting or diarrhea. These symptoms are the animal equivalent of a person's sneezing, runny nose, and watery eyes.

Pets with these kinds of allergic symptoms can be pretty miserable creatures, and unfortunately they can't be cured. Allergies are life-long, chronic problems. The good news is that there's a lot you can do to help your animal "children" feel better. The best way to start is to find out what your pet is allergic to, so you can keep the allergen out of his environment. Animal allergies generally fall under one of four main categories.

About This Chapter: "Allergies," reprinted with permission from http://www.healthypet.com, the website of the American Animal Hospital Association. Copyright © 2004, American Animal Hospital Association.

Contact Allergies

These are the least common type of allergy in animals. They happen when an animal's skin comes in contact with the material he's allergic to—if he rubs his face against a wool blanket, for example, and he's allergic to wool. The chemicals in flea collars can cause this problem as well. The skin at the point of contact will be irritated—it may itch, become thickened or discolored, have a strong odor, and/or lose hair due to constant biting or scratching. Contact allergies are generally not a hard problem to solve—they're usually confined to a specific area of an animal's body, and the allergen shouldn't take too much work to discover. You can try removing different materials that your pet touches until you find the one that irritates his skin.

Food Allergies

Diet can be a complicated factor in pet allergies. Most animals are not born with allergies to food; their immune systems develop an allergic response over time to some part of their diet, often one of the animal proteins. A food allergy can present in a lot of different ways, including the itching, digestive disorders, and respiratory distress already mentioned. They can be a real challenge to solve, however. You can try to figure out what's causing your pet's allergic reaction by feeding him different diets, but the allergic effects of food can stay in the system for eight weeks. You may have to keep your furry friend on a special hypoallergenic (non-allergy-causing) diet for eight to twelve weeks to see how he reacts, and you may have to do it several times with several different diets before you find one that doesn't cause an allergic reaction. And while you're feeding these test diets, you'll have to make very sure that your pet doesn't eat any treats, vitamins, leftovers or scraps, or even plants around the house. He has to eat the test diet exclusively for the entire eight to twelve weeks to determine whether he has an allergic reaction to it.

Inhalant Allergy

Inhalant allergies are the kind we humans are most used to. Just like us, our pets get hay fever, meaning they can be allergic to the pollen and mold that fills the outside air during the spring and fall. They can also be allergic to the dust mites, mildew, and mold that can be inside every home. These kinds of allergens usually produce severe itching in pets, which is usually concentrated in the ears, feet, groin, and armpits, though it can be spread across the entire body. Dogs in particular may develop hairless, irritated "hot spots" from constantly chewing on and scratching the affected skin.

Most animals that are allergic to airborne particles are usually allergic to more than one. Often, they will only experience itching during the pollen-heavy seasons of the year, just like humans with hay fever. If you find that your pet's allergies seem to be seasonal, you may be able to limit his outdoor time during allergy season. Your pet may be reacting to an indoor allergen, however, or an allergen that doesn't vary by season. In that case, there's not much you can do to keep him away from whatever he's allergic to, though an air filter might provide some relief.

Flea Allergies

This is an extremely common problem for pets, possibly the most common allergy of all. Animals aren't actually allergic to the fleas themselves, but to proteins that fleas secrete in their saliva when they bite. Your pet doesn't have to be a walking flea circus to suffer from an allergy, either. Affected animals can itch severely from a single bite for over five days! So, if you suspect your pet is allergic to fleas, you're going to have to work very hard to keep the little pests away. Frequent baths are a good idea, as are the prescription flea applications and pills. Consult your veterinarian when you chose a flea repellent for your pet, though; the wrong kind or too strong of a concentration could cause irritated skin, seizures, and even death in extreme cases. You will also want to treat your pet's environment, including any bedding or carpeting he comes in contact with.

Other Options

What makes allergies hard to deal with is that in many cases, you either won't be able to determine exactly what is causing the reaction or won't be able to remove it from your pet's environment. This is where your veterinarian comes into the picture. You and your veterinarian will probably have to work together to determine the best treatment, or combination of treatments, for your pet's allergy. You may have to go through a series of trying a possible solution, waiting to see how your pet reacts to it, and moving on to another solution. Your veterinarian may suggest one or more of the following things:

- **Testing:** Your veterinarian has a few different tools to help determine the source of your pet's allergy. Intradermal or "scratch" tests involve making small abrasions in an animal's skin and inserting small amounts of materials that the veterinarian suspects the pet might be allergic to. If the animal is allergic to one of the materials, say dust mites or ragweed pollen, the immune system will react to it and that particular scratch will become inflamed. There are also a number of blood tests your veterinarian can use to analyze the amount of certain chemicals that the immune system releases into the bloodstream when exposed to different allergens. These tests can be used to tell whether your pet is having an allergic reaction or whether the problem is caused by something else, and sometimes they can determine the source of the allergy.

  > **☞ Remember!!**
  >
  > Whatever treatment decision you and your veterinarian come to, rest assured that the patience and determination it can take to treat allergies is well worth it. Though it may take some time and effort, you can help your itchy, grouchy pet feel comfortable again.

- **Steroids:** These drugs work to suppress the immune system and make the allergic reaction less severe. Steroid treatment can help your pet even if you can't determine what he's allergic to or how he's being exposed. They can have several side effects, however, and they affect nearly every organ in the body. Steroid use can cause weight gain, increased thirst and urination, and increased aggression and other behavioral changes. They are generally used if the allergy occurs for a short amount of time, because long-term use makes animals more prone to infection, as well as susceptible to diabetes and seizures.

- **Immunotherapy:** This is one of the safest and most effective ways to treat allergies, but it also takes the longest amount of time to work. In immunotherapy, animals are given regularly—often weekly—vaccinations that contain small amounts of the substance they're allergic to. The same therapy is used for people who go in for allergy shots. It gradually desensitizes the immune system to the allergen, meaning that as time goes by, the immune system is reprogrammed and doesn't react to the allergen as strongly. Unfortunately, it takes some time for the immune system to readjust. It can sometimes be six to twelve months before animals show any improvement from the treatment.

- **Antihistamines:** These drugs, much like the allergy medication people take, work to block the chemicals released by the immune system, called histamines. They are effective at reducing itching and inflammation, and they are relatively safe to use. Their major drawback is that they cause sedation, and can make pets extremely drowsy and sluggish. Occasionally, they can change an animal's energy level enough to affect his quality of life.

- **Symptomatic treatment:** Even if none of the above treatments are effective, you can still give your pet a lot of relief by simply treating his symptoms as they come up. There are a number of soothing shampoos on the market that contain ingredients like oatmeal or Epsom salts. Your veterinarian may also be able to suggest ointments, ear treatments, or sprays that can make your pet more comfortable. Be cautious about using home remedies or herbal treatments on your pet, however. Consult with your veterinarian before trying any new treatment, because you could damage your pet's skin or aggravate the allergic reaction. Most of all, remember that while you can give these symptomatic treatments often, they will only provide temporary relief. If your pet still seems uncomfortable despite the baths or other treatments, you can talk to your veterinarian about long-term treatment.

Source: Reprinted with permission from http://www.healthypet.com, the website of the American Animal Hospital Association. Copyright © 2004, American Animal Hospital Association.

Part 5

Environmental, Chemical, And Drug Allergies

Chapter 40

Insect Venom Allergies

Heat, humidity, pollen and mold spores. If these aren't enough to make allergy sufferers dread the impending dog days of summer, here's one more thing to add to the list: insects.

Stinging insects, including bees, hornets, yellow jackets, wasps, and fire ants—and biting insects such as mosquitoes and "kissing bugs" (*Triatoma*)—are most plentiful in late July, August, and early September.

These uninvited guests in picnics, parks—and even in beds—send more than half a million people each year to hospital emergency rooms and cause at least 50 deaths, according to the American College of Allergy, Asthma and Immunology (ACAAI). Experts believe that many more deaths occur each year that are never identified as anaphylaxis caused by insect sting or bite allergies. At particular risk are the more than two million Americans who have had allergic reactions to bites or stings.

"Allergic reactions to insect stings and bites require immediate medical attention," said Richard D. deShazo, M.D., chair of the ACAAI Insect Hypersensitivity Committee and an allergist at University of Mississippi Medical

Center, Jackson, Miss. "People who know they are allergic should never be without an emergency kit containing epinephrine (adrenaline). If you experience any symptoms of an allergic reaction for the first time from an insect sting or bite, get to an emergency room right away."

These symptoms include hives, itchiness, swelling in areas other than the sting site, difficulty breathing, dizziness, hoarse voice and swelling of the tongue. In severe reactions, the person loses consciousness and can have cardiac arrest.

♣ It's A Fact!!

Five Allergy Myths That Can Sting

MYTH: Swelling at the site of an insect sting is a sign of an allergic reaction.

FACT: Swelling, which occurs even in a normal reaction to insect sting, does not necessarily indicate an allergic reaction. Sometimes the swelling will extend beyond the sting site. Allergic reactions are indicated by swelling in areas other than the sting site and involve additional symptoms such as hives and itchiness, tightness in the chest and difficulty breathing, dizziness or a sharp drop in blood pressure, and hoarse voice and swelling of the tongue.

MYTH: Like seasonal nasal allergies, insect sting allergies are very common and more of a nuisance than they are dangerous.

FACT: Insect sting allergies are much less common than seasonal nasal allergies but they are far more dangerous, even life-threatening. Approximately 2 million Americans are allergic to the venom produced by stinging insects such as yellow jackets, wasps, hornets and fire ants. Insect stings send more than 500,000 Americans to hospital emergency rooms and cause at least 50 known deaths each year.

Stinging Insects

"Once you've had an allergic reaction to an insect sting, it's important to see an allergist. You have a 60 percent chance of having another similar or worse reaction if you're stung again," Dr. deShazo said. "You should have an allergist prescribe an epinephrine kit and teach you and your family members how to administer the injection. You also should discuss whether you're a candidate for allergy shots, also known as immunotherapy, that desensitize you to insect stings.

MYTH: If you don't suffer a reaction within the first 24 hours after an insect sting, you probably are not allergic.

FACT: An allergic reaction often occurs immediately, but may appear as much as 24 hours later.

MYTH: A person can never be immune to insect sting allergies.

FACT: A person who is allergic to insect sting can gain immunity through a preventive treatment called allergy shots (also known as immunotherapy). The treatment, which has been shown to be 97 percent effective in preventing future allergic reactions to insect stings, works by injecting gradually increasing doses of purified insect venom.

MYTH: A person who experiences an allergic reaction to an insect sting is not very likely to have a future reaction.

FACT: Unfortunately, a person suffers an allergic reaction to an insect sting has a 60 percent chance of having another similar or worse reaction if stung again. Those who have had an allergic reaction to insect sting should see an allergist who can prescribe an emergency kit containing self-administered epinephrine (adrenaline) and provide instruction on how to use it.

Source: © 2005 American College of Allergy, Asthma, and Immunology (ACAAI). Reprinted with permission.

"People with venom allergies don't have to live in fear of insects. Studies have shown that allergy shots, which introduce tiny purified extracts of insect venom are 97 percent effective in protecting allergic people from potentially life-threatening reactions to insect stings," he said.

Insect repellents do not work against stinging insects, but there are ways to minimize your chances of being stung, without having to confine yourself to staying indoors.

"Don't look like a flower, smell like a flower or act like a flower," Dr. deShazo said. "Bees are attracted to flowers and they'll be attracted to you if you dress in bright colors and floral prints, wear strong perfumes and walk barefoot in the grass among the clover that bees love so much."

Most people are not allergic to insect stings and should recognize the difference between an allergic reaction and a normal or large local reaction.

Knowing how to avoid stings from fire ants, bees, wasps, hornets and yellow jackets leads to a more enjoyable summer for everyone. Here are some additional tips from the American College of Allergy, Asthma and Immunology:

- Keep food covered when eating outdoors.

- Don't drink soft drinks from cans. Stinging insects are attracted to the sweetness and may crawl inside the can.

✔ Quick Tip
What To Do If A Person Is Stung

1. Have someone stay with the victim to be sure that they do not have an allergic reaction.

2. Wash the site with soap and water.

3. The stinger can be removed using a four x four inch gauze wiped over the area or by scraping a fingernail over the area. Never squeeze the stinger or use tweezers. It will cause more venom to go into the skin and injure the muscle.

4. Apply ice to reduce the swelling.

5. Do not scratch the sting. This will cause the site to swell and itch more, and increase the chance of infection.

Source: Excerpted and reprinted with permission. Dawna L. Cyr and Steven B. Johnson, First Aid for Bee and Insect Stings, bulletin #2345 of the Maine Farm Safety Program (Orono, ME: University of Maine Cooperative Extension). © 1995, 2002.

- Garbage cans stored outside should be covered with tight-fitting lids.

- Keep window and door screens in good repair. Drive with car windows closed.

- Keep prescribed medications handy at all times and follow the attached instructions if you are stung. These medications are for immediate emergency use while en route to a hospital emergency room for observation and further treatment.

- Make sure your teachers, camp counselors, and other adult supervisors know that you have an emergency epinephrine kit.

If you have had an allergic reaction to an insect sting, it's important to see an allergist-immunologist to be evaluated for an allergy shot program that immunizes against future allergic reactions.

Fire Ants

Fire ants bite to hold on, and then can sting repeatedly.

According to Richard M. Weber, M.D., National Jewish Medical and Research Center, Denver, red fire ants have encroached on the territory of the black fire ant in northern portions of Mississippi and Alabama, and now extend over 310 million acres over 12 states including New Mexico, Arizona and California.

"Within even a few weeks' time, 50 percent of persons in fire ant-endemic areas will be stung," Dr. Weber said. "The sting of a fire ant causes an immediate burning sensation due to toxic oily alkaloids in the venom. Pustules develop 18 to 24 hours after the stings, and the lesions may persist for a week and may cause scarring. The ant can sting repeatedly, resulting in a ring of pustules."

Treatment for fire ant stings is aimed at preventing secondary bacterial infection, which may occur if the pustule is scratched or broken. Blisters should be cleaned with soap and water to prevent secondary infection. Topical corticosteroid ointments and oral antihistamines may relieve the itching associated with these reactions.

"Anaphylaxis occurs in 1 percent to 16 percent of fire ant stings, and is attributable to the soluble proteins comprising 1 percent of the venom weight. More than 80 deaths had been attributed to fire ants by 1998," Dr. Weber said.

"Kissing Bugs"

Although allergies to stinging insects are more common, according to John E. Moffitt, M.D., also an allergist at University of Mississippi Medical Center, Jackson, allergic reactions have been reported following many different types of arthropod bites, primarily *Triatoma*, flies, or mosquitoes.

♣ It's A Fact!!

Allergic Reactions To Bee Stings

Allergic reactions to bee stings can be deadly. People with known allergies to insect stings should always carry an insect sting allergy kit and wear a medical ID bracelet or necklace stating their allergy. See a physician about getting either of these.

There are several signs of an allergic reaction to bee stings. Look for swelling that moves to other parts of the body, especially the face or neck. Check for difficulty in breathing, wheezing, dizziness, or a drop in blood pressure. Get the person immediate medical care if any of these signs are present. It is normal for the area that has been stung to hurt, have a hard swollen lump, get red and itch. There are kits available to reduce the pain of an insect sting. They are a valuable addition to a first aid kit.

Source: Excerpted and reprinted with permission. Dawna L. Cyr and Steven B. Johnson, First Aid for Bee and Insect Stings, bulletin #2345 of the Maine Farm Safety Program (Orono, ME: University of Maine Cooperative Extension). © 1995, 2002.

"In the western and southwestern United States, *Triatoma* bites appear to be an important cause of anaphylaxis," Dr. Moffitt said. "Since their bite is usually painless and inflicted during sleep, the person may not be aware of the bite, and resulting allergic reactions may not be diagnosed or mistakenly attributed to other causes. The lack of commercial antigen limits diagnostic and treatment capabilities."

Management of *Triatoma* allergy is similar to that of anaphylaxis due to bites and stings of other insects for which no immunotherapy is available.

"Personal protection measures from kissing bugs involve avoidance where possible and use of pesticides approved for indoor use. Prevention of bug entry into homes may involve outdoor light management and sealing entry points around the home," said Dr. Moffitt.

"Blankets and sheets should be examined for *Triatoma*. Removal of piles of paper, clothing and other clutter from the bedroom may reduce hiding places. Since the bugs rarely bite covered skin, wearing of pajamas with long legs and sleeves is recommended. Some also recommend the use of insect repellants on exposed skin before sleep," he said.

Mosquitoes

Most people who get mosquito bites develop small, itchy skin reactions that last for a few hours or a few days. These reactions are caused by the saliva the mosquito injects into the skin at the time of the bite, according to F. Estelle R. Simons, M.D., professor and head, Division of Allergy and Clinical Immunology, University of Manitoba, Winnipeg, Canada.

"Increased IgE antibody to mosquito saliva develops in people with mosquito allergy, causing more severe reactions at the sites of the mosquito bites," said Dr. Simons. "These allergic reactions, such as a large red swelling, a skin blister, bruise, or hives, may last for a week or more. Rarely, severe acute allergic reactions involving many body systems may occur."

Steps to prevent mosquito allergy include avoiding mosquito-infested areas, wearing protective clothing, eliminating standing water on surrounding property, keeping window and door screens in good condition, avoiding scented products and using mosquito repellants.

"Personal repellants containing DEET work best. Repellants containing more than 10 percent DEET should not be used on infants or children under age six years," said Dr. Simons.

Chapter 41

Poison Ivy And Other Problematic Plants

Those nasty weeds! Poison ivy, poison oak, and poison sumac are the most common cause of allergic reactions in the United States. Each year 10 to 50 million Americans develop an allergic rash after contact with these poison plants.

Poison ivy, poison oak, and poison sumac grow almost everywhere in the United States, except Hawaii, Alaska, and some desert areas in the western U.S. Poison ivy usually grows east of the Rocky Mountains and in Canada. Poison oak grows in the western United States, Canada, Mexico (western poison oak), and in the southeastern states (eastern poison oak). Poison sumac grows in the eastern states and southern Canada.

A Poison Plant Rash

Poison plant rash is an allergic contact dermatitis caused by contact with oil called urushiol. Urushiol is found in the sap of poisonous plants like poison ivy, poison oak, and poison sumac. It is colorless or pale yellow oil that oozes from any cut or crushed part of the plant, including the roots, stems, and leaves. After exposure to air, urushiol turns brownish-black. Damaged leaves look like they have spots of black enamel paint making it easier to recognize and identify the plant. Contact with urushiol can occur in three ways:

- **Direct contact:** touching the sap of the toxic plant.

- **Indirect contact:** touching something on which urushiol is present. The oil can stick to the fur of animals, to garden tools or sports equipment, or to any objects that have come into contact with it.

- **Airborne contact:** burning poison plants put urushiol particles into the air.

When urushiol gets on the skin, it begins to penetrate in minutes. A reaction appears, usually within 12 to 48 hours. There is severe itching, redness, and swelling, followed by blisters. The rash is often arranged in streaks or lines where the person brushed against the plant. In a few days, the blisters become crusted and take ten days or longer to heal.

Poison plant dermatitis can affect almost any part of the body. The rash does not spread by touching it, although it may seem to when it breaks out in new areas. This may happen because urushiol absorbs more slowly into skin that is thicker such as on the forearms, legs, and trunk.

Who Is Sensitive And Who Is Not?

Sensitivity develops after the first direct skin contact with urushiol oil. An allergic reaction seldom occurs on the first exposure. A second encounter can produce a reaction which may be severe. About 85 percent of all people will develop an allergic reaction when adequately exposed to poison ivy. This

---

♣ It's A Fact!!

Poison Oak: In the west, this plant may grow as a vine but usually is a shrub. In the east, it grows as a shrub. It has three leaflets to form its leaves' "hairs."

Poison Ivy: Grows as a vine in the east, midwest and south, it grows as a vine. In the far northern and western United States, Canada and around the Great Lakes, it grows as a shrub. Each leaf has three leaflets.

Poison Sumac: Grows in standing water in peat bogs in the northeast and midwest and in swampy areas in parts of the southeast. Each leaf has seven to 13 leaflets.

sensitivity varies from person to person. People who reach adulthood without becoming sensitive have only a 50 percent chance of developing an allergy to poison ivy. However, only about 15 percent of people seem to be resistant.

Sensitivity to poison ivy tends to decline with age. Children who have reacted to poison ivy will probably find that their sensitivity decreases by young adulthood without repeated exposure. People who were once allergic to poison ivy may even lose their sensitivity later in life.

Recognizing Poison Plants

Identifying the poison ivy plant is the first step in avoiding the rash. The popular saying "leaves of three, beware of me" is a good rule of thumb for poison ivy and poison oak but is only partly correct. A more exact saying would be "leaflets of three, beware of me," because each leaf has three leaflets. Poison sumac, however, has a row of paired leaves. The middle or end leaf is on a longer stalk than the other two or more leaves. This differs from most other three-leaf look-alikes.

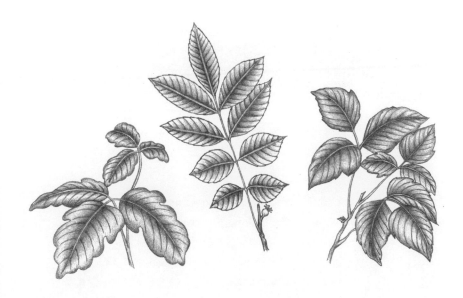

Figure 41.1. Poison Oak, left; Poison Sumac, middle; and Poison Ivy, right (illustration by Alison DeKlein).

Poison ivy has different forms. It grows as vines or low shrubs. Poison oak, with its oak-like leaves, is a low shrub in the East and can be a low or high shrub in the West. Poison sumac is a tall shrub or small tree. The plants also differ in where they grow. Poison ivy grows in fertile, well-drained soil. Western poison oak needs a great deal of water, and Eastern poison oak prefers sandy soil but sometimes grows near lakes. Poison sumac tends to grow in standing water, such as peat bogs.

These plants are common in the spring and summer. When they grow, there is plenty of sap and the plants bruise easily. The leaves may have black marks where they have been injured. Although poison ivy rash is usually a

✔ Quick Tip
Prevention Of Poison Ivy

Prevent the misery of poison ivy by looking out for the plant and staying away from it. You can destroy these weeds with herbicides in your own backyard, but this is not practical elsewhere. If you are going to be where you know poison ivy likely grows, wear long pants, long sleeves, boots, and gloves. Remember that the plant's nearly invisible oil, urushiol, sticks to almost all surfaces, and does not dry. Do not let pets run through wooded areas since they may carry home urushiol on their fur. Because urushiol can travel in the wind if it burns in a fire, do not burn plants that look like poison ivy.

Barrier skin creams such as a lotion containing bentoquatam offer some protection before contact with poison ivy, poison oak, or poison sumac. Over-the-counter products prevent urushiol from penetrating the skin. Ask your dermatologist for details.

summer complaint, cases may occur in winter when people burn wood to clear yards that has urushiol on it, or cut poison ivy vines for wreaths.

It is important to recognize these toxic plants in all seasons. In the early fall, the leaves can turn colors such as yellow or red when other plants are still green. The berry-like fruit on the mature female plants also changes color in fall, from green to off-white. In the winter, the plants lose their leaves. In the spring, poison ivy has yellow-green flowers.

Treatment

If you think you've had a brush with poison ivy, poison oak, or poison sumac, follow these simple steps:

- Wash all exposed areas with cold running water as soon as you can reach a stream, lake, or garden hose. If you can do this within five minutes, the water may keep the urushiol from contacting your skin and spreading to other parts of your body. Within the first 30 minutes, soap and water are helpful.

- Wash your clothing in a washing machine with detergent. If you bring the clothes into your house, be careful that you do not transfer the urushiol to rugs or furniture. You may also dry clean contaminated clothes. Because urushiol can remain active for months, wash camping, sporting, fishing, or hunting gear that was in contact with the oil.

- Relieve the itching of mild rashes by taking cool showers and applying over-the-counter preparations like calamine lotion or Burow's solution. Soaking in a lukewarm bath with an oatmeal or baking soda solution may also ease itching and dry oozing blisters. Over-the-counter hydrocortisone creams are not strong enough to have much effect on poison ivy rashes.

Prescription cortisone can halt the reaction if used early. If you know you have been exposed and have developed severe reactions in the past, consult your dermatologist. He or she may prescribe cortisone or other medicines that can prevent blisters from forming. If you receive treatment with a cortisone drug, you should take it longer than six days, or the rash may return.

Common Myths About Poison Ivy

Scratching poison ivy blisters will spread the rash.

False: The fluid in the blisters will not spread the rash. The rash is spread only by urushiol. For instance, if you have urushiol on your hands, scratching your nose or wiping your forehead will cause a rash in those areas even though leaves did not contact the face. Avoid excessive scratching of your blisters. Your fingernails may carry bacteria that could cause an infection.

Poison ivy rash is "catchy."

False: The rash is a reaction to urushiol. The rash cannot pass from person to person; only urushiol can be spread by contact.

Once allergic, always allergic to poison ivy.

False: A person's sensitivity changes over time, even from season to season. People who were sensitive to poison ivy as children may not be allergic as adults.

Dead poison ivy plants are no longer toxic.

False: Urushiol remains active for up to several years. Never handle dead plants that look like poison ivy.

Rubbing weeds on the skin can help.

False: Usually, prescription cortisone preparations are required to decrease the itching.

One way to protect against poison ivy is by keeping yourself covered outdoors.

True: However, urushiol can stick to your clothes, which your hands can touch, and then spread the oil to uncovered parts of your body. For uncovered areas, barrier creams are sometimes helpful. Learn to recognize poison ivy so you can avoid contact with it.

Chapter 42

Allergies And Cosmetics

Cosmetics and skin care products are part of most people's grooming habits. The average adult uses at least seven different skin care products each day. These include fragrances, astringents, moisturizers, sunscreens, skin cleansers, hair care items, deodorants/antiperspirants, colored cosmetics, hair cosmetics, and nail cosmetics.

The majority of people experience few problems from these products, however, problems can arise either with the first few applications, or after years of use. People usually know which product is causing the problem, but severe, chronic reactions may require the skills of a dermatologist.

What are the possible problems associated with the use of cosmetics and skin care products?

Reactions to skin care products can be simple irritations, depends on the condition of the skin, or a true allergy involving the immune system. Irritant contact dermatitis is the most common problem seen with cosmetics and skin care products.

What is irritant contact dermatitis?

Uninjured skin is an excellent barrier to most substances found in cosmetics and skin care products. If skin is very dry or injured, openings make that barrier less protective. Burning, stinging, itching, and redness may be signs that a product is irritating the skin. Bath soaps, detergents, antiperspirants, eye cosmetics, moisturizers, permanent hair-waving solutions, and shampoos are the most common skin irritants. Even water can irritate very dry skin.

♣ **It's A Fact!!**

Do cosmetics cause allergies?

Overuse of some cosmetics can cause allergies and other skin problems. Ingredients such as fragrance and preservatives can cause allergic reactions in some people. Skin reactions, which doctors call contact dermatitis, should be taken seriously. Even if you've used a cosmetic for years with no problems, you can develop an allergic reaction as you become sensitized to one or more of the ingredients.

Some cosmetics are labeled "allergy-tested" or "hypoallergenic," but products with these claims don't always offer a solution to cosmetic allergies. "Hypoallergenic" means only that the manufacturer feels that the product is less likely to cause an allergic reaction. Before placing this claim on the label, some companies conduct tests, and others simply don't include perfumes or other common problem-causing ingredients in their products. The claim "dermatologist-tested" on some cosmetic products only means that a skin doctor has tested the product to see if it will generally cause allergenic problems. Other label claims that carry no guarantee that they won't cause reactions include "sensitivity-tested" and "non-irritating."

"Natural" ingredients are extracted directly from plants or animal products as opposed to being produced synthetically. Natural ingredients can cause allergic reactions. If you have an allergy to certain plants or animals, you could have an allergic reaction to cosmetics containing those ingredients. For instance, "lanolin," extracted from sheep wool, is an ingredient in many moisturizers and is a common cause of allergies.

Source: Excerpted from "Cosmetics and Reality," U.S. Food and Drug Administration (FDA), *FDA Consumer*, May 1994.

What is allergic contact dermatitis?

Some people are allergic to a specific ingredient or ingredients in a product. They react whenever they are exposed to the ingredient, although it can take up to several days for the symptoms to appear. Signs include redness, swelling, itching, and fluid-filled blisters.

What are some of the ingredients that cause allergic reactions?

Fragrances and preservatives, ingredients commonly found in skin care products and cosmetics, are the most common cause of cosmetic allergic reactions.

Fragrances: Fragrances cause more allergic contact dermatitis than any other ingredient. More than 5,000 different fragrances are used in cosmetics and skin care products. Less "allergenic" fragrances have been developed to minimize the problem.

Remember that a product labeled "unscented" may really contain a fragrance which masks other chemical odors. A product must be marked "fragrance-free" or "without perfume" to indicate nothing has been added to make it smell good. Some fragrance reactions occur only when the skin is exposed to sunlight.

Preservatives: Preservatives in cosmetics and skin care products are the second most common cause of skin reactions. Preservatives prevent the growth of fungus and bacteria that can cause skin infections, and protect products from oxygen and light damage. Cosmetics that contain water must include some type of preservative.

Consumers who react to one preservative will not necessarily react to others. Examples of preservatives include paraben, imidazolidinyl urea, Quaternium-15, DMDM hydantoin, phenoxyethanol, methylchloroisothiazolinone, and formaldehyde, and should be listed as ingredients on product labels.

What are skin care products?

Skin care products are designed to maintain healthy skin. They include astringents, moisturizers, and sunscreens.

Astringents: Astringents remove oils and soap residue from the skin. They are generally drying and may contain water, alcohol, propylene glycol, witch hazel, or salicylic acid. These may cause itching, burning, or tingling in people with dry, sensitive, or irritated skin.

Moisturizers: Moisturizers prevent water loss by layering an oily substance over the skin to keep water in, or by attracting water to the outer skin layer from the inner skin layer. Dry skin causes cracks and fine wrinkles, losing its effectiveness as a barrier, and causing pain and itching. Substances that stop water loss include petrolatum, mineral oil, lanolin, and silicone. Substances that attract water to the skin include glycerin, propylene glycol, proteins, and some vitamins. These ingredients may cause an allergic reaction.

Sunscreens: Sunscreens contain chemicals that absorb, reflect, or scatter light. Light-absorbing chemicals include the PABA esters, avobenzone, and the cinnamates, that can cause an allergic reaction. Physical sunscreens contain fine powders of zinc oxide or titanium dioxide that reflect or scatter light. There are no known allergies to physical sunscreens.

What are personal care products?

Personal care products that help keep skin and hair clean and fresh smelling include skin cleansers, shampoos, conditioners, and deodorants/antiperspirants.

Skin Cleansers: Soaps, detergents, bath/shower gels, and bubble baths remove dirt, body oils, and bacteria. They prevent odor and infection but heavy use of these products can over dry the skin causing flaking, itching, and irritation. People with dry skin should choose a mild cleanser, bathe/shower with cool water, minimize water contact, and apply a moisturizer immediately after bathing while the skin is slightly wet.

There are several different varieties of soaps. Deodorant soaps have an antibacterial agent to eliminate odors. Beauty-bar soaps are generally less drying and irritating.

Shampoos: Shampoos remove dirt and oils from the scalp and leave the hair soft and shiny. Allergic reactions to shampoos are uncommon since their contact with the skin is brief but they can irritate and dry the skin when rinsed over the body.

There are several types of shampoos: mild baby shampoos do not irritate the eyes; conditioning shampoos cleanse lightly and leave hair soft; shampoos for oily hair remove oil; and shampoos for damaged hair are pH-adjusted to prevent more damage.

Conditioners: Conditioners are applied after shampooing to make hair shiny, easier to comb and style, and more manageable. They are not a common source of skin reactions themselves; they can have fragrance and preservatives.

Deodorants And Antiperspirants: Deodorants kill bacteria and leave a pleasant smell. Antiperspirants prevent sweating. The fragrance in deodorants and the aluminum salts in antiperspirants rarely cause problems. Skin irritation can occur if these products are used on already irritated skin, immediately after shaving, or if spread too widely around the armpit.

✎ What's It Mean?
What are cosmeceuticals?

Cosmeceuticals are skin care products designed to go beyond strictly coloring and adorning the skin. These products may improve the functioning of the skin and be helpful in preventing premature aging. Examples are alpha hydroxy acids such as glycolic acid, and beta hydroxy acid such as salicylic acid. These hydroxy acids increase skin exfoliation (the removal of dead skin cells) making aging skin appear smoother and feel softer. Some vitamins, such as vitamin A (retinol), may improve the appearance of aging skin by making the skin function better, but they may be drying or irritating and must be used appropriately. Dermatologists know how to use cosmeceutical ingredients and can advise their patients about the best ways to achieve healthy looking skin. Sunblocks prevent photo-aging and photo-carcinogenesis (cancer from the sun) and should be the cornerstone of any skin care regimen.

Source: © 2005 American Academy of Dermatology. Reprinted with permission from the American Academy of Dermatology. All rights reserved.

What are colored cosmetics?

Colored cosmetics are applied to the face, eyes, and lips to beautify and adorn the body.

Facial Cosmetics: Facial cosmetics ("make-up") are used to color the face. It is important to select make-up carefully since it remains in contact with the skin for a long time. Ideally, make-up should be hypoallergenic, non-comedogenic, and non-acnegenic—meaning it produces fewer allergies and will not plug pores or cause acne. Look for cosmetics with sunscreen which will help prevent skin cancer and wrinkles.

Eye Cosmetics: Eyelids are the most sensitive skin on the body. Eye cosmetics include eye shadow, eyeliner, and mascara. Lighter colored, matte-finish powdered eye shadows are less irritating. Water-based (soluble or washable) eye cosmetics are easier to remove. This is important because scrubbing or vigorous rubbing to remove eye cosmetics may cause irritation. Often irritating and allergenic substances can be introduced to the eye area by the fingers.

Eye cosmetics should never be shared and should be replaced every three to four months because of possible bacterial contamination.

Lip Cosmetics: Lip cosmetics include lipsticks and lip balms.

> **☞ Remember!!**
>
> Cosmetics and skin care products are part of grooming and daily hygiene. If a problem is suspected, a dermatologist can diagnose and treat the problem. Patch testing may be used to determine if there is an allergy to specific ingredients in these products. Dermatologists can tell you what should be avoided and personalize a skin care regime for you. They can also answer your questions and provide additional information about the safe use of cosmetics and skin care products.
>
> Source: © 2005 American Academy of Dermatology. Reprinted with permission from the American Academy of Dermatology. All rights reserved.

They moisturize dry, cracked lips, and provide sun protection. Some long-wearing lip stains have been linked to allergic contact dermatitis. Saliva is a common cause of irritant contact dermatitis.

What are hair cosmetics?

The appearance of hair can be altered by changing its color through dyeing, or its shape by permanent waving.

Dyes: Temporary hair dyes wash out after one shampoo. Gradual hair dyes produce a color change over a two to three week period. These dyes generally do not cause problems. Semipermanent hair dyes that wash out after four to six shampoos and permanent hair dyes that do not wash out can cause allergic reactions. These products should be tested on a small area of skin behind the ear or inside the elbow for 24 hours before using.

Permanent hair dyes make hair lighter or darker. Ammonium persulfate, sometimes used to lighten hair, can cause contact dermatitis. It can also cause an immediate allergic reaction like hives and wheezing.

Permanent Waving: "Permanents" make straight hair curly. A perm solution breaks the chemical bonds in straight hair to reform them in a curled position. This process can damage the hair. Hair should not be permed more often than every three months. If the perming solution is left on too long, is too strong, or is applied to hair already damaged by dyes, bleaches, or recent permanents, the hair could break. Scalp irritation may also occur.

What are nail cosmetics?

Nail cosmetics are used to color nails, increase nail strength, or to artificially add nail length.

Polishes: Nail polish can cause allergic contact dermatitis. A person allergic to nail polish may develop a rash on the fingers, eyelids, face, and neck—places the nail polish or fumes may have touched while it was drying. Formaldehyde is a common ingredient that causes allergies. People with nail polish allergies can try hypoallergenic polishes that are formaldehyde free. Red polishes may cause a harmless yellow discoloration of the nail.

Cuticles prevent infection and protect the nail-forming cells and should not be cut or removed.

Artificial Nails: The illusion of long nails can be created with plastic nails that cover the entire nail or nail tips. These artificial nails are attached with glue that may contain methacrylate, a common allergen. Methacrylate-free glues may cause the underlying nail to peel and crack. Nail repair kits also use these glues.

Sculptured Nails: Long-term use of sculptured nails, custom-made to fit permanently over natural nails, can cause severe and painful reactions, including infection of the skin around the nail, loosening or loss of nails, and dermatitis.

Women who have worn artificial or sculptured nails for a long time may notice their real nails are thin, dull, and brittle. Dermatologists recommend that regular artificial nail users take them off every three months to allow natural nails to rest.

Chapter 43

Fragrance Allergies

There are more than 5,000 different fragrances that are in use today. In any one product the number of fragrances used can be many. Fortunately only a small number of fragrances are actually common sensitizers and cause allergy in sensitive individuals.

What is fragrance mix and where is it found?

Fragrance mix is a mixture of eight individual fragrances that is used to screen for fragrance allergy. The eight listed are the most common allergy-causing fragrances that are used across many products for their fragrant and flavoring properties. The components of fragrance mix are described below:

Fragrance: Cinnamic Alcohol

- Odor of hyacinth

- Ester in natural fragrances such as Balsam of Peru, storax, cinnamon leaves, hyacinth oil and propolis

Used/Found In

- Fragrance in perfumes, cosmetics, deodorants, paper, laundry detergent products, toilet soap, personal hygiene products

About This Chapter: From "Fragrance Mix Allergy," This information is reprinted with the permission from DermNet, the website of the New Zealand Dermatological Society. Visit www.dermnet.org.nz for patient information on numerous skin conditions and their treatment. © 2004 New Zealand Dermatological Society.

- Flavoring in beverages (such as cola), chewing gums, toothpaste and mouthwash

Fragrance: Cinnamic aldehyde
- Warm spicy odor with a taste of cinnamon
- Constituent of cinnamon oil

Fragrance: Eugenol
- Powerful spicy odor of clove with a pungent taste
- Found in oils of clove and cinnamon leaf
- Also found in roses, carnations, hyacinths, and violets

Used/Found In
- Fragrance in perfume, cosmetics, colognes, toilet waters, hair cosmetics, aftershave, and personal hygiene products
- Flavoring in toothpaste, mouthwash, and food flavorings
- Used in dental cement and packing agents thus giving the characteristic odor of dental surgeries
- Inherent insecticidal and fungicidal properties—used to preserve meats and other foods
- Pharmaceutical creams and lotions for its antiseptic properties

Fragrance: Isoeugenol
- Odor of clove weaker than that of eugenol
- Constituent of nutmeg oil and ylang ylang oil
- Isomerization of eugenol

Fragrance: Geraniol
- Sweet floral odor of rose
- Constitutes a large portion of rose and palmarose oil, geranium oil, lavender oil, jasmine oil, and citronella oil
- Present in over 250 essential oils

Used/Found In
- Most widely used fragrance in perfumes, colognes, facial make-up, and skin care products

Fragrance: Alpha amyl cinnamic alcohol

- Intense odor of jasmine
- Synthetic essential oil

Used/Found In

- Found in perfumes, soaps, cosmetics, and toothpaste

Fragrance: Hydroxycitronellal

- Sweet fresh odor of lily of the valley
- Synthetic floral fragrance

Used/Found In

- Found in perfumes, soaps, cosmetics, eye cream, and aftershaves
- Also used in insecticides and antiseptics

Fragrance: Oak moss absolute

- Earthy, woody, masculine odor
- Essential oil produced by solvent extraction of tree lichen

Used/Found In

- Commonly used in colognes, aftershaves, and scented products for men

> ✔ **Quick Tip**
>
> *Treatment Of Dermatitis Caused By Fragrance Allergy*
>
> Once the dermatitis appears on the skin, treatment is as for any acute dermatitis/eczema: that is, topical corticosteroids, emollients, and treatment of any secondary bacterial infection (*Staphylococcus aureus*), etc.
>
> Source: © 2004 New Zealand Dermatological Society.

Fragrances may also be found in the workplace. Paints, cutting fluids, and metal working fluids may contain fragrances to mask offending odors. Fragrances may also be circulated through air conditioning.

What are the reactions to fragrance mix allergy?

Typical allergic contact dermatitis reactions may occur in individuals allergic to fragrance mix or any other chemically related substances. The rash is characteristically located on the face, hands and arms. There may be intense swelling and redness of the affected area within a few hours or the rash may appear after a day or two of the product being used. Sometimes symptoms may only be redness, dryness and itching.

Oral exposure may cause sore mouth (tongue) and rash of the lips or angles of the mouth. Flare-ups of dermatitis in fragrance-sensitive individuals may occur if they use or consume products containing fragrance allergens.

Am I allergic to fragrances?

Sensitivity to a perfume, cream, or lotion is usually the first indicator of an allergy to fragrance. Patch testing using fragrance mix and Balsam of Peru detects approximately 75% of fragrance allergy cases. A positive patch to fragrance mix indicates that you are allergic to one or more fragrance chemicals. An estimated 1–2% of the general population is allergic to fragrance.

Self-testing a product for fragrance allergy is possible but should be done only after first talking with your doctor. This should be done only with products that are designed to stay on the skin such as cosmetics and lotions. Apply a small amount (50 cent sized area) of the product to a small tender area of skin such as the bend of your arm or neck for several days in a row. Examine the area each day and if no reaction occurs, it is unlikely you are allergic to it. However, it may still not be suitable for you as it can still cause

✤ It's A Fact!!

Many teachers do not realize the adverse impact that exposure to strong odors, irritants, and allergens has upon allergic children. If no immediate, dramatic symptoms such as sneezing, profuse nasal discharge or eye itching, redness or swelling occur, they make the false assumption that no harm has been done. Whether or not an IgE (allergic) mediated reaction to perfume occurs, allergic children are still adversely affected. Strong odors such as perfume or cleaning solutions will further irritate the already inflamed air passages, causing additional troublesome symptoms. This may result in the need for more medication or increased days missed from school; all of which impact on the child's learning. Effects may be subtle but nonetheless dramatic.

Source: Excerpted from "Ask the Doctor," by Diane Schuller, M.D. Reprinted courtesy of Allergy & Asthma Network Mothers of Asthmatics (AANMA), 800-878-4403, www.breatherville.org, © 2005.

an irritant reaction. Products such as shampoos, conditioners, soaps and cleansers should not be tested in this way as they frequently cause an irritant dermatitis, which is not allergic, if they are covered or overused on tender areas.

What should I do to avoid fragrance allergy?

If you have a fragrance allergy the best way to avoid any problems is by avoiding all products that contain fragrances of any sort. Unfortunately, fragrance allergy is usually life-long and gets worse with continued exposure.

There are more than 5,000 different fragrances that are in use today. In any one product the number of fragrances used can be many. Fortunately only a small number of fragrances are actually common sensitizers and cause allergy in sensitive individuals.

Often products are only labeled as containing fragrance and do not identify the individual chemicals used to make up the fragrance. You should avoid all products that are labeled with any of the following names. These include other names for fragrances, individual fragrance allergens, and other related substances that you may also be allergic to.

Other Names For Fragrances

- Perfumes
- Toilet water
- Colognes
- Masking perfumes
- Unscented perfumes
- Aroma chemicals
- Essential oils

Individual Fragrance Allergens

- Amylcinnamic alcohol
- Anisyl alcohol
- Benzyl alcohol
- Benzyl salicylate
- Cinnamic alcohol
- Cinnamic aldehyde
- Coumarin
- Eugenol
- Geraniol
- Hydroxycitronellal
- Isoeugenol
- Musk ambrette
- Oak moss absolute
- Sandalwood oil
- Wood tars

Other Potential Allergens

- Balsam of Peru
- Cassia oil
- Cinnamon
- Cloves
- Citronella candles
- Ethylene bassylate

Be wary of products that are labeled "fragrance free" or "unscented" as these terms may not necessarily mean they do not contain fragrance chemicals, they just imply the product has no perceptible odor. These products may possibly contain a masking fragrance that is used to cover up the odor of other ingredients.

Note that clothes washed in scented laundry detergent can be a problem with prolonged skin contact of the garment in the presence of moisture and heat. It would be best to use fragrance-free laundry detergent.

Alert your doctor or dentist to the fact that you have an allergy to fragrance mix. If you are highly sensitive, your doctor may also recommend a special diet that eliminates foods to which these allergens or related allergens are added as flavoring.

Your dermatologist may have further specific advice, particularly if you are highly sensitive to fragrance mix.

Chapter 44

Allergy To Wool Alcohols (Lanolin)

What are wool alcohols?

Wool alcohols are the principle component of lanolin in which allergens are found. Lanolin is a natural product obtained from the fleece of sheep. Sebum is extracted from the wool, cleaned and refined to produce anhydrous lanolin. This comprises three parts, wool alcohols, fatty alcohols and fatty acids. Currently the wool alcohols are considered the main sensitizers in lanolin but whether they are the sole sensitizers, needs further investigation. Nowadays there is also chemically modified lanolin that may be less sensitizing than natural lanolin.

Wool alcohols, wool fat, anhydrous lanolin, lanolin alcohol, wool wax and wool grease are just some of the terms used interchangeably with lanolin. In this article we will use wool alcohols, as it is this fraction of lanolin that is the main cause of contact allergies.

What products contain wool alcohols?

Lanolin is a good emulsifier; this means it binds well with water thus it is particularly useful in the manufacture of pharmaceutical and cosmetic formulations. Wool alcohols are found in many pharmaceutical preparations, cosmetics and toiletries. They also have some industrial uses.

Pharmaceuticals

- Steroid-containing creams/ointments
- Hemorrhoidal preparations
- Medicated shampoos
- Veterinary products
- Liniments

Cosmetics/toiletries

- Hand creams
- Moisturizers
- Protective creams
- Self-tanners
- Sunscreens
- Glossy lipsticks
- Makeup removers
- Foundations, powders
- Eye makeup
- Hairspray
- Shaving creams
- Baby oils, diaper lotions

Industrial

- Printing ink
- Furniture and shoe polishers
- Textile finishers
- Lubricants, cutting fluids
- Paper
- Leather

♣ **It's A Fact!!**
Alternative Names
For Wool Alcohol

Wool alcohol is also known by several other names. These include the following:

- Adeps lanae anhydrous
- Aloholes lanae
- Amerchol
- Anhydrous lanolin
- Lanolin
- Wool fat
- Wool grease
- Wool wax

Avoid all of these. At work, request a material safety data sheet to help identify potential sources of exposure.

What are the reactions of allergy to wool alcohols?

Typical allergic contact dermatitis reactions may occur in individuals allergic to wool alcohols. The rash is characteristically located on the face, hands and arms. There may be intense swelling and redness of the affected area within a few hours or the rash may appear after a day or two of the product being used.

Am I allergic to wool alcohols?

Patch testing using 30% wool alcohol in petrolatum is what is routinely used to test for sensitivity to wool alcohols. Although wool alcohols are the main sensitizers in lanolin they may not always be the cause of the sensitivity and patch testing with natural lanolin from several sources is also recommended.

The development of chemically modified lanolin may help to reduce the incidence of skin reactions to natural lanolin. However, there have been cases where patients have shown marked sensitivity to modified lanolin, yet not to natural lanolin. Dermatitis caused by modified lanolin may be missed if patch testing is confined to testing with wool alcohols and natural lanolin only.

Since lanolin is a natural product, its constituents vary depending on its source. Therefore an individual may be allergic to some lanolin-containing products but not to others. Self-testing a product for allergy to lanolin-containing products is possible but should be done only after first talking with your doctor. This should be done only with products that are designed to stay on the skin such as cosmetics and lotions. Apply a small amount (50 cent sized area) of the product to a small tender area of skin such as the bend of your arm or neck daily for five to seven days. Examine the area each day and if no reaction occurs, it is unlikely you are allergic to it, although it may still act as an irritant. Products such as soaps, polishers and waxes should not be tested in this way.

How is dermatitis caused by wool alcohol allergy managed?

Once the dermatitis appears on the skin, the first thing to do is to remove the source. In most instances this would entail stopping the use of all products that contain lanolin.

Standard treatment with emollients and topical steroids must not contain lanolin.

✔ Quick Tip

What should I do to avoid wool alcohol allergy?

If you have wool alcohol allergy the best way to avoid any problems is by avoiding all products that contain wool alcohols. Check all product labels for the list of ingredients and do not use if they contain wool alcohols or any of the other names for wool alcohols. If you are unsure, ask your pharmacist for advice and a suitable alternative.

Alert your doctor to the fact that you have an allergy to wool alcohols. This is particularly important as some topical medications that your doctor may want to prescribe to you contain wool alcohols.

Your dermatologist may have further specific advice, particularly if you are highly sensitive to wool alcohols.

Chapter 45

Allergy To Paraphenylenediamine (Hair Dyes)

What is paraphenylenediamine and where is it found?

Paraphenylenediamine (PPD) is a chemical substance that is widely used as a permanent hair dye. It may also been found in textile or fur dyes, dark colored cosmetics, temporary tattoos, photographic developer and lithography plates, photocopying and printing inks, black rubber, oils, greases and gasoline.

The use of PPD as a hair dye is popular because it is a permanent dye that gives a natural look. Hair can also be shampooed without becoming decolored and perming to achieve waves or curls can be done without difficulty. PPD hair dyes usually come packaged as two bottles, one containing the PPD dye preparation and the other containing the developer or oxidizer. PPD is a colorless substance that requires oxygen for it to become colored. It is this intermediate, partially oxidized state that may cause allergy in sensitive individuals. Fully oxidized PPD is not a sensitizer thus individuals with PPD allergy can wear wigs or fur coats dyed with PPD safely.

About This Chapter: This information is reprinted with the permission from DermNet, the website of the New Zealand Dermatological Society. Visit www.dermnet.org.nz for patient information on numerous skin conditions and their treatment. © 2005 New Zealand Dermatological Society.

What are the reactions to PPD allergy?

Reaction caused by the use of hair dye in mild cases usually only involves dermatitis to the upper eyelids or the rims of the ears. In more severe cases, there may be marked reddening and swelling of the scalp and the face. The eyelids may completely close and the allergic contact dermatitis reaction may become widespread.

Severe allergy to PPD can result in contact urticaria and rarely, anaphylaxis.

People working with PPD such as hairdressers and film developers may develop dermatitis on their hands; patch testing usually reveals hypersensitivity to PPD. Occupational allergy to PPD has been found in a milk tester whom through laboratory work was in frequent contact with PPD solution. Dermatitis on the hands and occasional spreading to the arms and upper chest occurred.

♣ It's A Fact!!
Related Substances To PPD Which May Also Cause An Allergic Reaction

- Azo dyes: used in semi-permanent and temporary hair dyes, ballpoint pen inks, gasoline and diesel oil, and as coloring agent in foods and medications

- Benzocaine and procaine: these are local anesthetics used by doctors and dentists

- Sulfonamides, sulfones, sulfa drugs: PPD allergy may make you sensitive to the use of these drugs also, discuss with your doctor before changing or stopping your medication

- Para-aminobenzoic acid (PABA): this is used in sunscreens and creams that are readily available in over-the-counter preparations. You should only used sunscreens that are labeled "PABA-free." Ask your pharmacist for suitable alternatives.

- Para-aminosalicylic acid: used for tuberculosis

Your dermatologist may have further specific advice, particularly if you are highly sensitive to PPD.

Am I allergic to PPD?

Most hair color preparations, particularly those containing PPD, carry a warning on the packaging to the effect that a patch test should be done prior to use of the dye. There are basically two patch testing methods available to test for allergic sensitivity to PPD.

Patch Test Method 1: Uncovered

- Routine technique used by consumers for testing hair dye sensitivity

- Instructions for testing should be included with every package of hair dye preparation

- Essentially the test involves applying a spot of solution (for example, dye and developer mixed together) to either the neck (behind the ear) or the inner bend of the elbow. Allow to dry and leave uncovered for 48–72 hours. If no irritation or rash occurs during this time then the test is negative and one can assume that the risk of developing a rash will be much less when the dye is applied to the whole head.

- Any immediate signs of irritation or rash are more likely to be an irritant contact dermatitis (i.e. nonallergic)

- A 1+ to 2+ reaction (scale measuring PPD sensitivity) to PPD hair dye usually indicates that dermatitis will develop if the mixture is used

> ### ♣ It's A Fact!!
> **Alternative Names For Paraphenylenediamine**
> - PPD or PPDA
> - Phenylenediamine base
> - p-Phenylenediamine
> - 4-Phenylenediamine
> - 1,4-Phenylenediamine
> - 4-Benzenediamine
> - 1,4-Benzenediamine
> - para-Diaminobenzene (p-Diaminobenzene)
> - para-Aminoaniline (p-Aminoaniline)
> - Orsin™
> - Rodol™
> - Ursol™

Patch Test Method 2: Covered

- Diagnostic test used to determine PPD sensitivity

- Patch testing using 2% PPD in petrolatum

- A +/- reaction (scale measuring PPD sensitivity) to this patch test method usually means that these individuals can use PPD hair dyes without difficulty

- A 1+ to 3+ reaction indicates allergic dermatitis will most likely occur with use of hair dyes thus preventing their use

- Positive reaction from both methods provides confirmation that PPD is the cause of dermatitis and PPD containing products should be avoided

How is PPD dermatitis treated?

In acute severe cases of PPD hair dye dermatitis, wash the hair and scalp thoroughly with a mild soap or soapless shampoo to remove the excess dye. Apply a 2% hydrogen peroxide solution or compresses of potassium permanganate in a 1:5000 dilution to completely oxidase the PPD. To soothe, soften the crust and alleviate the tight feeling of the scalp, a wet dressing of cold olive oil and lime may be used. Further treatment with a topical application of an emulsion of water and water-miscible corticosteroid cream, or oral corticosteroids may be indicated.

Management of PPD dermatitis on other parts of the body may be treated as for any acute dermatitis/eczema; this may include treatment with topical corticosteroids and emollients.

What should I do to avoid PPD allergy?

If you have an allergy to PPD and have your hair dyed, you should avoid the use of all oxidation type hair dyes. These are usually recognized by coming in a 2-bottle preparation. Inform your hairdresser that you are allergic to PPD. Semi-permanent hair dyes may be a suitable alternative but approximately 10% of individuals who are allergic to PPD also react to these; patch testing to confirm sensitivity should be performed prior to their use. Metallic hair dyes and vegetable rinse hair dyes may be used but these do not provide permanent coloring. Currently there are no permanent oxidation type hair dyes that can be safely used by PPD allergic individuals.

In cases of occupational exposure, avoid contact with PPD by wearing suitable protective garments such as gloves and protective sleeves.

Alert your doctor or dentist to the fact that you have an allergy to PPD, this is particularly important if you a receiving treatment which may require the use of a local anesthetic.

Allergy to PPD may make you sensitive to other related compounds. As a precaution you should avoid using products containing any of these substances.

Chapter 46

Nickel Allergy

Nickel is a silvery-white metal that can be found in nature. It is usually mixed with other metals to produce alloys. For example, nickel-iron, which is used to manufacture stainless steel, is the most common nickel alloy. Other nickel alloys are used to make coins, costume jewelry (for example, earrings, watchbands, rings, necklaces, necklace clasps, bracelets), bra or girdle fasteners, zippers, snaps, buttons, suspender clips, hair-pins, studs, eyeglass frames, pens, handles, utensils, paper clips, keys, and tools. Nickel is tightly bound up is stainless steel, especially surgical stainless steel.

As one can see, nickel is found in many common, everyday items. Although one may be exposed to nickel in the workplace environment (if working with nickel, or live near industries using nickel), it is much more likely for the general population to come into contact with nickel through direct skin contact.

This is important because nickel appears to be a very common cause of allergic skin rashes, with nickel allergy being more common among women than men. Apparently, ear piercing (and probably any body piercing, in general), which women are more likely to do than men (although this has been changing), has put susceptible individuals at greater risk of becoming more easily sensitized to nickel.

A nickel allergy is a reaction that develops after initial and/or brief, or repeated and/or prolonged, exposure to nickel or nickel-containing items, depending on the individual's susceptibility. Degree of reaction also varies by person. Specifically, nickel allergy is a contact allergy, which is an allergic skin reaction in response to being exposed to a contact allergen or irritant, such as nickel. A nickel allergy can occur at any age, and typically manifests a few days after first contact as eczema (allergic contact dermatitis), which appears as an itchy, dry/crusty, and red/pigmented skin rash with watery blisters. The affected area is usually restricted to the site of contact, although it could also be found on other parts of the body. Once a nickel allergy has developed, it is usually a chronic condition, often being life-long.

One can be tested for nickel allergy by going to a dermatologist for patch testing. Patch tests are safe skin test procedures, which involve the direct application of tiny quantities of several suspected contact allergens, to the skin of the upper back using hypoallergenic tape. The concentrations of these allergens are low so that they won't cause irritation or reactions in non-allergic individuals, but are high enough to cause a positive response in sensitive individuals. The allergens are in contact with the skin for 48 hours, undisturbed, and then examined at 48, hours after application. An individual is allergic to nickel (or other contact allergen) if a positive reaction is noted. However, patch tests may produce vague or unclear results that may require further examination. This means that sometimes, the cause cannot be determined.

If one is allergic or sensitive to nickel, the best thing to do is to discontinue, whenever possible, exposure to nickel and nickel-containing items. It appears that this is the closest thing there is to a cure.

Here are some precautions to follow to avoid nickel. For clothing, choose fasteners made of plastic, coated or painted metal, or some other material. A nickel allergy does not mean jewelry cannot be worn. One just has to be much more selective in choices—make sure they are hypoallergenic, or made of stainless steel (although this contains nickel, it is so tightly bound that it cannot be leached out), solid gold (at least 12 carat), pure sterling silver, or polycarbonate plastic. However, if earrings must be worn that contain nickel, protect oneself with plastic covers made specifically for earring studs. Applying clear nail polish to earrings is another option of some use. Since perspiration dissolves nickel, some people have tried removing moisture by applying talcum powder to areas of the body in contact with nickel-containing items in the hopes of limiting the extent or degree of exposure. This is of little use.

Regarding treatments the following are only temporary solutions to a nickel allergy, since they do not desensitize one to nickel. Some nickel allergy treatments include topical steroids, which must be used as directed by a dermatologist; compresses made of Burow's solution diluted with water, which help dry up blisters; and/or, emollient creams, which help alleviate the dryness and itch of dermatitis when frequently applied.

☞ Remember!!

Regardless of one's nickel allergy status and/or exposure to nickel, when having piercing of ears, or other body parts, have it done only with a stainless-steel needle. More importantly, make sure the first pair of earrings have stainless steel or high quality 18-karat gold studs, which is worn until the skin is completely healed. These precautions will help reduce the risk for developing a nickel allergy in the future.

Chapter 47

Latex Allergies

Everyday we use products made of latex—balloons, rubber bands, condoms, rubber household gloves, rubber balls, and Band-Aids, for example. For some people, though, contact with these products can cause discomfort or painful reactions. In some rare cases, it can cause death.

Frequently Asked Questions About Latex Allergy

What is latex?

The term "latex" refers to the sap of the Brazilian rubber tree or the products made from that sap. The term is used to mean "natural rubber products."

What types of reactions are there?

You can have two different types of reaction from contact with latex. The most common reaction is contact dermatitis. This is a red, itchy rash that breaks out where latex has touched your skin. It appears 12 to 24 hours after contact.

Contact dermatitis usually is caused by frequent washing, harsh soaps and friction of putting on and taking off gloves. Sometimes it is caused by chemicals added to latex when products are made. This type of reaction is

About This Chapter: This chapter includes "Latex Allergy" and "Types of Latex Reactions," both reprinted with permission from the Asthma and Allergy Foundation of America, © 1998. All rights reserved. Reviewed in September 2005 by David A. Cooke, M.D.

often more severe, with blisters and crusted sores. Areas of the body not in contact with the latex product are not affected.

Poison ivy causes a similar reaction. In the past ten years, some people have begun to have an immediate hypersensitivity to latex. What happens is like an allergic reaction to an insect sting or to peanuts. Within minutes of contact, or even after inhaling glove dusting powder, an allergic person develops itching or hives, stuffy nose, sneezing, itchy eyes, or asthma symptoms.

In some cases, the allergy can cause anaphylactic shock. This is a dangerous condition in which the blood vessels widen so much that blood pressure plummets. Symptoms include sweating, paleness, panting, nausea, rapid pulse, faintness, confusion, and even passing out. With out speedy treatment, this intense allergic reaction can cause death.

What causes a reaction to latex?

The reaction is caused by allergens—proteins in the sap of the rubber tree. Most experts believe that the allergy has surfaced recently as a result of the increased use of latex to protect people from infectious agents. There may be other causes as well. Man-made latex is not a problem.

Who is likely to get a reaction?

Perhaps one in every 1,000 people develops a latex allergy. Although rare, the condition has become common in certain high-risk groups.

The highest risk is in children with spina bifida—a condition in which the spine failed to form completely before birth. About three of every five children with spina bifida are allergic to latex.

Also at high risk are any children who have frequent and repeated medical treatments or lengthy surgery that involve the use of latex products. Many medical supplies, from gloves to tubing to enemas tips, are made of latex.

From 5 percent to 15 percent of health care workers and others who regularly wear latex gloves are allergic to latex. Health care workers and children who have other allergies and get contact dermatitis when they use latex gloves are more likely to develop a latex allergy.

Sometimes people with latex allergies experience a reaction to many tropical fruits, nuts and vegetables, particularly avocado, banana, chestnut, hazelnut, kiwi, raw potato, tomato, peaches, papaya, stone fruits (such as plums), or celery.

What are the symptoms?

Common early symptoms include the following:

- Swelling, redness, and itching after contact with rubber. Itching or swelling of the lips after blowing up balloons or around Band-Aids suggests latex allergy.

- Swelling or itching of the mouth or tongue after a dental visit. Swelling and itching after medical exams such as vaginal and rectal exams or on contact with condoms or diaphragms.

- Redness or itching of the hands, stuffy nose, or asthma that occurs while wearing latex gloves or having frequent contact with latex products at work.

People highly allergic to latex may have severe reactions from contact with just a small amount of latex in the air. One person had a severe asthma attack after entering a room where children had blown up a few balloons.

Symptoms that suggest you may be allergic to latex should not be ignored. Constant contact with latex products—for example, intense exposure during surgery—can lead to more severe reactions. People also can develop chronic conditions such as occupational asthma.

How is a latex allergy diagnosed?

If you think you may be allergic to latex, see a doctor familiar with the condition. It can be diagnosed with a medical history, physical exam, and either a blood test or skin sensitivity test. The blood test involves looking for latex antibodies in a blood sample. For the skin test, an extract of latex is used to scratch or prick the skin. If you are allergic to the product, redness or swelling may appear at the scratch. Your doctor compares your test results with your history and physical exam to make a diagnosis of latex allergy.

What should I do if I am allergic to latex?

- Avoid latex. The only treatment for latex allergy is to prevent any contact with latex products. Medications may help control symptoms. They cannot be relied on to prevent symptoms from later contact with latex, though.

- To avoid airborne latex ask co-workers to wear only non-latex gloves or latex gloves that are not powdered.

- Avoid antihistamine medications which may hide problems with latex in the air.

- Always wear or carry a tag to identify your latex allergy in case you need emergency care.

- Obtain a letter about your allergy from your doctor. Latex allergy has been recognized only recently. Many health care workers may not have heard of it or know how to treat it.

- Ask doctors, dentists, and others whether routine exams or treatment will expose you to latex. You may want to carry latex-free exam gloves with you to give your dentist or doctor.

- Check labeling to make sure products contain no latex. Do not assume a product labeled "hypoallergenic" is latex-free.

- Always carry injectable epinephrine, such as Ana-Kit or EpiPen. These products are used to treat reactions to insect bites and foods. Injecting epinephrine can save your life if you have a severe reaction. Immediately seek medical care.

Be aware that people with latex allergy may also develop food allergies. The food allergy can occur unexpectedly, and even the first attack can be severe. Never eat fresh fruits or vegetables or nuts without having an injectable epinephrine syringe at hand.

Source: © 1998 Asthma and Allergy Foundation of America; reviewed by David A. Cooke, M.D., 2005.

Types Of Latex Reactions

There are three types of reactions to natural rubber latex: Irritant contact dermatitis, type IV (delayed) hypersensitivity, and type I (immediate) hypersensitivity. It is useful to occasionally review the differences between the three, since latex avoidance is critical to those who have latex allergy. While it's important to be aware of potential sources of natural rubber latex in the environment, understanding the difference between type IV and type I reactions can decrease the stress of vigilance.

Irritant Contact Dermatitis is a common reaction and is not an allergy. Itchy, dry, and irritated hands are the result of frequent hand washing and incomplete drying, use of hand sanitizers, and friction irritation from glove powder. Anyone who wears powdered latex gloves can develop this; however, in atopic individuals, contact dermatitis can be a sign of impending hypersensitivity if exposure to latex continues.

Type IV (delayed-type) Hypersensitivity is usually a sensitivity to chemicals used to make gloves, rather than to proteins from the natural rubber itself. Numerous chemicals are used in the manufacturing process, including antioxidants, emulsifiers, stabilizers, accelerators, stiffeners, colorants, and fragrances. Any of these can cause a contact dermatitis 24–48 hours after exposure, which can spread to other areas, including the face, if touched. Symptoms usually resolve spontaneously. Type IV hypersensitivity is also called allergic contact dermatitis, T-cell-mediated allergy, or chemical allergy. It is estimated that 80% of people who develop type I reactions experienced type IV reactions first. Approximately 7–18% of the population has type IV hypersensitivity.

Type I (immediate-type) Hypersensitivity is an allergy to natural rubber latex (*Hevea brasiliensis*) proteins that occurs as a response to exposure. Vasoactive mediators such as histamine are released, causing a spectrum of clinical symptoms including, among others, hives, nausea, abdominal cramping, and facial swelling with itchy, watery eyes.

Emergency treatment for anaphylaxis may be required, and anyone who has experienced a type I reaction attributable to latex exposure should wear a medical ID bracelet and carry an EpiPen. Type I reactions affect less than 1% of the population.

So how does one know what kind of reaction is occurring? Type IV reactions, so far, have not been life-threatening and tend to be localized near the area of contact. In contrast, type I reactions tend to be systemic and can be life-threatening. Chronic dermatitis may be a sign of chemical sensitivity to other components besides latex protein. Atopic individuals are susceptible to latex allergy, but they are also predisposed to other allergies. This may require further testing by an allergist, or a dermatologist who can prescribe topical medications to control chronic dermatitis.

Those with type I hypersensitivity should avoid latex allergen exposure and they should also be aware of chemical-induced delayed reactions that can be confused for reactions to latex proteins. Keeping a written record of reactions and their causes can help differentiate life-threatening Type 1 reactions from merely annoying Type IV reactions, and it can help physicians offer more targeted treatment.

✎ What's It Mean?

Latex: Latex refers to the natural rubber latex manufactured from a milky fluid that is primarily obtained from the rubber tree (*Hevea brasiliensis*). Some synthetic rubber materials may be referred to as "latex" but they do not contain the protein that produces latex allergy.

Source: Excerpted from "Safety and Health Topics: Latex Allergy," Occupational Safety and Health Administration, U.S. Department of Labor, May 2005.

Chapter 48

Drug Allergies

Most people have probably experienced an unwanted side effect to a medicine at some time in their lives. Many drugs commonly cause side effects, such as an upset stomach after taking aspirin or drowsiness after taking a cold medication. Adverse drug reactions also can be quite serious; they account for an estimated 106,000 deaths each year in the United States. As more medications are approved each year, the problem is expected to grow.

An adverse drug reaction is any effect not intended by proper administration of a medication. Reactions also can occur between medications, even nonprescription ones. Most adverse drug reactions—more than 90 percent—do not involve the immune system. When the immune system is involved, a person is said to have drug hypersensitivity. Allergy is one type of hypersensitivity reaction.

What Is Drug Hypersensitivity?

Medications can cause unwanted reactions in many ways. Sometimes, it's a direct effect of the drug on the body. Drug hypersensitivity reactions occur when the immune system responds to a medication or to the biologic products that result when the body breaks down a medication. In some cases, the immune system tries to attack the substance, causing symptoms of the drug reaction. Drugs also can cause allergic reactions similar to those caused by bee stings or other allergenic substances.

People who have a family history of allergic diseases may be more likely to have drug allergy, but are not at greater risk to develop non-allergic types of reactions. Fortunately, a family history of allergy to a particular drug does not increase a person's chance of being allergic to that same drug.

A person must have a previous exposure to a drug in order to have a true allergic reaction to it. Such reactions most often occur when a drug is administered intravenously or by injection, delivery methods that send the drug directly to the bloodstream. Reactions occur less frequently when drugs are taken by mouth. The chance of an allergic reaction increases when a medication is administered frequently or in large doses.

Certain medications are more likely to cause allergic reactions than others due to their chemical structure. Penicillin and other antibiotics are some of the most common culprits of allergic drug reactions. Penicillin, however, can also cause other types of immune reactions, as well as reactions that do not involve the immune system.

✦ It's A Fact!!

The penicillin antibiotics are popular and useful antimicrobial drugs because they are very effective and have low toxicity. However, they are also one of the most common causes of drug-induced anaphylactic reactions. Fatal penicillin-induced anaphylaxis has been reported at a rate of 0.002% among the general population, with 500 to 1,000 deaths per year.

Source: Excerpted from "Penicillin Allergy," by Mercedes E. Arroliga, M.D., © 2005 The Cleveland Clinic Foundation, 9500 Euclid Avenue, Cleveland, OH 44195, www.clevelandclinic.org. Additional information is available from the Cleveland Clinic Health Information Center, 216-444-3771, tollfree 800-223-2273 extension 43771, or at http://www.clevelandclinic.org/health.

Symptoms

The most common types of allergic reactions to a drug are as follows:

- Skin rash or hives
- Itchy skin
- Wheezing or other breathing problems
- Swelling of body parts
- Anaphylaxis, a life-threatening allergic reaction

While these are the most common symptoms of drug allergy, adverse reactions can occur in any organ or system of the body.

Allergic reactions can occur within minutes or hours of exposure to a medication. Drug reactions can even occur some time after a medication has been stopped. For example, a person may develop a rash or hives a week after stopping a medication.

A "pseudoallergic," or anaphylactoid, reaction does not involve allergic antibodies and can occur without prior exposure. Symptoms are similar to a true allergic reaction: a person may develop a rash or hives, have difficulty breathing, and experience swelling of body parts. Common causes of pseudoallergic reactions include aspirin and x-ray dye.

Diagnosis

Adverse drug reactions can be difficult to diagnose, because they often can look like other conditions. Further, although many common reactions to certain drugs are known, others may not have been identified yet.

It is important to distinguish an allergic (hypersensitivity) reaction from a non-allergic reaction. If drug hypersensitivity is suspected, your doctor may send you to a specialist in allergy and immunology.

If you suspect you are having, or had, an adverse reaction to a medication, take note of the circumstances. Your doctor will want to know when the medication was taken, when the symptoms started, what the symptoms were and how long they lasted, and any other medications you were taking at the

♣ It's A Fact!!

Severe allergic reactions during anesthesia are fortunately rare, occurring once in every 5,000 to 25,000 anesthetics. Unfortunately, these reactions can sometimes be fatal, with a 3.4% mortality.

The most severe form of allergic reaction is known as 'anaphylaxis.' The patient who is awake during an anaphylactic reaction may experience difficulty breathing, as air passages close up. Swelling of the face and mouth can occur, and a reddish skin rash is also sometimes seen. The heart and blood vessels are severely affected, and this is the hallmark of the condition: the heart rate increases and blood pressure can drop to dangerously low levels.

Anaphylaxis under general (asleep) anesthesia presents in a similar way but there are three unique features. First, the patient cannot tell us about light-headedness or breathlessness which might be early warning symptoms. Second, during a typical general anesthetic, many drugs are given, and it is hardly ever clear which of these drugs have caused the reaction. Third, during anesthesia there are many other potential causes for the blood pressure to be dropping or the air passages to be closing off. A diagnosis of anaphylaxis is therefore not always easy to establish.

Although severe allergic reactions may be a little more difficult to detect under anesthesia, a patient having an anaphylactic reaction under anesthesia is actually in a very good place to get treated. All the necessary equipment and medication to successfully treat the reaction is at hand in the operating room. Treatment may include insertion of a breathing tube, administration of intravenous fluid, and a variety of drugs, the most important of which is epinephrine (or adrenaline). Early and appropriate treatment is almost always successful.

Source: Excerpted from "Allergy to Anesthesia Drugs." Reprinted with permission from http://www.netwellness.com. Copyright ® 2005 University of Cincinnati.

time, including nonprescription medications. Bring copies of any treatment records of the reaction with you to the doctor's office. This information is important for the diagnosis and treatment of your condition.

Be sure to have the name of the exact medications you took to help the doctor identify which drugs should be tested for hypersensitivity. It also will allow the allergist to determine if there are alternative medications that would be safe for you to take—and which additional medications you should avoid in the future. If possible, bring the suspected medications with you.

Next, an allergist will perform a physical examination. This is necessary to check for different problems that may occur as part of an allergic reaction and to determine if there are other, non-allergic causes of the symptoms. The allergist will pay special attention to any symptoms of a reaction that you still have, such as a skin rash.

Allergy skin testing is available to test for allergic reactions to only a few drugs. Many experts recommend that testing not be done until there is a future, compelling need to use the same medication again. In some cases, an allergist will perform blood tests to identify antibodies against a medication. Blood tests tend to be less sensitive than skin tests, so a skin test will be used whenever possible.

Treatment

If a drug reaction is mild, treatment may be limited to stopping the medication. In many cases, discontinuing the drug is all that is needed.

To relieve the symptoms of a more serious or persistent reaction, an allergist may administer antihistamines, corticosteroids and other medications. Antihistamines work by counteracting the chemical histamine, which is released during the body's allergic response. Corticosteroids work by reducing inflammation.

In most cases, a person with drug hypersensitivity can safely be given alternative drugs, and the drug that caused the reaction is simply avoided. When no alternative medication exists, an allergist can undertake desensitization or graded challenge. These are methods of gradually introducing a medication into the body in small doses until a therapeutic dose is reached.

Anaphylaxis

Anaphylaxis is a severe, potentially life-threatening reaction that can occur within seconds or minutes of administration of a drug. Symptoms of anaphylaxis include swelling of body parts; shortness of breath or wheezing; a sudden drop in blood pressure, which may cause dizziness or loss of consciousness; and shock.

Anaphylaxis requires emergency treatment. Several drugs, including epinephrine, antihistamines and corticosteroids, are often administered. The patient may also receive oxygen and intravenous fluids.

If you take a medication and develop any of the symptoms of anaphylaxis, immediately call your local emergency phone number (911 in most locations in the United States and Canada). Although antihistamines are sometimes given to patients with anaphylaxis, antihistamines alone are not likely to be adequate treatment. If you are with someone who develops any symptoms of anaphylaxis, call your local emergency number. If he or she loses consciousness, lay the person down and elevate the feet.

If you have had a reaction to a drug:

- Make sure all of your doctors know the medication you took and the reaction you had;

- Talk to your primary care doctor or allergist about other medications you should avoid and which alternative medications are safe for you to take; and

- If the reaction is severe, wear a medical alert tag or bracelet in case of emergency.

Chapter 49

Chemical Sensitivities

A variety of vague and hard-to-pinpoint symptoms are experienced by an undetermined, but possibly sizable number of adults and children. Occasionally, they may suggest allergy or asthma, but most often the symptoms are much wider in scope.

Not much is currently known about what is referred to as "chemical sensitivity," but it is a subject that is often mentioned as a growing problem in the popular media. Since there are considered to be a variety of adverse health effects from so-called "chemical sensitivities," the public and their health care providers are rightly confused about what it is all about.

Why are chemical sensitivities gaining so much interest?

There are several reasons, among which are the following:

- A greater number of complex chemical compounds (polymers) in our natural environment than in the past.

- Less indoor air exchange in more highly insulated houses and buildings.

- Greater media coverage of news and opinions about chemical sensitivities and their possible ill effects on our health.

A few physicians who refer to themselves as "ecologically oriented" have proposed diagnoses such as the "Twentieth Century Disease," "Chemical AIDS," "multiple chemical sensitivities," or "Candida hypersensitivity." Intriguing as these labels may be to some whose symptoms seem to frustrate the attempts of a medical diagnosis and treatment, no single test or combination of tests has yet to clearly identify the causes of these symptoms.

♣ It's A Fact!!

Multiple Chemical Sensitivity

Multiple chemical sensitivity (MCS) is something of a medical mystery. The medical community is divided over whether or not MCS actually exists.

Some physicians acknowledge MCS as a medical disorder that is triggered by exposures to chemicals in the environment, often beginning with a short term, severe chemical exposure (like a chemical spill) or with a longer term, small exposures (like a poorly ventilated office building). After the initial exposure, low levels of everyday chemicals such as those found in cosmetics, soaps, and newspaper inks can trigger physical reactions in MCS patients. These patients report a range of symptoms that often include headaches, rashes, asthma, depression, muscle and joint aches, fatigue, memory loss, and confusion.

Others in the medical community, however, do not accept MCS as a genuine medical disorder. The Centers for Disease Control, for example, do not recognize MCS as a clinical diagnosis. There is no official medical definition of MCS, partially because symptoms and chemical exposures are often unique and are widely varied between individuals. Some physicians are skeptical of concluding that low concentrations of the same chemicals that are tolerated by everyone else can cause dramatic symptoms in MCS patients. The American Medical Association denies that MCS is a clinical condition because conclusive scientific evidence is lacking.

Source: Excerpted from "Allergies: Multiple Chemical Sensitivity," National Institute of Environmental Health Sciences, reviewed 1997.

Nevertheless, caring physicians are sensitive to patients with vague complaints. They endeavor to keep them from seeking in desperation care and "cures" that lack a medical-scientific basis or require much more study.

What are considered chemical sensitivities?

There are four general ways that we can classify chemical sensitivity:

Annoyance Reactions: These result from a heightened sensitivity to unpleasant odors, called olfactory awareness, in some susceptible individuals. Your ability to cope with offensive—but mostly nonirritating—odors has a lot to do with genetic or acquired factors, among which are infection and inflammation of the mucous membranes or polyps (growths of the nasal or sinus membranes), and abuse of tobacco and nasal decongestants.

Irritational Syndromes: These are caused by significant exposure to irritating chemicals that are more likely than others to penetrate the mucous membranes. These types of reactions can affect certain nerve endings and cause burning sensations in the nose, eyes and throat. They usually come and go, and can be reversed.

Immune Hypersensitivity: This is the basis of allergic diseases, such as allergic rhinitis (hay fever) and asthma. They are generally caused by naturally occurring organic chemicals found in pollens, molds, dust and animals. At present, only a relatively few industrial chemicals are known to have the capability of provoking a true immune system response. Among them are acid anhydrides and isocyanates and other chemicals that are able to bond to human proteins.

Intoxication Syndrome: In some cases, long-term exposure to noxious chemicals may cause serious illness, or even death. Permanent damage to health may be the outcome of such reactions, which are dependent on the nature and extent of the chemical exposure. Toxic pollutants are given off by a number of building products, such as furniture, cleaning fluids, pesticides and paints.

How does pollution affect my health?

Most people who believe they have symptoms from chemical sensitivity are concerned that they are related to their exposure to pollution, either outdoors or indoors. Outdoor pollution may result from natural causes (the eruption of volcanoes, dust storms, forest fires), or man-made causes (vehicle exhaust, fossil fuel combustion, petroleum refining). Other pollutants that may cause respiratory illness include the following:

Sulfur Dioxide: Substantial scientific evidence has linked specific air pollutants to increased respiratory illness and decreased pulmonary function, especially in children. People prone to allergy, especially those with allergic asthma, can be extremely sensitive to inhaled sulfur dioxide, for example. Symptoms may include bronchospasm, hives, gastrointestinal disorders and inflammation of the blood vessels (vasculitis-related disorder).

Ozone And Nitrogen Dioxide: Temporary or perhaps permanent bronchial hypersensitivity has been connected to inhaled ozone and nitrogen dioxide. Long-term exposure to nitrogen dioxide has been associated with the increased occurrence of respiratory illness.

Significant exposure to airborne pollution occurs inside homes, offices and non-industrial buildings. These settings have not received nearly the attention by pollution control agencies that they deserve.

Cigarette Smoke: One of the most disagreeable and potentially dangerous indoor pollutants is cigarette smoke. It is made up of a complex mixture of gases and particles that contain numerous chemicals. Indoor tobacco smoking substantially increases levels of carbon monoxide, formaldehyde, nitrogen dioxide, acrolein, polycyclic aromatic hydrocarbons, hydrogen cyanide, and many other substances and inhaled particles found in the air.

Formaldehyde is not only found indoors from cigarette smoke, but also outdoors from gasoline and diesel combustion. Data indicates that formaldehyde is capable of acting as a respiratory irritant. It also is known to cause an allergic skin rash. However, there is no convincing evidence that this pollutant is able to sensitize the respiratory system.

Wood Burning Stoves: There are more than 11 million wood burning units in American homes today. Wood burning usually occurs in cold, oxygen-poor conditions that heighten the emission of carbon monoxide and other inhaled chemicals and particles. Increased use of wood as a heating fuel has raised concern because of its ability to contaminate a home. Poorly ventilated stoves give off increased levels of carbon monoxide, nitrogen and sulfur oxides, formaldehyde, and benzopyrene.

Building-Related Illness: Poor air quality in today's tightly insulated homes and other buildings has been associated with a variety of syndromes, or group of symptoms. The term "building-related illness" or "sick-building syndrome" is applied to an office building in which one or more occupants develop a generally accepted, well-defined syndrome for which a specific cause related to the building is found.

There are a variety of illnesses broadly known as hypersensitivity pneumonitis—in which one or more organic dusts can create complex immune system reactions and symptoms, including mucous membrane irritation, coughing, chest tightness, headache and fatigue. These are well defined, and there are validated tests for diagnosing these conditions. Building occupants with these symptoms have been identified as having "multiple chemical sensitivities" or other forms of environmental illness.

One study, however, showed that the majority of nonspecific complaints by office workers had developed before the worker began working in the building suspected of causing their symptoms. Collaboration between the physician, industrial hygienist and building engineer may be necessary to clearly establish a cause-and-effect relationship between any indoor air quality level and disease.

How is chemical sensitivity diagnosed?

There are strategies that can produce reliable diagnoses with relatively low costs, reliable diagnoses at significant costs or questionable diagnoses at great expense. Obviously, the first alternative is preferable. It includes the following:

- A careful patient medical history that includes a review of all previous medical records and, when symptoms may be related to potentially hazardous substances in the workplace, reviewing a Materials Safety Data Sheet supplied by the employer.

- Upper respiratory tract and selective skin tests and a neurological examination.

- Routine laboratory studies, including nasal smear.

- Lung function measurements (spirometry and peak flow monitoring).

If these diagnostic procedures do not produce a definite diagnosis, more expensive—but worthwhile—evaluations may help. They include an industrial hygiene evaluation of the workplace, an evaluation of the home environment and psychiatric evaluations.

Diagnostic approaches are expensive and not effective in explaining suggested chemical sensitivity such as the RAST test, and tests for the Epstein-Barr virus, auto-immune disease, food allergies, and evaluations to determine airborne molds and bacteria.

Part 6

If You Need More Information

Chapter 50

Resources For More Information About Allergies

General Information About Allergies

Allergy Prevention Center
http://
www.allergypreventioncenter.com

Allergy Society of South Africa
P.O. Box 88
Observatory, 7935
Cape Town
South Africa
Phone: 011 27 021-4479019
Fax: 011 27 021-4480846
Website: http://allergysa.org

American Academy of Allergy, Asthma and Immunology
555 East Wells Street, Suite 1100
Milwaukee, WI 53202-3823
Toll-Free: 800-822-2762
Phone: 414-272-6071
Website: http://www.aaaai.org
E-mail: info@aaaai.org

American Board of Allergy and Immunology
510 Walnut, Suite 1701
Philadelphia, PA 19106
Phone: 215-592-9466
Fax: 215-592-9411
Website: http://www.abai.org
E-mail: abai@abai.org

About This Chapter: Information in this chapter was compiled many sources deemed reliable. All contact information was verified and updated in September 2005.

American College of Allergy, Asthma and Immunology
85 West Algonquin Road, Suite 550
Arlington Heights, IL 60005
Toll-Free: 800-842-7777
Phone: 847-427-1200
Fax: 847-427-1294
Website: http://www.acaai.org
E-mail: mail@acaai.org

American Osteopathic College of Allergy and Immunology
7025 E. McDowell Road, Suite 1B
Scottsdale, AZ 85257
Phone: 480-585-1580
Fax: 480-990-3184

Calgary Allergy Network
Website: http://www.calgaryallergy.ca

Canadian Society of Allergy and Clinical Immunology
774 Echo Dr.
Ottawa ON K1S 5N 8, Canada
Phone: 613-730-6272
Fax: 613-730-1116
Website: http://
www.csaci.medical.org
E-mail: csaci@rcpsc.edu

Joint Council of Allergy, Asthma, and Immunology
50 N. Brockway, Suite 3-3
Palatine, IL 60067
Phone: 847-934-1918
Website: http://www.jcaai.org
E-mail: info@jcaai.org

National Institute of Allergy and Infectious Diseases
6610 Rockledge Drive, MSC 6612
Bethesda, MD 20892-6612
Phone: 301-496-5717
Fax: 301-402-3573
Website: http://www.niaid.nih.gov

National Library of Medicine
MedlinePlus
8600 Rockville Pike
Bethesda, MD 20894
Toll-Free: 888-346-3656
Phone: 301-594-5983
Fax: 301-402-1384
Website: http://medlineplus.gov
E-mail: custserv@nlm.nih.gov

Pan-American Allergy Society
P.O. Box 700587
San Antonio, TX 78270-0587
Phone: 210-495-9853
Fax: 210-495-9852
Website: http://www.paas.org
E-mail:
panamallergy@sbcglobal.net

World Allergy Organization
555 East Wells Street, 11th Floor
Milwaukee, WI 53202-3823
Phone: 414-276-1791
Fax: 414-276-3349
Website: http://
www.worldallergy.org
E-mail: info@worldallergy.org

Allergic Skin Diseases

American Academy of Dermatology
P.O. Box 4014
Schaumburg, IL 60168-4014
Toll Free: 888-462-DERM
Phone: 847-330-0230
Fax: 847-330-0050
Website: http://www.aad.org

American Osteopathic College of Dermatology
1501 East Illinois Street
Kirksville, MO 63501
Toll-Free: 800-449-2623
Phone: 660-665-2184
Fax: 660-627-2623
Website: http://www.aocd.org
E-mail: info@aocd.org

Dermatology Consultants
1401 Harrodsburg Road, C-415
Lexington, KY 40504
Toll-Free: 800-447-3862
Phone: 859-278-9492
Fax: 859-277-3027
Website: http://
www.dermconsultants.com
E-mail: info@dermconsultants.com

National Eczema Association for Science and Education
4460 Redwood Highway, Suite 16-D
San Rafael, CA 94903-1953
Toll-Free: 800-818-7546
Phone: 415-499-3474
Fax: 415-472-5345
Website: http://
www.nationaleczema.org
E-mail: info@nationaleczema.org

National Institute of Arthritis and Musculoskeletal and Skin Diseases Information Clearinghouse
1 AMS Circle
Bethesda, MD 20892-3675
Toll-Free: 877-22-NIAMS (877-226-4267)
Phone: 301-495-4484
Fax: 301-718-6366
TTY: 301-565-2966
Website: http://www.niams.nih.gov
E-mail: naimsinfo@mail.nih.gov

New Zealand Dermatological Society
6 Knox Street
Hamilton
New Zealand
Phone: 011 67-7-838-1035
Fax: 011-67-7-838-2032
Website: http://dermnetnz.org

Asthma and Allergic Respiratory Diseases

American Academy of Otolaryngology—Head and Neck Surgery, Inc.
One Prince Street
Alexandria, VA 22314-3357
Phone: 703-836-4444
Fax: 684-4288
Website: http://www.entnet.org
E-mail: ServiceCentral@entnet.org

Allergy and Asthma Network Mothers of Asthmatics, Inc.
2751 Prosperity Avenue, Suite 150
Fairfax, VA 22031
Toll-Free: 800-878-4403
Fax: 703-573-7794
Website: http://www.aanma.org

Allergy/Asthma Information Association (AAIA)
Box 100
Toronto, ON M9W 5K9
Canada
Toll-Free: 800-611-7011
Phone: 416-679-9521
Fax: 416-679-9524
Website: http://www.aaia.ca
E-mail: national@aaia.ca

Allies Against Asthma
University of Michigan
School of Public Health
109 South Observatory Street
Ann Arbor, MI 48109-2029
Phone: 734-647-3179
Fax: 734-763-7379
Website: http://www.asthma.umich.edu
E-mail: asthma@umich.edu

American Academy of Otolaryngic Allergy
1990 M Street, NW, Suite 680
Washington, DC 20036
Phone: 202-955-5010
Fax: 202-955-5016
Website: http://www.entallergy.org
E-mail: info@aaoaf.org

American Association for Respiratory Care
9425 N. MacArthur Blvd., Suite 100
Irving, TX 75063-4706
Phone: 972-243-2272
Fax: 972-484-2720
Website: http://www.aarc.org
E-mail: info@aarc.org

American Lung Association
61 Broadway, 6th Floor
New York, NY 10006
Toll-Free: 800-LUNG-USA (800-586-4872)
Phone: 212-315-8700
Website: http://www.lungusa.org

Asthma and Allergy Foundation of America
1233 20th Street, NW, Suite 402
Washington, DC 20036
Toll-Free: 800-7-ASTHMA
(Hotline)
Phone: 202-466-7643
Website: http://www.aafa.org
E-mail: info@aafa.org

Asthma and Schools
Website: http://
www.asthmaandschools.org
E-mail: info@asthmaandschools.org

Asthma In Canada
Website: http://
www.asthmaincanada.com

Asthma Initiative of Michigan
403 Seymour
Lansing, MI 48933
Toll-Free: 866-395-8647
Phone: 517-484-7206
Website: http://
www.getasthmahelp.org
E-mail: info@GetAsthmaHelp.org

Asthma Resource Bank
Allies Against Asthma Resource Bank
University of Michigan School of
Public Health
109 S. Observatory St.
Ann Arbor, MI 48109-2029
Phone: 734-647-9047
Fax: 734-763-7379
Website: http://
www.asthmaresourcebank.org
E-mail: resourcebank@umich.edu

Asthma Society of Canada
130 Bridgeland Avenue, Suite 425
Toronto, ON M6A 1Z4, Canada
Toll-Free: 866-787-4050
Phone: 416-787-4050
Fax: 416-787-5807
Website: http://www.asthma.ca
E-mail: info@asthma.ca

Canadian Lung Association
1231 8th St., E
Saskatoon, SK S7H 0S5, Canada
Toll-Free: 888-566-LUNG
Website: http://www.lung.ca/
asthma

Canadian Network for Asthma Care
16851 Mount Wolfe Rd.
Bolton, ON L7E 5R7, Canada
Phone: 905-880-1092
Fax: 905-880-9733
Website: http://www.cnac.net

Childhood Asthma Foundation

Box 22033 Town & County Plaza
Niagara Falls, ON L2J 4J3
Canada
Toll-Free: 800-373-5697
Website: http://www.childasthma.com
E-mail:
asthmainfo@childhoodasthma.ca

Consortium on Children's Asthma Camps

490 Concordia Ave.
St. Paul, MN 44103
Phone: 651-227-8014
Website: http://asthmacamps.org/
asthmacamps

Environmental Protection Agency

Ariel Rios Building
1200 Pennsylvania Avenue, NW
Washington, DC 20460
Phone: 202-272-0167
Website: http://www.epa.gov

Global Initiative for Asthma

Website: http://www.ginasthma.com

National Allergy Bureau

555 East Wells Street, Suite 1100
Milwaukee, WI 53202-3823
Toll-Free: 800-9-POLLEN
Phone: 414-272-6071
Website: http://www.aaaai.org/nab
E-mail: info@aaaai.org

National Asthma Education Program

P.O. Box 30105
Bethesda, MD 20824
Phone: 301-592-8573
Website: http://www.nhlbi.nih.gov/
health/public/lung

National Center for Environmental Health

Centers for Disease Control and
Prevention
1600 Clifton Rd., NE MS E-17
Atlanta, GA 30333
Toll-Free: 888-232-6789
Phone: 404-639-2520
Fax: 404-693-2560
Website: http://www.cdc.gov/nceh

National Heart, Lung, and Blood Institute Information Center

P.O. Box 30105
Bethesda, MD 20824-0105
Phone: 301-592-8573
Fax: 240-629-3246
TTY: 240-629-3255
Website: http://www.nhlbi.nih.gov
E-mail: nhlbiinfo@nhlbi.nih.gov

National Institute of Environmental Health Sciences

Office of Communications
P.O. Box 12233
Research Triangle Park, NC 27709
Phone: 919-541-3345
Website: http://www.niehs.nih.gov/
airborne
E-mail: webcenter@niehs.nih.gov

National Jewish Medical and Research Center

1400 Jackson St.
Denver, CO 80206
Toll-Free: 800-222-5864
Phone: 303-388-4461
Fax: 303-270-2234
Website: http://
www.nationaljewish.org
E-mail: lungline@njc.org

Parents of Asthmatic/Allergic Children

748 S. Lemay Avenue, Suite A3
Box 109
Ft. Collins, CO 80524
Phone: 970-495-8153

Food Allergies and Anaphylaxis

Anaphylaxis Canada

416 Moore Ave., Suite 306
Toronto, ON M4G 1C9, Canada
Phone: 416-785-5666
Fax: 416-785-0458
Website: http://
www.anaphylaxis.org
E-mail: info@anaphylaxis.ca

Center for Food Safety and Applied Nutrition

Food and Drug Administration
5100 Paint Branch Parkway
College Park, MD 20740-3835
Toll-Free: 888- 463-6332 or 888-
723-3366
Website: http://www.cfsan.fda.gov

DEY, L.P. (EpiPen)

Website: http://www.allergic-
reactions.com

Food Allergy and Anaphylaxis Network

11781 Lee Jackson Highway, Suite 160
Fairfax, VA 22033-3309
Toll-Free: 800-929-4040
Fax: 703-691-2713
Website: http://www.foodallergy.org
E-mail: faan@foodallergy.org

Food Allergy Initiative
Website: http://
www.foodallergyinitiative.org

Institute of Food and Agricultural Services
University of Florida
Institute of Food and Agricultural
Science
Gainesville, FL 32611
Website: http://edis.ifas.ufl.edu
E-mail: EDIShelp@ifas.ufl.edu

International Food Information Council Foundation
1100 Connecticut Ave., NW, Suite 430
Washington, DC 20036
Phone: 202-295-6540
Fax: 202-296-6547
Website: http://www.ific.org
E-mail: foodinfo@ific.org

National Digestive Diseases Information Clearinghouse
2 Information Way
Bethesda, MD 20892-3570
Toll Free: 800-891-5389
Fax: 703-738-4929
Website: http://
www.niddk.nih.gov/health/digest/
nddic.htm
E-mail: nddic@info.niddk.nih.gov

Latex and Cosmetic Allergies

American Latex Allergy Association
3791 Sherman Road
Slinger, WI 53086
Toll-Free: 888-97-ALERT (888-
972-5378); Fax: 262-677-0324
Website: http://
www.latexallergyresources.org
E-mail:
alert@latexallergyresources.org

Center for Food Safety and Applied Nutrition
Food and Drug Administration
5100 Paint Branch Parkway
College Park, MD 20740-3835
Toll-Free: 888- 463-6332 or 888-
723-3366
Website: http://www.cfsan.fda.gov

Occupational Safety and Health Administration
U.S. Department of Labor
200 Constitution Ave., NW
Washington, DC 20210
Toll-Free: 800-321-OSHA (6742)
TTY: 877-889-5627
Website: http://www.osha.gov

Chapter 51

Additional Reading About Allergies

Books About Allergies

101 Questions about Your Immune System You Felt Defenseless to Answer ... Until Now
by Faith Hickman Brynie, Twenty-First Century Books, 2000.

Allergies A–Z: Practical Advice on Living with Allergies
by Myron A. Lipkowitz and Tova Navarra, Facts on File, Inc. 2001.

Allergies Sourcebook: Basic Consumer Information about Allergic Disorders, Triggers, Reactions, and Related Symptoms, Including Anaphylaxis, Rhinitis, Sinusitis, Asthma, Dermatitis, Conjunctivitis, and Multiple Chemical Sensitivity; Along with Tips on Diagnosis, Prevention and Treatment, Statistical Data, a Glossary, and a Directory of Sources for Further Help and Information
Edited by Annemarie S. Muth, Omnigraphics, 2002.

About This Chapter: This chapter includes a compilation of various resources from many sources deemed reliable. It serves as a starting point for further research and is not intended to be comprehensive. Inclusion does not constitute endorsement. Resources in this chapter are categorized by type and, under each type, they are listed alphabetically by title to make topics easier to identify.

Allergies
by Edward Edelson, Chelsea House, 2000.

Allergy Made Simple: For Those Who Are Allergic and for Those Who Might Become So
by Rudiger Wahl, Hogrefe and Huber, 2002.

Asthma and Allergy Action Plan for Kids: A Complete Program to Help Your Child Live a Full and Active Life
by Allen J. Dozor and Kate Kelly, Simon and Schuster, 2004.

Asthma Information For Teens: Health Tips about Managing Asthma and Related Concerns, Including Facts about Asthma Causes, Triggers, Symptoms, Diagnosis, and Treatment
Edited by Karen Bellenir, Omnigraphics, 2005.

Breathe Easy! A Teen's Guide to Allergies and Asthma
by Jean Ford, Mason Crest Publishers, 2005.

Caring for Your Child with Severe Food Allergies: Emotional Support and Practical Advice from a Parent Who's Been There
by Lisa Cipriano Collins, J. Wiley, Inc., 1999.

Complete Allergy Book
by Frank K. Kwong and Bruce W. Cook, Sourcebooks, Inc., 2002.

Complete Idiot's Guide to Food Allergies
by Lee H. Freund and Jeanne Rejaunier, Alpha, 2003.

Coping with Allergies
by Robert H. Schwartz and Peter M.G. Deane, Rosen Publishing, 1999.

Encyclopedia of Allergies
by Myron A. Lipkowitz, Tova Navarra, Facts on File, 2001.

Family Guide to Asthma and Allergies

by the American Lung Association and Norman H. Edelman, Little, Brown, and Co., 1998.

Food Allergies and Food Intolerance: The Complete Guide to Their Identification and Treatment

by Jonathan Brostoff and Linda Gamlin, Inner Traditions, 2000.

Food Allergies: The Complete Guide to Understanding and Relieving Your Food Allergies

by William E. Walsh, J. Wiley, 2000.

Food Allergy Field Guide: A Lifestyle Manual for Families

by Theresa Willingham, Savory Palate, Inc. 2000.

Guide to Your Child's Asthma and Allergies: Breathing Easy and Bringing up Healthy, Active Children

by the American Academy of Pediatrics, Random House, 2000.

My House Is Killing Me! The Home Guide for Families with Allergies and Asthma

by Jeffrey C. May, Johns Hopkins University Press, 2001.

Cookbooks For People With Allergies

Allergy Self-Help Cookbook: Over 325 Natural Foods Recipes, Free of All Common Food Allergens

by Marjorie Hurt Jones, Rodale Press, Incorporated, 2001.

Bakin' without Eggs: Delicious Egg-Free Dessert Recipes from the Heart and Kitchen of a Food-Allergic Family

by Rosemarie Emro, St. Martin's Press, 1999.

Complete Food Allergy Cookbook: The Foods You've Always Loved Without the Ingredients You Can't Have
by Marilyn Gioannini, Crown Publishing, 1997.

Dairy-Free Cookbook: Over 250 Recipes For People With Lactose Intolerance Or Milk Allergy
by Jane Zukin, Crown Publishing, 1998.

Food Allergy News Cookbook: A Collection of Recipes from Food Allergy News and Members of the Food Allergy Network
by Anne Munoz-Furlong, John Wiley and Sons, Inc., 1998.

Kid Friendly Food Allergy Cookbook: More Than 150 Recipes That Are: Wheat-Free, Gluten-Free, Dairy-Free, Nut-Free, Egg-Free, Low in Sugar
by Kevin A. Tracy, Rockport Publishers, 2004.

Milk Free Kitchen: Living Well without Dairy Products: 450 Family-Style Recipes
Beth Kidder, Henry Holt and Company, 1991.

My Kid's Allergic to Everything Dessert Cookbook: Sweets and Treats the Whole Family Will Enjoy
by Marry Harris and Wilma Nachsin, Chicago Review Press, 1996.

Special Foods for Special Kids: Practical Solutions and Great Recipes for Children with Food Allergies
by Todd Adelman and Jodi Behrend, Robert D. Reed Publishers, 2000.

Wheatless Cooking: Including Gluten-Free and Sugar-Free Recipes
by Lynette Coffey, Ten Speed Press, 1985.

Articles About Allergies

"Allergic Reactions to Insect Stings and Bites," by John E. Moffitt, *Southern Medical Journal*, November 2003, p. 1073(7).

"Allergy Epidemic: We've Conquered Most Childhood Infections, but Extreme Reactions to Everyday Substances Pose a New Threat," by Jerry Adler, *Newsweek*, September 22, 2003, p50.

"Allergy Shots: Liberation from Suffering," by Jen Waters, *World and I*, October 2004.

"Allergy-Proof Your Yard: The Source of Your Sneezes May Be Right Outside Your Window," *Prevention*, April 2005, p. 121.

"Diagnosing and Managing your Allergies," by Melinda Dennis, *Journal of the American Dietetic Association*, April 2003, p. S4(1).

"Elimination Diet, Food Challenge Tools for Patients with Allergies," by Barbara Schiltz, *Journal of the American Dietetic Association*, April 2003, p. S3(1).

"FAAN Launches Trick or Treat for Food Allergy Halloween Coin Collection Program," *Science Letter*, October 26, 2004, p. 546.

"First Biologic for Allergy-Related Asthma," *FDA Consumer*, September-October 2003 v37, p. 5(1).

"Food Allergies Under-Treated in Hospital Emergency Rooms," *Tufts University Health and Nutrition Letter*, April 2004, p. 3(1).

"Gesundheit: A Cat Allergy Is Nothing to Sneeze at," by Libby Tucker, *Science World*, February 7, 2005, p. 10(5).

"Handling Kids' Food Allergies," by Diane Lofshult, *IDEA Fitness Journal*, March 2005, p. 69(1).

"Help for Those with Severe Peanut Allergy," *Tufts University Health and Nutrition Letter*, January 2004, p. 2(1).

"How a Single Nut Can Wreak Havoc, " *New Scientist*, November 20, 2004, p. 19(1).

"Itching for Some Allergy Relief?" by Michelle Meadows, *FDA Consumer*, May-June 2002, p. 29(2).

"Kissing Allergies," *Pediatrics for Parents*, April 2002, p. 1(1).

"Lack of Allergy Specialists Drives Patients to Alternative Treatments," by Owen Dyer, *British Medical Journal*, June 28, 2003, p. 1415(1).

"Navigating the Food Allergy Minefield," by Linda Marienhoff Coss. *Pediatrics for Parents*, August 2004, p. 2(2).

"Patient Fact Sheet on Poison Ivy," *Patient Care*, May 2005, p. S12(1).

"Scratch, Sneeze, Sniffle; Allergy Shots Build Sufferers' Immunity," *Washington Times*, August 24, 2004 p. B01.

"Seafood Allergies: Common, Sudden, Deadly," *Consumer Reports*, June 2005, p. 48(1).

"Skin Products and Allergies," *Pediatrics for Parents*, April 2004, p.1

"Some Kids Outgrow Peanut Allergies," *Current Science*, November 21, 2003, p. 12(2).

"Take Allergy Drug and Sniff Flowers Safely?" *Consumer Reports*, June 2005, p. 48(1)

"Test Your Allergy Know-How," *Prevention*, June 2005, p. 62.

"Which Children Outgrow Milk Allergy?" *Nutrition Today*, May-June 2004, p. 117(1).

Selected Allergy-Related Web Documents And Tools

Airborne Allergies: Something in the Air
National Institute of Allergy and Infectious Diseases
http://www.niaid.nih.gov/publications/allergens/airborne_allergens.pdf

Allergies and Food Sensitivities: Links
Food and Nutrition Information Center
http://www.nal.usda.gov/fnic/etext/000004.html

Allergies to Pets
Humane Society of the United States
http://www.hsus.org/pets/pet_care/allergies_to_pets

Allergies: Common Questions, Quick Answers
Virtual Children's Hospital
http://www.vh.org/pediatric/patient/pediatrics/cqqa/allergies.html

Allergies: Health eHeadlines
American Academy of Allergy, Asthma, and Immunology
http://www.aaaai.org/news/SITEWare/output/html/default.stm

Allergies: Links
NOAH: New York Online Access to Health
http://www.noah-health.org/en/immune/allergies

Allergy Treatment Profiler
American Lung Association
http://www.lungusa.org (click under "Make Treatment Decisions")

Allergy Wizard
National Jewish Medical and Research Center
http://nationaljewish.org/disease-info/diseases/allergy/kids/wizard/
contents.aspx

Ask the Allergist
Asthma and Allergy Foundation of America
http://www.aafa.org/ask_allergist_online.cfm

Breatherville USA™
Allergy and Asthma Network Mothers of Asthmatics
http://www.aanma.org/breatherville.htm

Food Allergy News for Teens
Food Allergy and Anaphylaxis Network
http://www.fankids.org/FANTeen/index.html

Food Allergy: An Overview
National Institute of Allergy and Infectious Diseases
http://www.niaid.nih.gov/publications/pdf/foodallergy.pdf

Indoor Air Quality Topics
Environmental Protection Agency
http://www.epa.gov/iaq

MedlinePlus: Allergy (Links)
National Library of Medicine
http://www.nlm.nih.gov/medlineplus/allergy.html

MyAllergies.org
HealthScout Network
http://www.myallergies.org

Special Allergy Alerts
Food Allergy and Anaphylaxis Network
http://www.foodallergy.org/alerts.html

Your Lung Health: 60 Second Check Up
American Association for Respiratory Care
http://www.yourlunghealth.org/60_second_checkup

Index

Index

Page numbers that appear in *Italics* refer to illustrations. Page numbers that have a small 'n' after the page number refer to information shown as Notes at the beginning of each chapter. Page numbers that appear in **Bold** refer to information contained in boxes on that page (except Notes information at the beginning of each chapter).

A

AAAAI *see* American Academy of Allergy, Asthma and Immunology
AANMA *see* Allergy and Asthma Network Mothers of Asthmatics
ACAAI *see* American College of Allergy, Asthma, and Immunology
Access Media Group, LLC, conjunctivitis publications 109n, 114n
Accolate 47
acne, described **120**
Actifed (triprolidine hydrochloride) 49, 90
acupuncture, described 62
acute sinusitis, described 102–3, 104
acute urticaria, described **138**
ADA *see* Americans with Disabilities Act
A.D.A.M., Inc., angioedema publication 131n
Adams, Kenneth 66, 67
adenoids
    nasal congestion 87
    rhinitis 94
adeps lanae anhydrous **342**
adrenaline, food allergies 159
Advair 44
Afrin 42

airborne allergens
    described **296**
    overview 245–64
    urushiol 322
"Airborne Allergens: Something in the Air" (NIAID) 245n
airborne allergies
    management **259**
    pets 306–7
airborne particles, allergies 5
air conditioners
    airborne allergens 260
    hay fever 267
    mold allergies 279
air filters, pollen allergies 273
Alamast 47
albumin 181, 208
alcohol use, migraine headache 142
alkylamines, described 49
"All About Eczema" (Nemours Foundation) 119n
Allegra (fexofenadine) 42, 89, 98
Allegra-D 44, 90
allergenic, defined **246**
allergen immunotherapy *see* allergy shots; immunotherapy

allergens
  allergy tests 34–35
  contact dermatitis **130**
  defined **14, 246**
  described 3, **10**, 15, 117
  dust mites 288
  food labels 219–20
  headaches 140
  hives 133
allergic conjunctivitis, described 109
allergic contact dermatitis
  described 117, 127–28, 329
  urushiol 321
"Allergic Contact Dermatitis" (AOCD) 127n
allergic diseases
  cognitive impairment 143–46
  immune system 32
"Allergic Diseases and Cognitive
  Impairment" (ACAAI) 143n
allergic reactions
  described 4, 149–51, 247
  responses **239**
allergic rhinitis (hay fever)
  allergy shots 37, 39, **40**
  cognitive impairment 144
  described **8**, 93
  immunotherapy 262
  nasal congestion 88–90
  statistics 11
  symptoms **144**
allergic salute, described 248
allergic shiners, described 248
allergic tension fatigue syndrome 161
allergic urticaria **138**
allergies
  alternative medicine 61
  animals 305–9
  versus colds 9, **86,** 249
  defined **14**
  described **15, 248**
  development, depicted *32*
  diagnosis **34**
  discovery **6**
  nasal congestion 88–90
  overview 3–12
  research 65–72, 262–64
  symptoms **210**
  treatment **146**
"Allergies" (American Animal Hospital
  Association) 305n

"Allergies: Pet Allergies" (Wood) 295n
allergists
  described 36
  filters 260
  immunotherapy 38, 98
  insect stings 315
  skin tests 256
Allergy and Asthma Network Mothers of
  Asthmatics (AANMA)
  animal allergies publications 295n
  contact information 378
  Web site address 389
Allergy/Asthma Information Association,
  contact information 378
allergy immunization *see* allergy shots;
  immunotherapy
"Allergy Medications" (Cleveland
  Clinic) 41n
allergy medications, overview 41–52
Allergy Prevention Center, Web site
  address 375
allergy quiz
  answers **12**
  questions **4**
allergy shots
  asthma prevention **40**
  described 9, **40**
  food allergies 163
  overview 37–40
  see also immunotherapy
Allergy Society of South Africa, contact
  information 375
"Allergy Statistics" (NIAID) 3n
allergy tests
  eczema 122
  hives 134
  overview 33–36
Allies Against Asthma, contact
  information 378
Alocril 47
aloholes lanae **342**
Alomide 47
alpha amyl cinnamic alcohol 337
Alrex 45
Alternaria 69, 253, 275
alternative tests, allergies 35
alternative therapies
  allergy treatment 59–63
  sinusitis **105**

"Alternative Therapies" (Asthma and
Allergy Foundation of America) 59n
Alupent 46
amerchol 342
American Academy of Allergy, Asthma
and Immunology (AAAAI)
contact information 375
Web site address 388
American Academy of Dermatology
contact information 377
publications
cosmetics 327n
eczema 119n
American Academy of Otolaryngic
Allergy, contact information 378
American Academy of Otolaryngology -
Head and Neck Surgery, Inc., contact
information 378
American Animal Hospital Association,
allergies publication 305n
American Association for Respiratory Care
contact information 378
Web site address 390
American Board of Allergy and
Immunology, contact information 375
American College of Allergy, Asthma,
and Immunology (ACAAI)
contact information 376
publications
cognitive impairment 143n
drug allergies 361n
headaches 139n
insect venom allergies 313n
urticaria 138n
American Latex Allergy Association,
contact information 382
American Lung Association
contact information 378
hay fever publication 265n
Web site address 389
American Osteopathic College of
Allergy and Immunology, contact
information 376
American Osteopathic College of
Dermatology (AOCD)
contact dermatitis publication 127n
contact information 377
Americans with Disabilities Act (ADA;
1990), companion animals 304

anaphylactic reactions
anesthesia 364
food allergies 159–60
insect stings 5
latex allergy 356
penicillin 362
symptoms 79–80
treatment 78, 228
urticaria 134
anaphylaxis
defined 84
described 4–5, 82
drug allergies 366
egg allergy 178
epinephrine 53
fire ants 318
kissing bugs 319
milk allergy 186
myths 81–84
nut allergies 197–98
overview 75–84
paraphenylenediamine 346
seafood allergies 203
Anaphylaxis Canada, contact
information 381
anesthesia, anaphylactic
reaction 364
angioedema
described 8
overview 135–37
"Angioedema" (A.D.A.M., Inc.) 131n
angioneurotic edema see angioedema
anhydrous lanolin 341, 342
animal allergies
companion animals 304
described 7, 255, 258
overview 295–304
persistence 298
recommendations 300
research 70–72
rhinitis 96
school settings 301–4
animal dander
allergies 5
allergy research 71
dog breeds 297
hay fever 267
"Animals in School" (Goldberg) 295n
annoyance reactions, described 369

antibiotics
  allergies 5
  lactose intolerance 190
  sinusitis 104
antibodies
  defined **246**
  described **20**
  food allergies 165
  immunotherapy 9
antigens
  defined **14**
  depicted *25*
  immune system 15, 19
antihistamines
  airborne allergens 261
  allergy shots 39
  anaphylactic reaction 80–81
  cognitive impairment 145
  defined **43**
  described 41–42
  eye allergies 111–13
  food allergies 160
  hay fever 268
  mold allergies 278
  nasal congestion 89–90
  OTC medications 48–52
  pets allergies 309
  prick skin test 33
  rhinitis 98
anti-inflammatory medications
  defined **43**
  rhinitis 97
antiperspirants, allergies 331
AOCD *see* American Osteopathic
  College of Dermatology
arthritis, food allergies 161
art therapy, described 62
aspartame
  described 142
  food labels 228–29
Aspergillus 69, 253–54, 275
Astelin (azelastine) 98
asthma
  allergic reactions 249
  allergy shots 37, **40**
  food allergies 151, **157**
  hay fever 266
  latex allergy 357
  sinusitis **107**

Asthma and Allergy Foundation of
  America
  contact information 379
  publications
    alternative therapies 59n
    dust mites 287n
    latex allergy 355n
    mold allergy 275n
    over the counter medications 41n
  Web site address 389
Asthma and Schools, Web site address 379
Asthma in Canada, Web site address 379
Asthma Initiative of Michigan, contact
  information 379
Asthma Resource Bank, contact
  information 379
Asthma Society of Canada, contact
  information 379
astringents, allergies 330
Atarax 42
Atkins, Dan **112**, 171n, 203, 206
atopic dermatitis
  described **8**, 117, 119–20, **121**
  statistics 11
  see also eczema
Atrohist (chlorpheniramine) 49
Atrovent (ipratropium bromide) 98
aura, described **142**
Aureobasidium 253, 275
autoimmune diseases, described 15
avoidance
  allergens 6–7, 9–10, 257–60
  eye allergies 111
  food allergies 158–59
  latex allergy **358**
  milk allergy 186
azelastine 98
Azmacort 44
azo dyes, described **346**

B

bacteria, immune system 27
bacterial conjunctivitis, described 109
Baker's asthma 209–10
basophils
  defined **14, 246**
  depicted *22*
  described 23

B cells
  depicted *28*
  described **19**
  immune system 19, 23, 27
beclomethasone 97
Beclovent 44
Beconase (beclomethasone) 44, 97
Beconase AQ (beclomethasone) 97
Benadryl (diphenhydramine hydrochloride)
  42, 44, 49, 80–81, 89
benzocaine, described **346**
Better Health Channel, hives publication
  131n
biofeedback, described 62
blood platelets, described 23
blood tests
  allergies 35, 257
  food allergies 156
  latex allergy 357
body piercings *see* piercings
bone marrow, immune system 15
brain infections, sinusitis **102**
breastfeeding, food allergies 160–61
Brethaire 46
Bromfed (brompheniramine maleate) 49
brompheniramine maleate 49
bronchodilators
  defined **43**
  described 45–47
  food allergies 160
building-related illness, described 371

C

calcium, lactose intolerance 193
Calgary Allergy Network, Web site
  address 376
"Camping with a Food Allergy" (Food
  Allergy and Anaphylaxis Network) 233n
camps, food allergies 238–40
Canadian Lung Association, contact
  information 379
Canadian Network for Asthma Care,
  contact information 379
Canadian Society of Allergy and Clinical
  Immunology, contact information 376
canine allergies *see* animal allergies
CAP system FEIA (CAP FEIA) 173–74
carrageenan **205**

cat allergies *see* animal allergies
CAT scan *see* computed tomography
celiac disease
  overview 211–14
  symptoms **212**
Center for Food Safety and Applied
  Nutrition, contact information 381, 382
cerebral allergy, food allergies 161–62
cetirizine 98
chef cards
  depicted **234**
  described 233–34
chemicals
  allergic reactions 248
  allergies 6
  avoidance 259–60
  immune system 14, 18
chemical sensitivities
  described **256**
  overview 367–72
  see also multiple chemical sensitivity
chemokines, described 24
Childhood Asthma Foundation, contact
  information 380
childhood hyperactivity, food allergies 162
children
  allergic diseases 143
  alternative medicine 60
  atopic dermatitis 11
  celiac disease 212
  eczema 116
  egg allergy 177–78
  fevers research 67–68
  food allergies 160–61, 219
  fragrance allergy **338**
  latex allergy 356
  nasal congestion 87–88
  pollen allergies 269
  sinusitis 105
chiropractic spinal manipulation,
  described 62
chlorpheniramine 49
Chlor-Trimeton (chlorpheniramine) 42,
  49, 89, 90
chromates, contact dermatitis 130
chronic sinusitis
  described 103, 104–6
  hay fever 266
  statistics 11

"Chronic Sinusitis Sufferers Have Enhanced
    Immune Responses to Fungi" (NIAID) 65n
chronic urticaria **138**
cigarette smoke, allergic
    reactions 370
cinnamic alcohol 335–36
cinnamic aldehyde 336
Cladosporium 69, 253, 275
Clarinex (desloratadine) 42, 89, 98
Claritin (loratadine) 42, *50*, 89, 98
Claritin-D 42, 44, 90
classic migraine, described **142**
clemastine fumarate 49
Cleveland Clinic, publications
    allergy medications 41n
    food intolerance 165n
cockroach allergy
    described **284**
    house dust 255
    overview 283–86
Cohen, Martin A. 301
colds
    versus allergies 9, **86, 249**
    infections 85–87
common cold *see* colds
"Commonly Asked Questions
    about Anaphylaxis" (Wood) 75n
common migraine,
    described **142**
"Common Myths about
    Anaphylaxis" (Wood) 75n
complement
    defined **14**
    immune system 27
complement cascade
    defined **14**
    depicted *25*
    described 24–25
complement system, described 24–25
computed tomography (CAT scan;
    CT scan), rhinitis 95
conditioners, allergies 331
conjunctivitis
    defined **246**
    overview 109–14
"Conjunctivitis (Pink Eye)" (Access
    Media Group, LLC) 109n
Consortium on Children's Asthma
    Camps, contact information 380

contact dermatitis
    defined **128**
    described **8**
    latex allergy 355–56
    overview 127–30
    see also allergic contact dermatitis;
        irritant contact dermatitis
contact lenses, eye allergies 113–14
corticosteroids
    defined **43**
    described 44–45
    eye allergies 113
cosmeceuticals, described **331**
cosmetics
    allergic reactions 241–42
    allergies **328**
    allergy overview 327–34
    eczema **122**
    safety concerns **332**
Crolom 47
cromolyn sodium 47, 52, 97, 261, 271
cross-contamination, food allergies
    229–31
cross-reactivity, described **151**, 205
CTL *see* cytotoxic T lymphocytes
CT scan *see* computed tomography
cytokines
    allergic reactions 248
    described 23–24
    sinusitis 69
cytotoxicity tests, food allergies 162
cytotoxic T lymphocytes (CTL),
    described 20

D

dating, food allergies **236**, 237–38
"Dating and Food Allergies: Do
    They Go Hand-in-Hand?" (Food
    Allergy and Anaphylaxis Network)
    233n
DBPCFC *see* double-blind
    placebo-controlled food
    challenge
"Dealing with Allergies"
    (Nemours Foundation) 3n
"Decoding Food Labels: Tools
    for People with Food Allergies"
    (Gollub; Simonne) 219n

decongestants
    airborne allergens 261–62
    cognitive impairment 145
    described 42–43
    eye allergies 111–13
    mold allergies 278
    OTC medications 51–52
    pollen allergies 271
    rhinitis 98
    sinus headaches 141
    sinusitis 104
Deltasone (prednisone) 45
deodorants, allergies 331
dermatitis
    fragrance allergy 338
    wool alcohol 343–44
    see also atopic dermatitis; contact
        dermatitis
dermatitis herpetiformis, described
    213–14
dermatologists
    allergic contact dermatitis 128
    makeup decisions 122
    nickel allergy 352
Dermatology Consultants, contact
    information 377
deShazo, Richard D. 313–16
desloratadine 98
deviated septum
    nasal congestion 87
    rhinitis 94
Dexamethasone 45
DEY, L.P.
    contact information 381
    EpiPen publications 53n, 57n
Diaz-Sanchez, David 66
diesel fumes, allergy research 65–67
diet diary, food allergies 155
Dimetane (brompheniramine maleate)
    42, 49
Dimetapp (brompheniramine
    maleate) 49
"Dining Out with a Food Allergy"
    (Food Allergy and Anaphylaxis
    Network) 233n
diphenhydramine hydrochloride 49
dog allergies see animal allergies
"Don't Let the Bugs Bite Allergists Say"
    (ACAAI) 313n

double-bind food challenge, described
    157–58
double-blind placebo-controlled food
    challenge (DBPCFC), described 172–73
drug allergies, overview 361–66
"Drug Reactions" (ACAAI) 361n
dust mite allergy
    described 5, 254–55
    overview 287–94
dust mites
    allergy shots 37
    bedding 7
    carpeting 292
    described 287–88
    management 290
    rhinitis 96
"Dust Mites" (Asthma and Allergy
    Foundation of America) 287n

E

"Early Fevers Associated with Lower
    Allergy Risk Later in Childhood"
    (NIAID) 65n
echinacea, allergies 63
eczema
    defined 121
    described 8, 116
    food allergies 151
    makeup decisions 122
    overview 119–26
    see also atopic dermatitis
egg allergy
    described 222
    infants 161
    management 180
    overview 177–81
electrostatic precipitators, described 260
elimination diet
    food allergies 155–56
    hives 134
ELISA see enzyme-linked
    immunosorbent assay
Emadine 42
emotional stress, eczema 121
endoscopy, lactose intolerance 191
environmental allergens, described 5
environmental control, allergy shots 38
environmental illness, food allergies 162

Environmental Protection Agency
   contact information 380
   Web site address 390
enzyme-linked immunosorbent assay
   (ELISA), food allergies 156
eosinophils
   depicted *22*
   described 23
Epicoccum 253, 275
epinephrine
   allergies 7
   anaphylactic reaction 80–81
   auto-injector information **56, 80**
   defined **84**
   described **78**
   egg allergy 179, 180
   food allergies 159, **220**
   nut allergies 198–99
   overview 53–57
EpiPen
   described **78, 80**
   latex allergy 360
   overview 53–57
"EpiPen and EpiPen JR: Dosing"
   (DEY, L.P.) 53n
epithelial cells, immune system 27
ethanolamines, described 49
cthmoid sinuses, described 100
ethnic factors
   cockroach allergy 285
   lactose intolerance 190
ethylenediamines, described 49
eugenol 336
exercise induced food allergy
   anaphylaxis 77–79
   described **158**
   wheat 210
eye allergies
   described 110–14
   quiz **110**
   treatment **112**
"Eye Allergies" (Access Media
   Group, LLC) 109n
eye cosmetics, allergies 332

F

facial cosmetics, allergies 332
"Facts about Hay Fever" (American
   Lung Association) 265n

FALCPA *see* Food Allergen Labeling and
   Consumer Protection Act
Fauci, Anthony 65, 67, 70
FD&C Yellow No. 5, food labels 229
feline allergies *see* animal allergies
fexofenadine 98
Filley, Warren V. **280**
financial considerations
   alternative medicine 60
   sinusitis statistics 11
fire ants, described 317–18
fish allergies
   carrageenan **205**
   described 227
   iodine **205**
   management **204**
   overview 203–6
   see also shellfish allergies
"Fishing For Answers: Seafood Allergies
   Impact Few, But Can Be Deadly If
   Undiagnosed" (National Jewish Medical
   and Research Center) 203n
flea allergies, pets 307
Flonase (fluticasone) 44, 97
Flovent 44
flunisolide 97
fluticasone 44, 97
food additives
   allergies 227–29
   intolerances 153
Food Allergen Labeling and Consumer
   Protection Act (FALCPA) 220
food allergies
   anaphylactic reactions 76, **220**
   asthma **157**
   common items **153**
   coping strategies 215–18
   dating **236**
   described 5, **150**
   eczema 120
   exercise **158**
   versus food intolerances 165–69, 221–22
   guidelines **164**
   overview 149–64
   pets 306
   public awareness **197**
   social settings 233–40
   statistics 11–12, **167**
   students **217**

Food Allergy and Anaphylaxis Network
   contact information 381
   publications
      anaphylaxis 75n
      cosmetics 241n
      social life 233n
   Web site address 389, 390
Food Allergy Initiative, Web site address 382
"Food Allergy: An Overview" (NIAID) 149n
Food and Nutrition Information Center,
   Web site address 388
food challenges
   allergies 35
   described 157–58, **172–73**
   food allergies 171–75
"Food Challenges: Why Bother?" (Atkins)
   171n
food intolerances
   described 151–54
   versus food allergies 165–69
   statistics **167**
   treatment **169**
food labels
   examples **230**
   interpretation 219–32
   nut allergies 199
   required information **229**
formaldehyde 370
4-phenylenediamine **347**
benzenediamine **347**
fragrance allergies
   dermatitis **337**
   described 329
   overview 335–40
"Fragrance Mix Allergy" (New Zealand
   Dermatological Society) 335n
"Frequently Asked Questions About Dust
   Mite Allergy" (Asthma and Allergy
   Foundation of America) 287n
frontal sinuses, described 100
Fusarium 253, 275

G

genes
   defined **246**
   GSTM1 66
   GSTP1 66
   GSTT1 66

geraniol 336
giant papillary conjunctivitis
   (GPC), described 110
glaucoma, antihistamines 51
gliadin 208
Global Initiative for Asthma,
   Web site address 380
globulin 181, 208
glutenin 208
gluten intolerance
   described 154
   versus wheat allergy 207–14
Goldberg, Ellie 295n
Gollub, Elizabeth A. 219n
GPC *see* giant papillary
   conjunctivitis
granules, defined **246**
granulocytes
   depicted *22*
   described 23

H

hair cosmetics
   allergies 333
   paraphenylenediamine 345–49
hand eczema
   dermatologists **126**
   described 124–26
"Hand Eczema" (American
   Academy of Dermatology) 119n
handwashing, animal allergies 297
hay fever, overview 265–69
   see also allergic rhinitis
"Headaches" (ACAAI) 139n
headaches, allergies 139–42
health insurance *see* financial
   considerations; insurance
   coverage
HealthScout Network,
   Web site address 390
Hefle, Susan L. 241n
Helminthosporium 253, 275
helper cells
   depicted *21*
   described 20
HEPA filters *see* high-efficiency
   particulate air filters
herbal supplements, allergies **63**

heredity
  allergies 5
  celiac disease 207
  drug allergies 362
  eczema 120
  eye allergies 110
  food allergies 150, **166**
  hay fever 265
  immunity 30
  migraine headaches 141
  mold allergies 276
  pollen allergies 269
high-efficiency particulate air filters
  (HEPA filters)
  airborne allergens 260
  animal allergies 297, 299
  house dust 258
  mold allergies 279
histamine
  animal allergies 70
  defined **132**
  described 4, 23
  mast cells 133
  milk allergy 184
histamine sensitivity,
  described 221–22
histamine toxicity,
  described 152
hives
  chemicals 6
  described **8, 138**
  food allergies 151
  overview 131–35
  statistics 12
  see also urticaria
"Hives Explained" (Better Health
  Channel) 131n
hormonal rhinitis, described 95
house dust
  avoidance 258–59
  described 254–55
house dust mites *see* dust mites
"How to Create a Dust-Free Bedroom"
  (NIAID) 287n
Humane Society of the
  United States, Web site
  address 388
humidifiers, mold allergies 279
hydrogen breath test, described 191

hydroxycitronellal 337
hypersensitivity
  latex allergy 359
  medications 361–62
hyphae, described 252
hypnosis, described 62
hypoallergenic, described 295, **328**

I

idiopathic anaphylaxis, described 79
IgA *see* immunoglobulin A
IgD *see* immunoglobulin D
IgE *see* immunoglobulin E
IgG *see* immunoglobulin G
IgG subclass assay, food allergies 163
IgM *see* immunoglobulin M
immune cells
  depicted *18*
  described *19*
immune complex assay,
  food allergies 162–63
immune hypersensitivity,
  described 369
immune response
  depicted *26*
  described 26–30
immune system
  defined **246**
  drug allergies 361
  food intolerances 165, 167–68
  nut allergies 195–97
  overview 13–32
  urticaria **138**
immune system organs, depicted *16*
immune tolerance, described 31
immunity, described 30–31
immunoglobulin A (IgA)
  celiac disease 213
  described **20**
  immune system 27
immunoglobulin D (IgD)
  described **20**
immunoglobulin E (IgE)
  allergies 4, 247
  described **20**
  egg allergy 177
  food allergies 149–50
  milk allergy 184
  pollen allergies 273

immunoglobulin G (IgG)
  celiac disease 213
  described **20**
immunoglobulin M (IgM), described **20**
immunotherapy
  airborne allergens 262
  allergic diseases 146
  animal allergies 299–300
  defined **38**
  eye allergies 113
  mold allergies 279
  overview 37–40
  pets allergies 308–9
  pollen allergies 273
  rhinitis 98
  see also allergy shots
infants
  atopic dermatitis 11
  celiac disease 212
  food allergies 160–61
  immune responses 30–31
infectious rhinitis, described 94
inflammation, defined **246**
inflammatory response, defined **14**
ingredient labels, food allergies **242**
insect stings
  allergy shots 37, **40**
  allergy statistics 12, 313
  anaphylaxis 77
  described 5
  myths **314–15**
  overview 313–20
Institute of Food and Agricultural
  Services, contact information 382
insurance coverage, alternative
  medicine 60
Intal 47
interleukins
  described 24
  sinusitis 69
International Food Information Council
  Foundation, contact information 382
intoxication syndrome, described 369
intradermal skin tests, described 34
iodine **205**
ipratropium bromide 98
irritant contact dermatitis
  described 116, 327–28
  latex allergy 359

irritants, rhinitis 96–97
irritational syndromes, described 369
isoeugenol 336

J

Johnson, Christine C. 68
Joint Council of Allergy, Asthma, and
  Immunology, contact information 376

K

killer cells, depicted *21*
killer T cells, described 20
kissing bugs, described 318–19
Kita, Hirohito 69–70

L

labels *see* food labels; ingredient labels
lactase, described 189
lactose intolerance
  described 152
  management **192**
  overview 189–93
lanolin 341, **342**
laser therapy, described 62
latex
  anaphylaxis 77
  contact dermatitis 129
  defined **360**
latex allergy
  coping methods **358**
  overview 355–60
  statistics 11
"Latex Allergy" (Asthma and Allergy
  Foundation of America) 355n
leukotriene modifiers, described 47–48
leukotrienes, allergic reactions 248
lip cosmetics, allergies 332–33
livetin 181
Livostin 42
loratadine *50*, 98
lymphatic system, immune system
  16–17
lymph nodes, depicted *17, 18*
lymphocytes
  defined **246**
  immune system 15–19

lymphoid organs, immune system 15
lysozyme 181

M

macrophages
  depicted *22*
  described 23
  immune system 27
major histocompatibility complex
  molecules (MHC molecules) 22
makeup *see* cosmetics
"Managing Food Allergies and
  Outdoor Activities" (Food
  Allergy and Anaphylaxis
  Network) 233n
massage therapy, described 62
mast cells
  allergic reactions 248
  antihistamines 42
  defined **14, 132, 246**
  depicted *22*
  described 23
  histamines 133
mast cell stabilizers
  described 47
  eye allergies 111–13
Maxair 46
maxillary sinuses, described 100
McClellan, Mark B. **50**
MCS *see* multiple chemical sensitivity
mechanical obstruction, rhinitis 94
MedicAlert bracelet
  anaphylaxis **78**
  latex allergy 360
medical history
  allergy tests **34**
  food allergies 154–55
  hives 134
  rhinitis 95
medications
  airborne allergens 260–62
  allergies 5, 7–9, 41–52
  anaphylactic reaction 80–81
  anaphylaxis 76–77
  eye allergies 111–13
  mold allergies 278–79
  prescription pointers **46**
  quick tips **49**

memory cells
  defined **14**
  immunity 31
Metaprel 46
MHC molecules *see* major
  histocompatibility complex molecules
microbes, immune system 26–27
migraine headaches
  described **142**
  food allergies 161
  overview 141–42
milk allergy
  described 223
  food contents **188**
  food labels 187, **188**
  management **185**
  overview 183–88
Moffitt, John E. 318–19
moisturizers, allergies 330
mold allergies
  described 251–54
  hay fever 267
  overview 275–81
"Mold Allergy" (Asthma and Allergy
  Foundation of America) 275n
mold count, described **278**
molds
  allergy shots 37
  avoidance 257
  described **276**
  inhalation **280**
molecules, defined **246**
mometasone 97
monocytes
  depicted *22*
  described 23
monokines, described 23
monosodium glutamate (MSG) 142,
  153, 228
mosquitoes, described 319–20
Mucor 253, 275
mucus
  immune system 26–27
  infections 87
  sinusitis 101
multiple chemical sensitivity (MCS),
  described **368**
  see also chemical sensitivities
music therapy, described 62

N

nail cosmetics, allergies 333–34
Naphcon 44
Nasacort (triamcinolone) 44, 97
Nasacort AQ (triamcinolone) 97
nasal congestion, overview 85–91
Nasalcrom (cromolyn sodium) 47, 52,
    146
nasal polyps
    hay fever 266
    nasal congestion 87
    rhinitis 95
    sinusitis 105–6
nasal sprays
    airborne allergens 261
    allergic diseases 146
    sinusitis 105
nasal steroids, airborne allergens 261
nasal wash, rhinitis 98
Nasarel (flunisolide) 97
Nasonex (mometasone) 44, 97
National Allergy Bureau, contact
    information 380
National Asthma Education Program,
    contact information 380
National Cancer Institute (NCI),
    immune system publication 13n
National Center for Environmental
    Health, contact information 380
National Eczema Association for
    Science and Education, contact
    information 377
National Heart, Lung, and
    Blood Institute (NHLBI),
    contact information 380
National Institute of Allergy
    and Infectious Diseases
    (NIAID)
    contact information 376
    publications
        airborne allergens 245n
        allergies research 65n
        allergy statistics 3n
        dust mites 287n
        food allergies 149n
        immune system 13n
        pollen allergy 265n
    Web site address 388, 389

National Institute of Arthritis and
    Musculoskeletal and Skin Diseases
    (NIAMS), contact information 377
National Institute of Diabetes and
    Digestive and Kidney Diseases
    (NIDDK), contact information 382
National Institute of Environmental
    Health Sciences, contact information 381
National Jewish Medical and Research
    Center
    contact information 381
    seafood allergies publication 203n
    Web site address 389
National Library of Medicine
    contact information 376
    Web site address 390
natural killer cells, described 22
NCI see National Cancer Institute
nedocromil 97
Nemours Foundation, publications
    allergies overview 3n
    eczema 119n
Neo-Synephrine 42
neutrophils
    depicted 22
    described 23
New Zealand Dermatological Society
    contact information 377
    fragrance allergies publication 335n
NHLBI see National Heart, Lung, and
    Blood Institute
NIAID see National Institute of Allergy
    and Infectious Diseases
nickel
    allergy 351–53
    contact dermatitis 128–29
NIDDK see National Institute of
    Diabetes and Digestive and Kidney
    Diseases
nitrogen dioxide, allergic reactions 370
NK cells, immune system 27
NOAH: New York Online Access to
    Health, Web site address 389
Nolahist (phenindamine tartrate) 51
non-allergic rhinitis, described 94
non-allergic urticaria, described **138**
nonself marker molecules, described 15
nonsteroidal anti-inflammatory drugs
    (NSAID), eye allergies 113

"Novel Therapy Tested in Mice
    Could Chase away Cat Allergies"
    (NIAID) 65n
NSAID *see* nonsteroidal
    anti-inflammatory drugs
nut allergies
    anaphylaxis 76
    described 226
    food names **198**
    hidden sources **196, 201**
    overview 195–201
    statistics 12

O

oak moss absolute 337
Occupational Safety and Health
    Administration (OSHA), contact
    information 382
Ocu-Hist 42
OFC *see* open food challenge
1,4-phenylenediamine **347**
open food challenge (OFC), described
    172
Opticrom 47
Optivar 44
organism, defined **246**
organ transplantation, immune
    system 22
Orsin **347**
OSHA *see* Occupational Safety and
    Health Administration
OTC *see* over the counter medications
ovalbumin 181
"Over-the-Counter Medications"
    (Asthma and Allergy Foundation
    of America) 41n
over the counter medications (OTC)
    allergies 48–52
    cognitive impairment 144–45
    hay fever 269
    quick tips **49**
    sinusitis **104**
ovoglobulin 181
ovomucin 181
ovomucoid 181
ovotransferrin 181
ovovitella 181
ovovitellin 181

ozone
    allergic reactions 370
    electrostatic precipitators 260

P

PABA *see* para-aminobenzoic acid
Pan-American Allergy Society, contact
    information 376
para-aminoaniline **347**
para-aminobenzoic acid (PABA),
    described **346**
para-aminosalicylic acid, described **346**
para-diaminobenzene **347**
paraphenylenediamine (PPD; PPDA)
    alternative names **347**
    contact dermatitis 129–30
    overview 345–49
parasites, immune system 30
Parents of Asthmatic/Allergic Children,
    contact information 381
"Participating in Specialty Camps" (Food
    Allergy and Anaphylaxis Network) 233n
Patanol 44
patch tests
    allergic contact dermatitis 128
    allergies 35
    nickel allergy 352
    paraphenylenediamine 346, 347–48
pathogens, described 26
"Patient Insert" (DEY, L.P.) 53n
peanut allergy
    anaphylaxis 84
    described 226
    hidden sources **196, 201**
    infants 161
    overview 195–201
penicillin
    allergic reactions 362
    allergy statistics 12
    anaphylactic reaction **362**
    molds **252**
Penicillium 69, 253, 275
perennial, defined **246**
pet allergies *see* animal allergies
phagocytes
    depicted *22*
    described **19**
    immune system 18, 27

phenindamine tartrate 51
pheniramine maleate 49
phenylenediamine base **347**
phenylethylamine 142
physical examinations
    allergy tests **34**
    eczema 121
    hives 134
    lactose intolerance 191
    rhinitis 95
piercings, nickel allergy **353**
pink eye *see* conjunctivitis
placebo effect, alternative
    medicine 61
plants
    contact dermatitis 130
    pollen allergies 249–51
    urushiol 321–26
plasma cells, immune system 19
platelets, described 23
Plaut, Marshall 68
poison ivy
    contact dermatitis 130
    depicted *323*
    described **322**
    overview 321–26
    prevention **324**
    treatment 117
poison oak
    depicted *323*
    described 321–25, **322**
poison sumac
    depicted *323*
    described 321–25, **322**
pollen
    allergic reactions 249–51
    allergies 5, 265–74
    allergy shots 37
    avoidance 257, *274*
    bloom times 266–67, *268*
    nasal congestion 88–89
    sources **251**
    types *270*
    see also hay fever
pollen count, described *272*
pollinosis *see* hay fever
postnasal drip, sinusitis 101
PPD *see* paraphenylenediamine
PPDA *see* paraphenylenediamine

p-phenylenediamine **347**
prednisone 45, 105
preservatives, allergies 329
prick skin test, described 33
"Problem Foods: Is It An Allergy Or
    Intolerance?" (Cleveland Clinic) 165n
procaine, described **346**
prolamin 208
Proventil 46
provocative challenge, food allergies 162
pseudoallergic reaction, described 362
pseudoephedrine 98
psychological triggers, described 154
Pulmicort 44
pyrilamine maleate 49

Q

"Questions about Allergies" (Nemours
    Foundation) 3n
"Questions and Answers About Pollen
    Allergy" (NIAID) 265n

R

RadioAllergoSorbent Test (RAST)
    animal allergies 299
    described *35*
    food allergies 156, 210
rashes
    fragrance allergy 337
    overview 115–17
    poison plants 321–26
    prevention **116**
    urticaria 131
RAST *see* RadioAllergoSorbent Test
"The Real Truth about Cats and Dogs"
    (Wood) 295n
relaxation therapy, described 62
rhinitis
    defined **94**, **246**
    nasal congestion 90–91
    overview 93–98
    treatment 95, 97
rhinitis medicamentosa, described 94
Rhinocort (flunisolide) 44, 97
Rhizopus 253, 275
Rodol **347**
rush immunotherapy, described 39

S

Saxon, Andrew 71–72
SBPCFC *see* single-blind
  placebo-controlled food
  challenge
"Scientists Identify Genes that
  Regulate Allergic Response to
  Diesel Fumes" (NIAID) 65n
scratch skin test *see* skin tests
seafood allergies
  described 227
  overview 203–6
seasonal allergic rhinitis *see* hay fever
seasonal allergies, asthma **8**
self marker molecules, described 15
Semprex-D 44
sensitivity
  described 267
  poison plants 322–23
shampoos, allergies 330–31
shellfish allergies
  carrageenan **205**
  iodine **205**
  management **204**
  see also fish allergies
sick-building syndrome,
  described 371
silici albuminate 181
Simonne, Amy H. 219n
Simons, F. Estelle R. 319–20
Simplesse 181
single-blind placebo-controlled
  food challenge (SBPCFC),
  described **172–73**
Singulair 47
sinuses
  defined **100**, **246**
  described 100
sinus headache, described 140–41
sinusitis
  asthma **107**
  defined **100**
  fungus immune response 68–70
  nasal congestion 87
  overview 99–108
skin
  allergies **120**
  immune system 26

skin care products *see* cosmetics
skin cleansers, allergies 330
skin prick test, described 33
skin tests
  egg allergy 179
  food allergies 156
  IgE antibody levels 256
  milk allergy 184–85
sleep disruption, cognitive
  impairment 144
snacks, eggs **178**
sneezing, described **88–89**
"Solving Problems Related to the
  Use of Cosmetics and Skin Care
  Products" (American Academy of
  Dermatology) 327n
soy allergy, described 224–25
sphenoid sinuses, described 100
spina bifida, latex allergy 356
spleen, immune system 17
spores, described 175, 252, 253, 267
sputum, defined **246**
statistics
  adverse drug reactions 361
  airborne allergens 245
  allergic drug reactions 12
  allergies 11–12
  cockroach allergy 283, 285
  dust mite allergy 287
  hay fever 265
  hives **8**
  lactose intolerance 190
  latex allergy 77, 356
  nut allergies 197
  rhinitis 93
  sinusitis 99
  wheat allergy 209
Steinman, Harris 207n
stem cells, described *19*
steroids
  pets allergies 308
  sinusitis 105
"Storage/Transport/How Supplied"
  (DEY, L.P.) 53n
stuffy nose
  described **91**
  overview 85–91
Sudafed (pseudoephedrine) 42,
  89, 98

sulfites
  food intolerances 153–54
  food labels 228
sulfonamides, described **346**
sulfur dioxide, allergic reactions 370
sunscreens, allergies 330

T

tartrazine, food labels 229
Tavist (clemastine fumarate) 42, 49
T cells
  depicted *21, 29*
  described **19**
  immune system 15, 19–23, 27
tests
  allergies 33–36, *34, 35, 36*
  angioedema 136
  animal allergies 299
  celiac disease 213
  chemical sensitivities 371–72
  cockroach allergy 286
  ELISA 156
  food allergies 156–58
  fragrance allergy 338–39
  lactose intolerance 191
  latex allergy 357
  mold allergy 254
  nickel allergy 352
  paraphenylenediamine 346, 347–48
  pets allergies 308
  RAST *35*, 156, 210, 299
  rhinitis 95
  wheat allergy 210
  wool alcohol 373
theophylline, defined **43**
thymus, immune system 15
Tilade 47
tissues, defined **246**
Tornalate 46
triamcinolone 97
Triaminic (pheniramine maleate) 49
Triaminic (pyrilamine maleate) 49
Triatoma see kissing bugs
triprolidine hydrochloride 49
Tylenol 44
"Types of Latex Reactions" (Asthma and
  Allergy Foundation of America) 355n
tyramine 142

U

ultraviolet light therapy, eczema 122
"Understanding the Immune System"
  (NIAID; NCI) 13n
upper respiratory tract, defined **246**
Ursol **347**
urticaria
  defined **132**
  described **8, 138**
  overview 131–35
  paraphenylenediamine 346
  statistics 12
  see also hives
urushiol 321–26

V

vaccines, immunity 31
Vancenase (beclomethasone) 97
Vancenase AQ (beclomethasone) 97
Vasocon 44
vasomotor rhinitis, described 90–91, 94
venom immunotherapy
  described 9
  insect stings 315–16
Ventolin 46
viral conjunctivitis, described 109
Virtual Children's Hospital, Web site
  address 388
viruses, immune system 27
Visine 42
vitellin 181
Volmax 46

W

Weber, Richard M. 317–18
"What You Need to Know about Allergy
  Medications" (Cleveland Clinic) 41n
wheals, described 131
"Wheat, Gluten Allergy, Gluten
  Intolerance and Gluten Enteropathy"
  (Steinman) 207n
wheat allergy
  described 223–24
  versus gluten intolerance 207–14
wheat-dependent exercise induced
  reactions, described 210

wheat intolerance, described **208**
"Will Food Proteins in Cosmetics
    and Bath Products Cause Reactions?"
    (Hefle) 241n
Wood, Robert A. 75n, 295n, 297–99
wood burning stoves, allergic reactions
    370–71
wool alcohol
    allergies 341–44
    alternative names **342**
    reaction prevention **344**
wool fat 341, **342**
wool grease 341, **342**
wool wax 341, **342**
World Allergy Organization, contact
    information 376

X

Xopenex 46
x-rays, rhinitis 95

Y

yoga, described 62

Z

Zaditor 44
Zyflo 47
Zyrtec (cetirizine) 42, 89, 98
Zyrtec-D 44

WITHDRAWAL